HEALTH SYSTEMS RESEARCH

Edited by K. Davis and W. van Eimeren

Detlef Schwefel Reiner Leidl Joan Rovira
Michael F. Drummond (Eds.)

Economic Aspects of AIDS and HIV Infection

With 66 Figures and 69 Tables

Springer-Verlag Berlin Heidelberg New York
London Paris Tokyo Hong Kong

Professor Dr. Detlef Schwefel
GSF-Institut für Medizinische Informatik und Systemforschung
Ingolstädter Landstraße 1, 8042 Neuherberg, FRG

Dr. Reiner Leidl
GSF-Institut für Medizinische Informatik und Systemforschung
Ingolstädter Landstraße 1, 8042 Neuherberg, FRG

Professor Dr. Joan Rovira
Department de Teoria Econòmica, Universitat de Barcelona
Av. Diagonal 690, Barcelona 0834, Spain

Professor Dr. Michael F. Drummond
Health Services Management Centre, The University of Birmingham
Park House Edgbaston Park Road, Birmingham, B15 2RT, UK

Publication No. EUR 12565 of the Scientific and Technical Communication Unit, Commission of the European Communities, Directorate-General Telecommunications, Information Industries and Innovation, Luxembourg

---

ISBN 3-540-52135-6 Springer-Verlag Berlin Heidelberg New York
ISBN 0-387-52135-6 Springer-Verlag New York Berlin Heidelberg

Library of Congress Cataloging-in-Publication Data
Economic aspects of AIDS and HIV infection / Detlef Schwefel ... [et al.], eds. p. cm.–(Health systems research) "On behalf of the Concerted Action Committee (COMAC) on Health Services Research (HSR), the GSF-Institut für Medizinische Informatik und Systemforschung (MEDIS) convened an international conference ... in Munich, 16–18 March 1989"–Pref. Includes bibliographical references. ISBN 0-387-52135-6 (U.S. : alk. paper) 1. AIDS (Disease)–Economic aspects–Congresses. I. Schwefel, Detlef. II. Commission of the European Communities. Concerted Action Committee on Health Services Research. III. Institut für Medizinische Informatik und Systemforschung (Gesellschaft für Strahlen- und Umweltforschung) IV. Series. RA644.A25E33 1990 362.1'969792–dc20

Printed in Germany

Printing and Bookbinding: Druckhaus Beltz, Hemsbach/Bergstraße
2119/3145-543210 – Printed on acid-free paper

Preface

From the early days of its recognized occurrence, AIDS has been perceived as posing tremendous threats, burdens and challenges to human beings. Individuals, societies and, in a global point of view, mankind are affected by the effects of the HIV infection, the nature and extent of which is still unclear in many ways. In the beginning only biomedical and epidemiological analyses of the problem were the top research priorities, the former laden with great hopes that it may soon be possible to stop the spread of the disease and to overcome its physical impact. Yet it soon became clear that AIDS would be something to be reckoned and coped with on a long-term basis, making a thorough investigation of its impact absolutely mandatory.

AIDS has serious economic consequences. Taken seriously, they cannot be confined to predictions of costs intended to support the AIDS issue in the struggle for resources. Besides cost calculations – a methodologically tricky and wide-ranging topic in itself – and their application to cost-effectiveness and other analyses, economic issues include identifying and assessing patterns of care, analyzing problems of financing, exploring impacts on markets other than health care, and modelling scenarios for future developments and strategies. At present, the economic aspects of AIDS still constitute a very recent topic in European health economics and health systems research. Many projects are just about to start, and there must be a better exchange of information between research groups.

On behalf of the Concerted Action Committee (COMAC) on Health Services Research (HSR), the GSF-Institut für Medizinische Informatik und Systemforschung (MEDIS) convened an international conference on "Economic Aspects of AIDS and HIV Infection" in Munich, 16-18 March 1989. The conference forms a major part of a study contracted by COMAC-HSR to Professor Schwefel of GSF-MEDIS. In conducting the study, Professor Schwefel was assisted by Dr. Leidl. The full study comprises the examination of research groups and issues (which was conducted in the study phase prior to the Munich meeting), the conference, and support for stimulating concerted European research action in this field.

The participants of the workshop were invited according to a number of criteria. The topics relevant to European countries were to be represented adequately, and there was to be balanced representation of researchers from the various European countries. Furthermore, researchers and experts working in international organizations were asked

to participate. Finally, each participant was asked to play an active role by giving a lecture and writing a paper.
Researchers from nearly all the countries of the European Communities accepted the invitation; some workers from neighboring countries like Sweden, Switzerland, and the United States of America also participated. Within the groups of EC countries, however, some were slightly overrepresented, others slightly underrepresented at the conference. This was due to the selection criteria and the response rate.
The papers given at the conference form the basis of this publication. Some contributions not presented at the conference were also accepted. All papers submitted passed through an editorial review process. The review was supported by Professor Rovira, who was reponsible for the sections 'Exploring Spread and Context' and 'Patterns of Health Care and Social Support Systems', Professor Drummond who commented on the section 'Costs of AIDS', and Dr. Leidl who took care of the sections 'Financial Aspects', 'Scenarios and Policies', and 'Prospects'.
Besides the COMAC-HSR study, other activities in the European region are also concerned with the economic aspects of AIDS. To avoid unnecessary duplication and to coordinate the planning of international research, an exchange between these projects has been arranged. One study focuses more on the methodological aspects, especially of costing issues; it was initiated by the World Health Organization, Regional Office for Europe. Another project, promoted by the same institution, is concerned with scenarios on the social and economic impact of AIDS.
The focus of the COMAC conference and of this book is on the exploration of economic aspects, on empirical approaches, on case studies, and, last but not least, on modelling techniques for economic scenarios. We hope this collection provides an up-to-date overview of the state of economic research on AIDS in Europe, and that it may stimulate further work to come.
Finally, we are greatly indebted to our colleagues at the MEDIS Institute whose steady and thorough team work transformed the pile of manuscripts into a camera-ready publication. In the editorial assistance, Mrs. Ursula Weber managed the technical production of texts, graphics, references, and the general bibliography. Mr. Darwin Santo took over the tremendous task of processing all the manuscripts into their final form. Mrs. Frauke Hörnig supplemented some of the graphics. Dr. Walter Satzinger and Dr. Andreas Mielck assisted in the editing of a number of papers.

October 1989 The Editors

Contents

Preface V

Introduction

Social Sciences, Economics and AIDS
D. Schwefel 3

Exploring Spread and Context of AIDS and HIV Infection

Patterns of AIDS and HIV Infection in Europe
A.M. Downs, R.A. Ancelle-Park, I. de Vincenzi, J-B. Brunet 19

Demographic Impact of Mortality from AIDS in France: Projection for 1991
M. Guiguet, A.J. Valleron 38

Social and Political Aspects of AIDS
J. Santos Lucas 43

Economic Aspects of AIDS
J. Rovira 49

Patterns of Health Care and Social Support Systems

The US Hospital AIDS Survey: Structure and Substance
D.P. Andrulis 59

Description and Analysis of Patterns of Outpatient Care for AIDS Patients and HIV Infected Persons
G. Brenner 67

Social Support Systems for People Affected by AIDS. Observations from West Germany
W. Satzinger 80

Use of Sentinel Systems in the Evaluation of the Impact of AIDS and HIV Infection
G. Thiers, M. Denayer, A. Stroobant 90

Services for the Management of HIV Infection: Problems for Planners
A.M. Johnson 98

Costs of AIDS and HIV Infection

Economic Evaluation of Programmes for AIDS and HIV Infection: Methodological Issues
M. Drummond, L. Davies 107

The Economic Analysis of Prevention of HIV Infection: Evaluation of Programmes and Decision Support for Priority Setting in Health Policy. Case Study. Sweden
M. Lagergren 118

The Cost of AIDS and HIV Infection: Public Expenditures for AIDS Prevention in the Federal Republic of Germany
A. Jenke, A.-M. Reinkemeier 127

The Costs of Hospital Care of AIDS Patients at the Teaching Hospital of the University of Amsterdam
P.R.E. Bijlsma 136

Direct and Indirect Costs of AIDS in Belgium: A Preliminary Analysis
J. Lambert, G. Carrin 151

Hospital Costs for AIDS Patients
B. Olesen, P. Gøtzsche, I. Bygbjerg, L. Møller, V. Faber . . 160

Comparing Inpatient and Outpatient Costs for HIV, LAS and AIDS: Methodology, Results and Consequences from a Study in Germany
R. Hanpft, F. Reinecke, F. Beske 164

Medical Services and Costs of AIDS Patients in an Outpatient Clinic for Infectious Diseases, Frankfurt University Hospital
I. Gschrey-Düver, H. Exner-Freisfeld, A. Koock-Walewski, C. zur Lippe, R. Müller, S. Staszewski, W. Stille 172

AIDS/HIV Costs in England: The Case of the Oxfordshire District
M. Rees 187

The Regional Costs of AIDS in Spain
J. Ginestal Gómez 195

Indicators and Trends of Direct and Indirect Costs of AIDS on a National Level: Results from Switzerland
M.R.H. Pedergnana 203

Costs of AIDS in a Developing Area: Indirect and Direct Costs of AIDS in Puerto Rico
D.S. Shepard 226

Financial Aspects

Some Implications of AIDS for Permanent Health Insurance
A.D. Wilkie 241

Scenarios and Policies

Planning for AIDS or HIV Related Services in Greece: First Steps towards Operational Schemes
M. Diomidis, A. Sissouras 251

Epidemiological Models and Socioeconomic Information: Methodological Aspects of AIDS/HIV Scenario Analysis
J.C. Jager, M.J. Postma, F.M. van den Boom, D.P. Reinking, J.C.C. Borleffs, S.H. Heisterkamp, J.A.M. van Druten, E.J. Ruitenberg 262

Model-Based Scenarios to Describe Economic Impacts of AIDS: The Role of Case-Mix
R. Leidl 282

Scenarios as a Tool to Support Health Planning and Management
R.F. Schreuder 295

Main Policy Issues of the Social and Economic Impact of AIDS from the Perspective of a Health Ministry
X. Scheil-Adlung 302

Prospects

The Economic Evaluation of Care Programmes for Patients with HIV-AIDS
A. Maynard 311

International Research Needs for AIDS
S. Wayling, H. Zöllner 328

Future Research Policies
H. Stein 344

References 349

Contributors

R.A. Ancelle-Park
WHO Collaborating Centre on AIDS, Institut de Médecine et d'Epidémiologie Africaines et Tropicales, Hôpital Claude Bernard, 10 Avenue Porte d'Aubervilliers, 75019 Paris, France

Dr. Dennis P. Andrulis
President of The National Public Health & Hospital Institute, 1001 Pennsylvania Avenue NW, Suite 635, Washington, DC 20004, USA

Prof. Dr. med. Fritz Beske
Institut für Gesundheits-System-Forschung, Weimarer Strasse 8, 2300 Kiel 1, FRG

Dr. Frans van den Boom
Netherlands Institute of Mental Health, Da Costakade 45, 3521 VS, Utrecht, The Netherlands

J.C.C. Borleffs
University Hospital Utrecht, 3521 VS, Utrecht, The Netherlands

Dipl.-Kfm. Gerhard Brenner
Zentralinstitut für die kassenärztliche Versorgung in der BR Deutschland, Herbert-Lewin-Strasse 5, 5000 Köln 41, FRG

J.B. Brunet
WHO Collaborating Centre on AIDS, Institut de Médecine et d'Epidémiologie Africaines et Tropicales, Hôpital Claude Bernard, 10 Avenue Porte d'Aubervilliers, 75019 Paris, France

I. Bygbjerg
Department of Infectious Diseases, Rigshospitalet, 1124 Copenhagen, Denmark

Dr. P.R.E. Bijlsma
Academic Medical Center, Teaching Hospital of the University of Amsterdam, BEB/Prog. Buro, Merbergdreef 9, 1105 AZ Amsterdam, The Netherlands

Prof. Guy Carrin
University of Antwerp, Prinsstraat 13, 2000 Antwerp, Belgium

Linda Davies
Health Services Management Centre, The University of Birmingham, Park House, Edgbaston Park Road, Birmingham B15 2RT, United Kingdom

Dr. M. Denayer
Institut d'Hygiène et d'Epidémiologie, Rue Juliette Wytsman 14, 1050 Bruxelles, Belgium

Dr. Marianna Diomidis
Ministry of Health and Social Welfare, P.O. Box 14156, 11510 Athens, Greece

Dr. Angela M. Downs
WHO Collaborating Centre on AIDS, Institut de Médecine et d'Epidémiologie Africaines et Tropicales, Hôpital Claude Bernard, 10 Avenue Porte d'Aubervilliers, 75019 Paris, France

Prof. Dr. M.F. Drummond
Health Services Management Centre, The University of Birmingham, Park House, Edgbaston Park Road, Birmingham B15 2RT, United Kingdom

J.A.M. van Druten
Department of Medical Statistics, Nijmegen, The Netherlands

V. Faber
Department of Infectious Diseases, Rigshospitalet, 1124 Copenhagen, Denmark

Dr. Helga Exner-Freisfeld
Landesversicherungsanstalt Hessen, Städelstrasse 28, 6000 Frankfurt am Main 70, FRG

Dr. Jaime Ginestal Gómez
Facultad de Ciencias Económicas y Empresariales, Catedra de Hacienda Publica, Universidad del País Vasco, Avenida del Ejercito, 83, 48015 Bilbao, Spain

P. Gøtzsche
Department of Infectious Diseases, Rigshospitalet, 1124 Copenhagen, Denmark

Dr. Irene Gschrey-Düver
Zentrum der Inneren Medizin, Infektiologie, Klinikum der Johann-Wolfgang-Goethe-Universität, Theodor-Stern-Kai 7, 6000 Frankfurt am Main 70, FRG

M. Guiguet
Centre Coopérateur de Données sur l'Epidémiologie de l'Immunodéficience Humaine et de l'Unité de Recherche Biomathématiques et Biostatistiques, INSERM/URBB 263, Université Paris 7, Tour 53, 7, Place Jussieu, 75251 Paris Cedex 05, France

Dr. Reinhard Hanpft
Institut für Gesundheits-System-Forschung, Weimarer Strasse 8, 2300 Kiel 1, FRG

S.H. Heisterkamp
National Institute of Public Health and Environmental Protection, P.O. Box 1, 3720 BA Bilthoven, The Netherlands

Dr. J.C. Jager
National Institute of Public Health and Environmental Protection, P.O. Box 1, 3720 BA Bilthoven, The Netherlands

Axel Jenke
Institut für Gesundheits-System-Forschung, Weimarer Strasse 8, 2300 Kiel 1, FRG

Dr. Anne M. Johnson
Academic Department of Genito Urinary Medicine, James Pringle House, 73-75 Charlotte Street, London W1N 8AA, United Kingdom

Dr. Anita Koock-Walewski
Zentrum der Inneren Medizin, Infektiologie, Klinikum der Johann-Wolfgang-Goethe-Universität, Theodor-Stern-Kai 7, 6000 Frankfurt am Main 70, FRG

Mårten Lagergren, Ph.D.
Department of Social Medicine, Karolinska Institute, 172 83 Sundbyberg, Sweden

Dr. Julien Lambert
Department of Dermatology, University of Antwerp, Universiteitsplein 1, 2610 Antwerp, Belgium

Dr. Reiner Leidl
GSF-Institut für Medizinische Informatik und Systemforschung (Medis), Ingolstädter Landstrasse 1, 8042 Neuherberg, FRG

Dr. med. Dipl. rer. pol. C. zur Lippe
Kuratorium AIDS der Paul-Ehrlich-Gesellschaft, Vogelweidstrasse 8, 6000 Frankfurt am Main 70, FRG

Prof. Dr. Alan Maynard
University of York, Centre for Health Economics, Heslington, York, Y01 5DD, United Kingdom

L. Møller
Department of Infectious Diseases, Rigshospitalet, 1124 Copenhagen, Denmark

Ruth Müller
Kuratorium AIDS der Paul-Ehrlich-Gesellschaft, Vogelweidstrasse 8, 6000 Frankfurt am Main 70, FRG

Dr. Bente Olesen
Abenra 35, 2. th., 1134 Copenhagen K, Denmark

Maurice R.H. Pedergnana, lic. oec. HSG
Management Zentrum St. Gallen, Rosenbergstrasse 38, 9001 St. Gallen, Switzerland

M.J. Postma
National Institute of Public Health and Environmental Protection, P.O. Box 1, 3720 BA Bilthoven, The Netherlands

Malcolm Rees
109 High Street, Amersham, HP7 ODY, United Kingdom

F. Reinecke
Institut für Gesundheits-System-Forschung, Weimarer Strasse 8, 2300 Kiel 1, FRG

Andrea-Marina Reinkemeier
Institut für Gesundheits-System-Forschung, Weimarer Strasse 8, 2300 Kiel, FRG

D.P. Reinking
Netherlands Institute of Mental Health, Da Costakade 45, 3521 VS, Utrecht, The Netherlands

Prof. Dr. Joan Rovira
Departament de Teoria Econòmica, Facultat de Ciències Econòmiques, Universitat de Barcelona, Av. Diagonal, 690, 08034 Barcelona, Spain

E.J. Ruitenberg
National Institute of Public Health and Environmental Protection, P.O. Box 1, 3720 BA Bilthoven, The Netherlands

Dr. Joao Santos Lucas
Department of Human and Social Sciences, National School of Public Health, Av. Padre Cruz, 1699 Lisboa Codex, Portugal

Dr. Walter Satzinger
GSF-Institut für Medizinische Informatik und Systemforschung (Medis), Ingolstädter Landstrasse 1, 8042 Neuherberg, FRG

Dr. Xenia Scheil-Adlung
Bundesministerium für Jugend, Familie, Frauen und Gesundheit, Postfach 200220, 5300 Bonn 2, FRG

R.F. Schreuder
Steering Committee of Future Health, Scenarios (STG), Ministry of Welfare, Health and Cultural Affairs (WVC), P.O. Box 5406, 2280 HK Rijswijk, The Netherlands

Prof. Dr. Detlef Schwefel
GSF-Institut für Medizinische Informatik und Systemforschung (Medis), Ingolstädter Landstrasse 1, 8042 Neuherberg, FRG

Prof. Dr. Donald S. Shepard
Harvard Institute for International Development, One Eliot Street, Cambridge, MA 02138, USA

Prof. Dr. Aris Sissouras
University of Patras, O.R. Department, Unit of Health Services Research, 26500 Patras, Greece

Dr. S. Staszewski
Zentrum der Inneren Medizin, Infektiologie, Klinikum der Johann-Wolfgang-Goethe-Universität, Theodor-Stern-Kai 7, 6000 Frankfurt am Main 70, FRG

MinR Dr. Hans Stein
Bundesministerium für Jugend, Familie, Frauen und Gesundheit, Postfach 200220, 5300 Bonn 2, FRG

Prof. Dr. W. Stille
Zentrum der Inneren Medizin, Infektiologie, Klinikum der Johann-Wolfgang-Goethe-Universität, Theodor-Stern-Kai 7, 6000 Frankfurt am Main 70, FRG

Dr. A. Stroobant
Institut d'Hygiène et d'Epidémiologie, Rue Juliette Wytsman 14, 1050 Bruxelles, Belgium

Dr. Godfried Thiers
Institut d'Hygiène et d'Epidémiologie, Rue Juliette Wytsman 14, 1050 Bruxelles, Belgium

Prof. Dr. A.J. Valleron
Centre Coopérateur de Données sur l'Epidémiologie de l'Immunodéficience Humaine et de l'Unité de Recherches Biomathématiques et Biostatistiques, INSERM/URBB 263, Université Paris 7, Tour 53, 7, Place Jussieu, 75251 Paris Cedex 05, France

J. de Vincenzi
WHO Collaborating Centre on AIDS, Institut de Médecine et d'Epidémiologie Africaines et Tropicales, Hôpital Claude Bernard, 10 Avenue Porte d'Aubervilliers, 75019 Paris, France

Steven Wayling
University of North Carolina, 6212 Braes Meadow Ct, Raleigh, NC 27612, USA

Prof. Dr. A. D. Wilkie
R. Watson & Sons, Consulting Actuaries, Watson House, London Road, Reigate, Surrey RH2 9PQ, United Kingdom

Dr. Herbert Zöllner
Regional Office for Europe, World Health Organization, 8, Scherfigsvej, 2100 Copenhagen, Denmark

Introduction

Social Sciences, Economics and AIDS

D. Schwefel

Threats can be challenges. But AIDS, today still, seems to be only a threat rather than a positive challenge - individually, socially as well as professionally.

- Since the hope for individual survival of the disease is practically non-existent for the time being, coping with the unalterable is the main option for people afflicted with AIDS; there is little room for other ways out of this life destroying catastrophe.
- Being members of social minorities, infected and affected people generally tend not to get the human affection they need, but are most probably socially stigmatized; the challenge to bridge the gap between strong majorities and weak minorities is not yet taken seriously other than rhetorically in TV spots and newspaper advertisements.
- The different professions and academic disciplines, up to now, have rarely met the challenge of bringing biomedical and socioeconomic research, medical and psychosocial care together in concerted action.
- Some joint statements, rather than actions, have however evolved at national levels; ministers of health from many a country convene rather often to discuss policies. At least at this level, the threat of AIDS has been taken as a challenge towards extended international understanding in health affairs.

This rather pessimistic outlook on individual, social and professional responses to the threat of AIDS was thus complemented in the eighties by a slowly growing international understanding of the global challenges to be met - a first marker for hope.

1. Social sciences and AIDS

To overcome the threat of AIDS, effective vaccination and/or treatment is indeed needed. But the prospects for that are rather dim. Therefore prevention is crucial, and the alleviation of hopelessly dying must also be at the top of the agenda. Even if vaccination and treatment are available soon, prevention through behavioural changes and policies, management and/or alleviation through socioeconomic and psychosocial (coping) strategies, and the widest possible extension of the best care by the most cost-effective measures will be of highest importance.

Through its task force on AIDS, the Concerted Action Committee (COMAC) on Health Services Research (HSR) of the European Community has tried to open avenues for social science research in this field. It identified four main areas which so far have been lacking sufficient scientific attention and public funding:

- Studies on risky and risk avoiding behaviour before and after preventive interventions are being conducted in some places now to test their effectiveness and acceptance. Nevertheless, coordination and concerted actions in this field are still needed and would benefit patients, professionals and politicians alike. Behavioural studies should also include the behaviour of providers, professionals and politicians and not only that of "ordinary" people and patients. Sociology could and should play a role in this field as well as in analysing and interpreting social responses to this threat.
- The existing incurability of AIDS imposes severe emotional burdens on the affected and their fellows. The risk of infection during service adds another load onto the helping professions. Mass reactions in terms of social psychology are real and to be anticipated. Psychology could and should bring information, knowledge and advice.
- Policies quite often reflected prejudices rather than results of analyses (which were not available, one has to add). So far policy responses have rarely relied on sound analyses of initiatives, their implementation and impacts. In this double sense, policy sciences could and should support regional and national prevention strategies and health policy planning.
- Being relatively weak in the range of social science approaches to health and health care, these three disciplines - sociology, psychology and political science - are being outpaced by health economics. Direct and indirect costs of AIDS and HIV infection were estimated or calculated relatively early; remarkable differences in approaches, results and implications make a more extensive and intensive economic analysis of AIDS advisable.

Other aspects should certainly not be disregarded. Ethical questions have to be addressed as well as legal ones, questions which are interwoven with the approaches mentioned. The social sciences mentioned can support concerted actions on AIDS and HIV infection quite a bit - concerted actions between patients and professionals, between helping professions, between academic disciplines and between bio- and sociomedical endeavours. Concerted actions bridging bio- and sociomedical approaches may be far ahead of us. COMAC-HSR's task force on AIDS therefore advocated first of all sound disciplinary responses in the fields of social sciences - sociology, psychology, political sciences and economics - as a starting point.

2. Economics of AIDS

One of the project proposals - the one on economic aspects of AIDS and HIV infection - got approval by COMAC-HSR first. It intended to study direct and indirect costs of AIDS and HIV infection for individuals, families, health services and societies and to try to prepare concerted actions for further research in this field.

At the beginning, direct and indirect costs of AIDS and HIV infection seemed to be relatively high. First estimates in USA (Hardy et al., 1986; Scitovsky et al., 1986; Scitovsky and Rice, 1987; Hatziandreou et al., 1987) differed quite considerably regarding the costs involved, methodology of cost estimations, underlying treatment pattern, etc. Most of them stressed - in addition to the high direct personal costs - the importance of indirect costs in terms of lost life years (quality adjusted life years or QALYs, productive life years, etc.) and of lost output due to a reduction of productivity caused by premature morbidity and mortality. Beyond these direct and indirect costs wider impacts of AIDS and HIV infection are to be considered when exploring the socioeconomic context of this topic: impacts on demography, on markets and the like.

Recent thoughts and calculations (Reinhardt, 1988; Pedergnana, 1988) hint at cost levels much lower than expected at the beginning. Only very few studies tried to compare the cost of AIDS with costs of other diseases (Hatziandreou et al., 1987). Only rarely does a study - as far as we know - stress the political and social context of cost and financing of AIDS (Fox, 1986). These three points indicate that we still know too little in this field, in absolute, relative and contextual terms. But we are quite sure that all over the world, and in Europe, social scientists are beginning to deal with such questions. This is why a study contracted by COMAC-HSR first of all tried to explore what is going on in this field of research and action.

2.1 Exploration

First, a worldwide literature survey and a European project survey were undertaken by the Institute for Medical Informatics and Health Systems Research MEDIS of GSF - National Center for Radiation and Environmental Research Munich, to explore the field. The literature survey covered the wide field of social science approaches dealing with AIDS and HIV infection. There has obviously been a steep increase in the number of relevant publications, starting quite late in the eighties. Nevertheless, since many of the projects are still going on and have not rendered publications yet, an additional project survey was required that involved sending a questionnaire to as many health systems researchers in Europe as possible and discussing with many researchers results, studies and research plans.

2.2 Pattern of concerns

Taking into consideration some of the more recent representative and relevant publications in this field, a quite diversified pattern of research emerges:

1. General aspects
   - overview of topics (7,8,34,46,48,55)
   - bibliographies (38,57), e.g. on cost studies (6)
   - review of cost studies (20,21,25,31,74,82,83)
   - patterns of care (5,20,36,43,51)

2. Cost studies
   - hospital costs (5,36,37,39,43,51,63,65,72,76,78)
   - regional and national costs (26,27,44,49,77)
   - patient costs (12,14,28,29,31,39,42,66,67)
   - general aspects and cost projections (31,59,68,80,81,82,83)
3. Other economic aspects
   - financial aspects (2,8,22,32,68,82,83), e.g., for insurers
   - resource allocation considerations (83)
   - evaluations, e.g. of treatments (21,45)
   - cost-effectiveness approaches (1,12,64,68)
   - effectivity measures, e.g. QALYs (21,30,67,73,86)
4. Wider approaches
   - policy studies (4,24,25,61,68)
   - behavioural studies (40,75)
   - cognition, attitudes and perceptions (4,10,13,16,17,23,41,50,52,53,54,56,79)
   - general remarks (58)
5. Projections and scenarios
   - disease projections (3,15,18,21,32,33,35,60,69,70,71,84)
   - scenarios (47,62)
6. Impact studies
   - impacts on care (19,85)
   - demographic impacts (15,86)
   - social impacts (11)
   - ethical aspects (9)
   - global impacts (87)

This picture takes into account literature reviews, results of previous research and preliminary results of ongoing socioeconomic research on AIDS and HIV infection. This pattern of concerns shows clearly that social research is available for policy makers to learn from. Some aspects, though, deserve special support: wider impact analyses - especially asked for in the original COMAC-HSR proposal for studying economic aspects of AIDS and IV infection - and cost-effectiveness analyses, for example, are certainly not being conducted in sufficient number and intensity.

A preliminary analysis of the results of our research survey showed the following pattern of research concerns in terms of research groups dealing with the topics indicated:

- patterns of care		8 groups
- direct costs		15 groups
of hospitals	4 groups	
of districts, regions, nations	7 groups	
of insurances	4 groups	
of patients, families	8 groups	
- indirect costs		12 groups
- cost-effectiveness (benefit/utility) analysis		9 groups

- financing problems 4 groups
- methodological issues 10 groups
- impacts on demography 4 groups
- other impacts 2 groups
- prediction and scenarios 12 groups

2.3 Lessons

This pattern of published and ongoing research shows several remarkable features when interpreted and compared with already published studies.

- First, the main track of research is and will be cost studies. Studies on hospital costs are a rather dominant starting point for economic analyses - the most feasible one.
- Second, financing problems are quite less a prominent research topic in European research as compared to the American one. This may reflect the wide spread coverage of public insurances for health and of social security systems for the majority in European countries, a major feature with important implications for AIDS and HIV infection as well.
- Third, other impacts of AIDS and HIV infection are rarely taken up as research topics; this is valid for forgone and ongoing research. Some of these aspects are taken into consideration, nevertheless, in the drafting of scenarios, a rather prominent approach in Europe.
- Scenario approaches are still linked very much to basic epidemiological questions and based on the development and adaptation of mathematical tools. Economics is coming in hesitantly.
- A fifth point is that cost-effectiveness or cost-utility studies are still rare, and that comparative effectivity measures need further research and application.
- Sixth, methodological approaches could and should be supported much more, so should approaches which compare AIDS and HIV infection with other killers and cripples, and those that compare the social and economic contexts of treatment patterns of other diseases.
- Finally, research in these areas seems to be a bit isolated from research in biomedical environments except for cost studies in hospitals. This not only reflects isolation, but also that applied health economics research addresses its messages to much wider audiences than to the clinical establishment, since social and not only clinical management is the focus.

These aspects of the actual and emerging pattern of research on some economic aspects of AIDS and HIV infection should be taken into consideration when trying to bridge existing gaps between the research of different professions, disciplines and countries.

3. Outlook

We do not know enough about the socioeconomic context of diseases and patterns of treatment and care. Too often rather narrow approaches were used to look into incidences and prevalences alone, but not into life years lost, productive life years lost, quality adjusted life years lost, labour and human productivity lost, welfare and well-being lost. The psychosocial and socioeconomic context of diseases is much wider than mostly analyzed. In this sense socioeconomic research on AIDS and HIV infection bears the challenge of applying such a wider view. AIDS is too awful a threat as to analyse its incidences and prevalences only. It is the social, psychological, economical and political context of this disease which plays an important role, and to neglect this would mean to close the eyes where twilight should stimulate rather than prevent research. The same may be true for the psychosocial and the socioeconomic context of actions to alleviate the burden for the affected and their fellow-men and to prevent AIDS as far and fair as possible. Socioeconomic research on AIDS and HIV infection, if it accepts these challenges, could also be fruitful for preventing and treating, effectively and efficiently, other patterns of disease. Social sciences, including economics, could and should try to turn the threat of AIDS to hopeful challenges.

References

1. Abreu Cruz, M.A. (1986). Avaliação económica de um programa de prevenção - SIDA - análise custo-benefício. Escola nacional de saúde pública. Cadeira de economia da saúde, curso III.

2. Aerni, R. (1988). Die Auseinandersetzung der Lebens- und Krankenversicherer mit AIDS (unter spezieller Berücksichtigung der gesellschaftlichen Verantwortung). Vorgelegt an der Hochschule St. Gallen für Wirtschafts- und Sozialwissenschaften.

3. Alderman, M.H., Drucker, E., Rosenfield, A., and Healton, C. (1988). Predicting the future of the AIDS epidemic and its consequences for the health care system of New York. Bulletin of the New York Academy of Medicine 64(2), 175-183.

4. Altman, D. (1987). AIDS in the mind of America. Anchor Press, Doubleday, Garden City, New York, 59-81, 111-113.

5. Andrulis, D.P., Beers, V.S., Bentley, J.D., and Gage, J.D. (1987). The provision and financing of medical care for AIDS patients in US public and private teaching hospitals. Journal of the American Medical Association 258, 1343-1346.

6. Annotated Bibliography (1987). The costs of AIDS. Health Policy 8, 29-31.

7. Arno, P.S. (1987). The economic impact of AIDS. Journal of the American Medical Association 258, 1376-1377.

8. Arno, P.S. and Lee, P.R. (1986). Economic costs of AIDS. In: AIDS. Facts and Issues (eds. V. Gong and N. Rudnick). Rutgers University Press, New Brunswick, London, 167-178.

9. Barry, M. (1988). Ethical considerations of human investigation in developing countries: the AIDS dilemma. The New England Journal of Medicine 319(16), 1083-1086.

10. Bayer, R. (1986). AIDS, power, and reason. The Milbank Quaterly 64, Suppl. 1, 168-182.

11. Carballo, M. and Carael, M. (n.y.). Impact of AIDS on social organization. Manuscript, Global Programme on AIDS, World Health Organization, Geneva.

12. Cunningham, D. and Griffith, S.F. (1987). AIDS: counting the costs. British Medical Journal 295, 921-922.

13. Dab, W., Moatti, J.P., Bastide, S., Abenhaïm, L., and Pollak, M. (1988). La perception sociale du SIDA en région Île-de-France. Bulletin épidémiologique hebdomadaire 12, 45-46.

14. Davachi, F., Baudoux, P., Ndoko, K., Ngoie, K., N'Galy, B., and Mann, J. (n.y.). The economic impact on families of children with AIDS in Kinshasa, Zaire. Unpublished manuscript.

15. Daykin, C.D. (n.y.). The impact of AIDS on the UK population. Directing Actuary (Social Security). Unpublished manuscript, London.

16. DiClemente, R.J., Zorn, J., and Temoshok, L. (1986). Adolescents and AIDS: a survey of knowledge, attitudes and beliefs about AIDS in San Francisco. American Journal of Public Health 76(12), 1443-1445.

17. Doherty, J.P. (1986). AIDS: one psychosocial response. Quality Review Bulletin 12(8), 295-297.

18. Downs, A.M., Ancelle, R.A., Jager, J.C, and Brunet, J.-B. (1987). AIDS in Europe: current trends and short-term predictions estimated from surveillance data, January 1981-June 1986. AIDS 1(1), 53-57.

19. Drucker, E. and Einstein, A. (1987). AIDS and addiction in New York City: the transformation of a chronic social problem into a public health catastrophe. Paper presented at the Collogue 'SIDA, Droit et Liberté (AIDS, Law and Liberty)', Paris, 11-12 December.

20. Drummond, M. and Davies, L. (1988). Treating AIDS: the economic issues. Health Policy 10, 1-19.

21. Eastwood, A. and Maynard, A. (1987). Treating AIDS patients: Is it ethical to be efficient? Paper presented at the IRISS Conference 'Quality of Life: Perspectives and Policies', University of York, 11-12 November.

22. Eden, J. (1988). AIDS and health insurance. An OTA Survey. A staff paper in OTA's Series on AIDS-Related Issues, Washington D.C.

23. Eskola, A., Jylhä, M., and Weckroth, K. (1988). On the 'logic' of AIDS. Paper presented at the First International Conference on The Global Impact of AIDS, Barbican Centre, London, 8-10 March.

24. Fox, D.M. (1986). AIDS and the American health polity: the history and prospects of a crisis of authority. The Milbank Quaterly 64, Suppl. 1, 7-33.

25. Fox, D.M. and Thomas, E.H. (1987/88). AIDS cost analysis and social policy. Law, Medicine & Health Care 15(4), 186-211.

26. Ginestal, J., Barrenechea, E., and de la Sierra, M.P. (1988). Marco de planificación y evaluación del SIDA en la C.A.P.V. Universidad del País Vasco, Bilbao.

27. Gutzwiller, F., Martin, J., Mombelli, G., Somaini, B., and Steffen, R. (eds.) (1989). AIDS in der Schweiz. Die Epidemie, die Folgen, die Maßnahmen. Ein Bericht der Eidgenössischen Kommission für AIDS-Fragen und des Bundesamtes für Gesundheitswesen, 66-74.

28. Hanpft, R., Reinecke, F., and Beske, F. (1988). Ausgaben für und Kosten der Diagnostik und Therapie HIV-infizierter Patienten. Paper presented at: Deutscher AIDS-Kongreß, München, 8 January.

29. Hardy, A., Rauch, K. et al. (1986). The economic impact of the first 10,000 cases of acquired immunodeficiency syndrome in the United States. Journal of the American Medical Association 255, 209-211.

30. Hatziandreou, E., Graham, J.D., and Stoto, M.A. (1987). AIDS and biomedical research funding: a comparative analysis. Reviews of Infectious Diseases 10(1), 159-167.

31. Hellinger, F.J. (1988). Forecasting the personal medical care costs of AIDS from 1988 through 1991. Public Health Reports 103(3), 309-319.

32. Institute of Actuaries (ed.) (1987). AIDS working party. Bulletin No. 1, London.

33. Institute of Actuaries (ed.) (1987). AIDS working party. Bulletin No. 2, London.

34. Institute of Medicine (ed.) (1986). Confronting AIDS. Directions for public health care and research. National Academy Press, Washington D.C., 155-175.

35. Institute of Medicine (ed.) (1988). Approaches to modeling disease spread and impact. Report of a workshop on mathematical modeling of the spread of human immunodeficiency virus and the demographic impact of acquired immune deficiency syndrome, 15.-17. Oktober 1987. National Academy Press, Washington D.C.

36. Jager, J.C, Borleffs, J.C.C., Geels, R.M.A., Heisterkamp, S.H., Jong, J.T.L., and Ruitenberg, E.J. (1988). A method for monitoring hospital costs related to AIDS and HIV-infection. Poster presentation at the IV International Conference on AIDS, Stockholm.

37. Jager, J.C, Borleffs, J.C.C., Geels, R.M.A., Jong, J.T.L., and Ruitenberg, E.J. (1988). Quantitative estimation of hospital costs for patients with AIDS and infection with HIV. Poster presentation at the First International Conference on The Global Impact of AIDS, Barbican Centre, London, 8-10 March.

38. Jager, J.C., Borleffs, J.C.C., Geels, R.M.A., Jong, J.T.L., and Ruitenberg, E.J. (1988). References concerning AIDS and economy. Annex to: Quantitative estimation of hospital costs for patients with AIDS and infection with HIV. Poster presentation at the First International Conference on The Global Impact of AIDS, Barbican Centre, London, 8-10 March.

39. Johnson, A.M., Adler, M.W., and Crown, J.M. (1986). The acquired immune deficiency syndrome and epidemic of infection with human immunodeficiency virus: costs of care and prevention in an inner London district. British Medical Journal 293, 489-492.

40. Johnson, A. M., Wadsworth, J., Elliott, P. et al. (1989). A pilot study of sexual lifestyle in a random sample of the population of Great Britain. Unpublished Manuscript.

41. Kaplan, H.B., Johnson, R.J., Bailey, C.A., and Simon, W. (1987). The sociological study of AIDS: a critical review of the literature and suggested research agenda. Journal of Health and Social Behavior 28, 140-157.

42. Koock-Walewski, A., Wilke, K., Wegner, R., and Stille, W. (1988). Kostenanalysen von LAS- und AIDS-Patienten in der Universitätsklinik Frankfurt. Deutscher AIDS-Kongress, München, 8./9.1., Programm und Abstracts, 60.

43. Lafferty, W.E., Hopkins, S.G., Honey, J., Harwell, J.D., Shoemaker, P.C., and Kobayashi, J.M. (1988). Hospital charges for people with AIDS in Washington State: utilization of a statewide hospital discharge data base. American Journal of Public Health 78(8), 949-952.

44. Lakhani, A. et al. (1988). West Lambeth Health Authority - Human Immunodefieciency Virus (HIV) and AIDS related services projected expenditure 1987/8 plus requirements 1988/9. Paper presented at the First International Conference on The Global Impact of AIDS, Barbican Centre, London, 8-10 March.

45. Lehmann, P., Hausser, D., Somaini, B., and Gutzwiller, F. (1987). Campaign against AIDS in Switzerland: evaluation of a nationwide educational programme. British Medical Journal 295, 1118-1120.

46. Leidl, R. (1988). AIDS - Ökonomische Aspekte einer Epidemie. Unpublished manuscript, GSF - Institut für medizinische Informatik und Systemforschung (Medis), Neuherberg.

47. Leidl, R. (1988). Methods to assess the dynamics of the economic impact of AIDS: a PC-based scenario-approach. Paper presented at the EC-Workshop 'Quantitative Analysis of AIDS', Bilthoven, 4-6 July.

48. Leidl, R. (1989). Ökonomische Aspekte. In: AIDS und HIV-Infektionen. Diagnostik, Klinik, Behandlung. Handbuch und Atlas für Klinik und Praxis (ed. H. Jäger). Ecomed, Landsberg, IX-3, 1-14.

49. Majnoni d'Intignano, B. (1988). 18 milliards. La facture du SIDA en 1990? Informations Professionelles, No. 4202, 12 Decembre.

50. McCombie, S.C. (1986). The cultural impact of the 'AIDS' test: the American experience. Social Science and Medicine 23(5), 455-459.

51. Meyran, S., Sabatini, J., Barlet, P., and Vedrinne, J. (1988). Une approche économique de la prise en charge de l'infection par le virus de l'immunodéficience humaine (HIV 1) en milieu hospitalier. VIIIième Journées d'Economie Sociale, Dijon, 22-23 Septembre.

52. Moatti, J.-P. and Dab, W. (1988). The social perception of AIDS in the Île-de-France. Initial findings of the survey. METROPOLIS, International Committee on Major Hazards, Madrid, January.

53. Moatti, J.P., Le Galès, C., Manesse, L., Pagès, J.P., and Fagnani, F. (1988). La perception sociale du SIDA dans l'opinion publique française. Le Concours Médical 110(15), 1231-1236.

54. Moatti, J.P., Manesse, L., Le Galès, C., Pagès, J.P., and Fagnani, F. (1988). Social perception of AIDS in the general public: a French study. Health Policy 9, 1-8.

55. Moja Jauregui, F. (1987). Consideraciones sobre los costes sociales causados por el SIDA. Economía y Salud, Año 1(1), 10-11.

56. Morin, S.F. and Balchelor, W.F. (1984). Responding to the psychological crisis of AIDS. Public Health Reports 99(1), 4-9.

57. National Center for Health Services Research and Health Care Technology Assessment (NCHSR) (ed.) (1987). Selected bibliography on AIDS for health services research. Program note. Rockville MD, September.

58. National Center for Health Services Research and Health Care Technology Assessment (NCHSR) (ed.) (1988). HIV-related illnesses: topics for health services research. Program note. Rockville MD, October.

59. National Center for Health Services Research and Health Care Technology Assessment (NCHSR) (ed.) (1988). Research Activities No. 106.

60. National Institute of Public Health and Environmental Protection (RVIM) (ed.) (1988). Abstracts. EC Workshop on Quantitative analyses of AIDS, Bilthoven, July 6th-8th.

61. National Working Party on Health Service Implications of HIV Infection (1987). Report. Scotland, May.

62. Nederlands centrum Geestelijke volksgezondheid (NcGv) (ed.) (1988). Feasability study for scenario project: the sociocultural and economic impact of AIDS on society.

63. Office of the New York State Comptroller (ed.) (1987). Projected costs of the treatment of acquired immune deficiency syndrome in New York City. Report 11-88, July 8.

64. Ohi, G., Kai, I., Kobayashi, Y., Hasegawa, T., Takenaga, N., Takata, S., Takaku, F., Yoshikura, H., and Yoshimura, T. (1987). AIDS prevention in Japan and its cost-benefit aspects. Health Policy 8, 17-27.

65. Olesen, B., Gøtzsche, P.C., Bygbjerg, I.C., Møller, L.H., and Faber, V. (1988). Hospitalsomkostninger ved diagnostik og behandling af AIDS-patienter. Ugeskr Læger 150/38, 2250-2252.

66. Over, M., Bertozzi, S., and Chin, J. (1988). Guidelines for making a preliminary estimate of the direct and indirect cost of HIV infection in developing countries. Paper presented at the III International Conference on AIDS and Related Cancers in Africa, Arusha, Tanzania, September 16.

67. Over, M., Bertozzi, S., Chin, J., N'Galy, B., and Nyamuryekung'e, K. (1988). The direct and indirect cost of HIV-infection in developing countries: the cases of Zaire and Tanzania. Paper presented at the IV International Conference on AIDS, Stockholm.

68. Pascal, A. (1987). The costs of treating AIDS under medicaid: 1986-1991. RAND Corporation, Santa Monica, May.

69. Pedergnana, M.R.H. (1988). Morbidität und Mortalität als indirekte Kosten von AIDS: Möglichkeiten und Grenzen ihrer Messung im Lichte der Prognosen über die Ausbreitung von AIDS bis 1995. Diplomarbeit an der Hochschule St. Gallen für Wirtschafts- und Sozialwissenschaften.

70. Pedergnana, M., Schmid, H. et al. (eds.) (1988). AIDS: Zur Entwicklung in der Schweiz bis 1995. Hans Huber, Bern, Stuttgart, Toronto, 5-8, 131-136.

71. Rees, M. (1987). Describing the AIDS epidemic. The Lancet, July 11, 98-99.

72. Rees, M., Hawkins, D.A., Gazzard, B.G., Roberts, B. (1988). The impact of AIDS/HIV on the activities and costs of St. Stephen's Hospital, London. IV International Conference on AIDS, Stockholm (abstract 9601).

73. Rees, M. and Roberts, B. (1988). Quality adjusted life years (QUALYs) and the cost of AIDS patients. IV International Conference on AIDS, Stockholm (abstract 9586).

74. Reinhardt, U.E. (1987). What 'staggering' costs? We can afford AIDS care. Washington Post, October.

75. Robertson, J.R., Skidmore, C.A., and Roberts, J.J.K. (1988). HIV infection in intravenous drug users: a follow-up study indicating changes in risk-taking behaviour. British Journal of Addiction 83, 387-391.

76. Rocha Nogueira, J.M. (1987). Hospitalização por SIDA em Portugal. Custos actuais e previsão para 1992. Escola Nacional de Saúde Pública, curso II. Unpublished manuscript.

77. Rovira Forns, J., Badia Llach, X. (1988). Informe preliminar y propuesta de estudio de los costes del SIDA en Cataluña. Dictamen encargado por el programa para la prevención y el control del SIDA en Cataluña. Barcelona, agosto.

78. Ruiz González, C. and Ponce de León, S. (1987). Perfil socioeconómico y costo del tratamiento de pacientes con síndrome de inmunodeficiencia adquirida atendidos en el Instituto Nacional de la Nutrición "Salvador Zubirán". La Revista de Investigación Clínica 39, Suplemento, 139-141.

79. Santos Lucas, J. (1987). Os portugueses e a SIDA. Inquérito Nacional sobre conhecimentos, atitudes e comportamentos associados com a SIDA. Revista Portuguesa de Saúde Pública 5(3-4), 89-100.

80. Scitovsky, A.A., Cline, M. et al. (1986). Medical care costs of patients with AIDS in San Francisco. Journal of the American Medical Association 256, 3103-3106.

81. Scitovsky, A.A. and Rice, D.P. (1987). Estimates of the direct and indirect costs of acquired immunodeficiency syndrome in United States 1985, 1986 and 1991. Public Health Reports 102, 5-17.

82. Sisk, J.E. (1987). The costs of AIDS and other HIV infections: review of the estimates. Staff paper, Health Program, Office of Technology Assessment, US Congress, Mimeo, Washington DC, May.

83. Sisk, J.E. (1987). The costs of AIDS: a review of the estimates. Health Affairs, Summer, 5-21.

84. Tennison, B.R. and Hagard, S. (1988). AIDS: predicting cases nationally and locally. British Medical Journal 297, 711-713.

85. United Hospital Fund (ed.) (1987). Blueprint. The Newsletter of the United Hospital Fund, New York, Fall.

86. Valleron, A.J. and Flandre, P. (1988). Demographic impact of mortality from AIDS in France: projection in 1990. Paper presented at the First International Conference on The Global Impact of AIDS, Barbican Centre, London, 8-10 March.

87. World Health Organization and London School of Hygiene and Tropical Medicine (eds.) (1987). Abstract book & final programme. First International Conference on The Global Impact of AIDS, Barbican Centre, London, 8-10 March 1988.

Exploring Spread and Context of AIDS and HIV Infection

Patterns of AIDS and HIV Infection in Europe

A.M. Downs, R.A. Ancelle-Park, I. de Vincenzi, J.-B. Brunet

1. Introduction

Since 1983, countries belonging to the WHO European region have participated in the surveillance of AIDS in Europe by reporting to the WHO Collaborating Centre on AIDS in Paris. Data are supplied to the Centre, at regular intervals and according to agreed standardized formats, by a single, nationally recognized source per country, each source being responsible for the quality of the data provided.

To date, surveillance has been primarily concerned with cases of AIDS, diagnosed in accordance with successive updates of the Centers for Disease Control (CDC) case definition. However, the clear need for good quality data on the prevalence and incidence of HIV infection has recently lead to increased activity in this important area. Some recent results from both of these aspects of surveillance are presented and discussed below. Further details may be found in the regular quarterly reports issued by the Centre and available on request.

2. AIDS surveillance data

By 31st December 1988, a total of 19,058 cases of AIDS had been reported by 31 countries (see Table 1), with an increase of 87% (8,877 newly reported cases) since December 1987 (WHO Collaborating Centre on AIDS, Paris, 1988). The cumulative incidence per million population remained highest in Switzerland (106.4) and France (101.7), followed by Denmark (70.2). Countries in the eastern part of the region reported much lower numbers of cases, with rates of less than 3 per million population. The equivalent rate in the USA was 339.5 per million at 2nd January 1989 (Centers for Disease Control, 1989).

Considering all cases diagnosed in adults or adolescents (over 12 years of age), the male:female sex ratio was 7.7. This ratio was however much closer to unity among intravenous (IV) drug users (3.1), persons presumed infected by heterosexual contact (1.6) and transfusion recipients (1.3) (see Table 2).

Among the 18,603 cases in adults/adolescents, 53% were diagnosed in homosexual or bisexual men and 26% among IV drug users (a further 2% being both homo- or

Table 1. Cumulative AIDS cases reported by 31 European countries and estimated cumulative incidence rates per million population

Country	Date of report:					
	Dec. 87	Mar. 88	June 88	Sept. 88	Dec. 88	Rate per million
Albania	-	0	0	0	0	0.0
Austria	139	158	191	191*	191*	25.1
Belgium	277	336	368	408	424	42.8
Bulgaria	1	1	3	3	3	0.3
Czechoslovakia	8	10	11	12	12	0.8
Denmark	228	262	292	319	358	70.2
Finland	24	27	32	37	41	8.4
France	3,073	3,628	4,211	4,874	5,655	101.7
German Dem. Rep.	6	6	6	6	11	0.7
Germany, Fed. Rep.	1,669	1,906	2,210	2,488	2,779	45.6
Greece	88	106	127	151	170	17.0
Hungary	8	11	13	14	17	1.6
Iceland	4	5	6	7	10	50.0
Ireland	33	37	49	64	74	21.1
Israel	47	58	65	67	76	17.3
Italy	1,411	1,736	2,094	2,556	3,008	52.4
Luxemburg	9	10	12	13	13	32.5
Malta	7	10	12	12	14	35.0
Netherlands	420	487	539	605	694	47.5
Norway	70	81	88	91	100	23.8
Poland	3	3	3	3	5	0.1
Portugal	90	123	139	173	199	19.3
Romania	3	4	8	9	10	0.4
San Marino	-	0	0	0	0	0.0
Spain	789	1,126	1,471	1,850	2,165	55.5
Sweden	163	181	205	223	256	30.5
Switzerland	355	439	502	605	702	106.4
Turkey	-	-	-	10	17	0.3
United Kingdom	1,227	1,429	1,598	1,794	1,982	34.9
USSR	3	3	4	4	7	0.0
Yugoslavia	26	38	40	58	65	2.8
Total	10,181	12,221	14,299	16,647	19,058	

Source: WHO Collaborating Centre on AIDS, Paris, 1988

* June 1988 data

bisexual and IV drug users), while 8% were presumed to be infected through heterosexual contact. Among the 2,134 adult female cases, more than half (54.5%) were IV drug users. There is however a considerable between-country variation in the distribution of cases by transmission group, as shown in Fig. 1. Whereas, in five northern European countries, over 70% of all cases have occurred in homo-/bisexual

Table 2. Cumulative AIDS cases by transmission group for 31 European countries* (as reported by 31st December 1988)

Transmission group	Adults/adolescents		Paediatric	Total	
	Male	Female	< 13 years	No.	%
Homo-/bisexual	9,812	-	-	9,812	51.5
IV drug user	3,641	1,163	-	4,804	25.2
Homosexual IV drug user	415	-	-	415	2.2
Haemophilia/coag.disorder	637	7	48	644	3.4
Transfusion	389	289	55	678	3.6
Heterosexual contact	882	550	-	1,432	7.5
Mother-to-child	-	-	350	350	1.8
Other/unknown	693	125	2	818	4.3
Total	16,469	2,134	455	19,058	100.0

Source: WHO Collaborating Centre on AIDS, Paris, 1988

* Albania, Austria, Belgium, Bulgaria, Czechoslovakia, Denmark, Finland, France, German DR, Germany FR, Greece, Hungary, Iceland, Ireland, Israel, Italy, Luxemburg, Malta, Netherlands, Norway, Poland, Portugal, Romania, San Marino, Spain, Sweden, Switzerland, Turkey, United Kingdom, USSR, Yugoslavia

men, in Italy and Spain 65% and 60% of cases respectively have occurred among heterosexual IV drug users. Amongst the 455 paediatric cases reported (Table 3), mother-to-child transmission was the main mode of transmission (77% of cases); within this group, 55% of the mothers were IV drug users.

The overall proportion of adult cases diagnosed among heterosexual IV drug users has increased sharply over the last four years, from 1% in December 1984 to 26% in December 1988 (see Fig. 2). These cases are concentrated particularly in southern Europe, with 85% of them reported from Italy, Spain or France. The seriousness of this situation has been repeatedly stressed (Ancelle-Park et al., 1987; Ancelle-Park and De Vincenzi, 1988), particularly in regard to the potential spread of HIV in the heterosexual population and to the increase in vertical (mother-to-child) transmission of HIV. In the latter context, it should be noted (Table 3) that 74% of all cases attributed to mother-to-child transmission have been reported from Italy, Spain or France.

The proportionate increase in cases among IV drug users has been accompanied by other changes in the characteristics of reported AIDS cases in Europe. In particular, the distribution by age and sex (Fig. 3) shows percentage increases in women and in younger men; between December 1984 and December 1988, female cases increased from 8% to 12% of the total, while, amongst all adult male cases, the percentage under

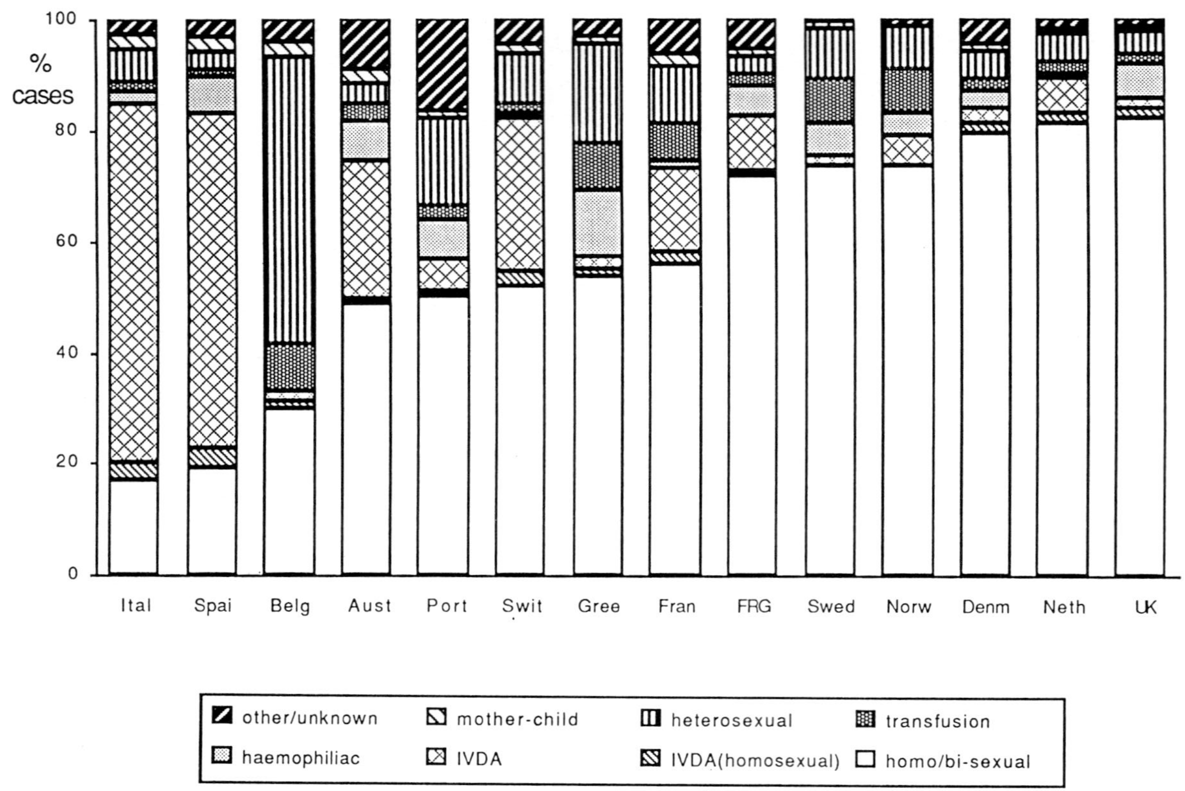

Fig. 1. Percentage distribution of cumulative AIDS cases among transmission groups, by country of diagnosis, at 31st December 1988 (see Table 1 for total numbers of cases)

Table 3. Cumulative paediatric AIDS cases* by country of diagnosis and transmission group as reported by 31st December 1988

Country of diagnosis	Mother with AIDS or at risk for AIDS				Haemo-	Trans-	Other/	
	IVDU	Trans	Hetero	Oth/Unk	philiac	fusion	unknown	Total
Austria	4	0	0	1	1	1	0	7
Belgium	0	0	12	0	1	0	0	13
Denmark	1	0	1	0	0	0	0	2
France	44	4	60	13	3	25	1	150
Germany FR	15	1	4	4	3	7	0	34
Greece	0	0	0	2	3	1	0	6
Ireland	3	0	1	0	0	0	0	4
Italy	57	0	21	4	5	4	0	91
Netherlands	1	1	1	1	0	6	0	10
Portugal	0	0	1	0	2	0	0	3
Spain	56	0	1	0	21	5	1	84
Sweden	0	0	3	0	1	0	0	4
Switzerland	7	0	1	5	0	1	0	14
Turkey	0	0	0	0	1	0	0	1
United Kingdom	3	5	8	3	6	5	0	30
USSR	0	0	1	0	0	0	0	1
Yugoslavia	0	0	0	0	1	0	0	1
Total	191	11	115	33	48	55	2	455

Source: WHO Collaborating Centre on AIDS, Paris

* under 13 years; IVDU: Intravenous drug user; Trans: Transfusion recipient; Hetero: Heterosexual contact; Oth: Other; Unk: Unknown.

No paediatric cases were reported in: Albania, Bulgaria, Czechoslovakia, Finland, German DR, Hungary, Iceland, Israel, Luxemburg, Malta, Norway, Poland, Romania, San Marino.

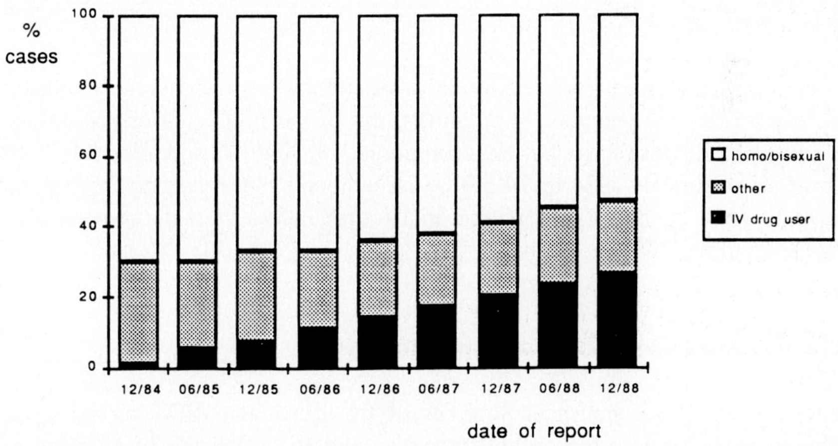

Fig. 2. Percentage distribution of cumulative AIDS cases among the main transmission groups, by date of report; 31 European countries

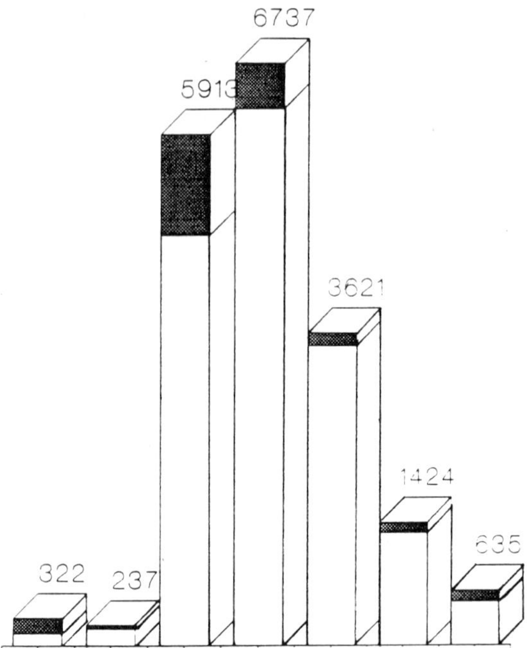

	0-9	10-19	20-29	30-39	40-49	50-59	60 & over
Females	180	40	1167	530	149	118	129
Males	142	197	4746	6207	3472	1306	506

Fig. 3. Distribution of cumulative AIDS cases by age and sex at 31st December 1988; 31 European countries

30 years of age increased from 16% to 30%. A change has also been observed in the distribution by disease category at diagnosis; the proportion of cases presenting with opportunistic infections alone (i.e. unaccompanied by Kaposi's sarcoma) has increased from 64% at December 1984 to 74.5% by December 1988, reflecting the significantly lower occurrence of Kaposi's sarcoma in IV drug users than in homosexual men (Ancelle-Park et al., 1987).

3. Trend analyses and short-term predictions

Since December 1985, statistical analyses of the European AIDS surveillance data have been carried out at 6-monthly intervals, with the dual aim of monitoring and comparing the evolution of the epidemic, within individual countries and within the principal transmission groups, and of providing short-term predictions. The method adopted (Downs et al., 1987, 1988) is based on fitting an exponential model to half-yearly incidence data over successive periods of 3 years, in order to obtain successive estimates of average doubling times over the chosen time windows. Despite the crudeness of this approach, we believe that it has proved particularly useful in providing early indicators of trends within particular geographical or behavioural sub-populations. Since doubling times in given subpopulations are generally found to be lengthening, forward extrapolation on the basis of latest estimated doubling times is expected to produce overestimates of future cases. Nevertheless, short-term predictions, for up to two years ahead, can be of some value, provided that the exponential model fits sufficiently well over the most recent 3-year period.

As the analysis is based on the numbers of incident cases by period (half-year) of diagnosis, and not by period of report, the data must first be adjusted for delays in reporting. This is done using a maximum likelihood approach (Heisterkamp et al., 1988, 1989), with data from successive surveillance reports.

Table 4. Estimated average doubling times of cumulative AIDS cases over the period January 1986 - December 1988, by country of diagnosis and transmission group (at least 50 reported cases)

Country	All cases	Homo/bi	IVDU	Hetero
Denmark	23.2	24.1	-	-
FR Germany	23.0*	23.3*	***	***
United Kingdom	22.8	24.3	-	14.2*
Netherlands	20.4*	23.5*	11.6*°	-
Switzerland	16.0	24.8*	10.8	8.2**
France	15.6	18.6	10.5	13.7
Spain	12.4	16.0*	10.5	9.7
Italy	10.8	15.9	10.4	7.3
Greece	11.9*			
Austria +	10.9 +			
Portugal	10.9			
Yugoslavia	8.8			
Ireland	8.2			
Belgium	***			
Israel	***			
Norway	***			
Sweden	***			
E.C.	15.6	20.4	10.8	12.5

\+ June 1988 estimate
E.C.: European Community (pooled data)

° 45 reported cases only
* $0.80 < R^2 < 0.90$
** $R^2 = 0.76$
*** $R^2 < 0.70$
in all other cases:
$R^2 > 0.90$

Selected results from the analysis of data reported by 31st December 1988 are presented in Fig. 4 - 6 and Table 4. Fig. 4 is based on pooled data from the countries of the European Community (which together account for 92% of all European cases) and shows the evolution in estimated doubling times in the two principal transmission groups and for all groups combined. The overall epidemic doubling time has lengthened steadily from around 7 months in the early stages of the epidemic (only 21 cases are reported to have been diagnosed before 1981) to a latest estimate (for the period 1986 - 1988) of 15.6 months. As most of the early cases were among homo-/bisexuals, the early evolution was in large part a reflection of the trends in this group. However, since the onset of a separate epidemic among IV drug users, with an

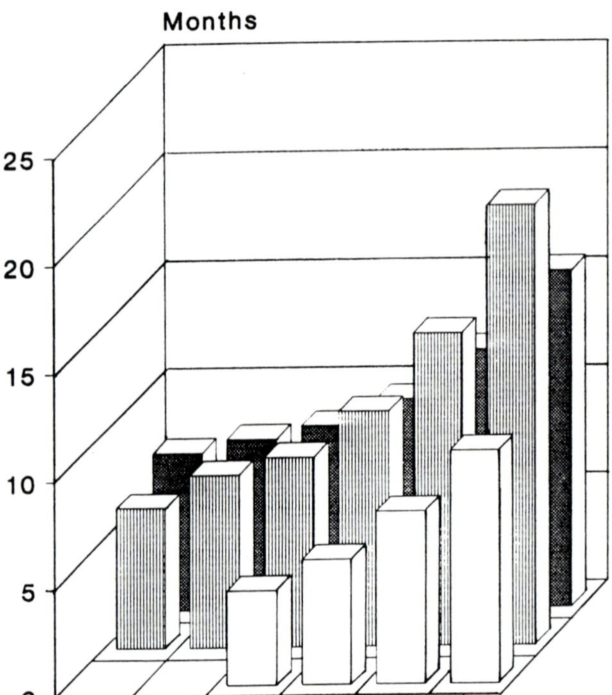

DIAGNOSED BETWEEN YRS:	81 83	82 84	83 85	84 86	85 87	86 88
ALL	7.3	7.9	8.5	9.7	12	15.6
HOMO	6.5	8	8.8	10.9	14.5	20.4
IVDU			4.4	5.8	8	10.8

Fig. 4. Trends in the AIDS epidemic among homosexuals (HOMO), among IV drug users (IVDU) and for all transmission group combined (ALL), in the countries of the European Community (pooled data). Estimated average doubling times of diagnosed AIDS cases over successive 3-year periods, are indicated in months

estimated initial doubling time (4.4 months) much shorter than that ever observed in the homo-/bisexual group, overall doubling times have been intermediate between those in these two groups. Although both groups show lengthening doubling times, the more rapid rise in incidence among IV drug users is confirmed by the consistently shorter estimates for this group (10.8 months versus 20.4 months over the last three years). The estimated doubling time for cases attributed to heterosexual transmission has remained relatively stable at around 12 - 13 months since 1984 (latest estimate: 12.5 months).

Extrapolation on the basis of the above estimates would predict a cumulative incidence of 64,600 cases in the EC by the end of 1990 (Fig. 5). As discussed above, this figure is probably an over-estimate. Due to delays in reporting, the number of cases actually reported by the end of 1990 can in any case be expected to be considerably less than the projection given here, which relates to diagnoses and not to reports (typically, around 75% of cumulated diagnosed cases are estimated to be reported at any given moment). Nevertheless, since the resources needed for the care of AIDS patients would seem not to depend on whether or not they have been reported to the surveillance system, this seems a more useful quantity for planning purposes. Extrapolations in the separate transmission groups suggest that incident cases among IV drug users could well exceed those among homo-/bisexual males from mid-1989 onwards, with equality in terms of cumulative cases towards the end of 1990 (28,400 IVDU cases v. 26,100 homo-/bisexual cases projected to be diagnosed by the end of 1990).

Epidemic trends within individual European countries show considerable variation. A large part of this variation can be explained by differences in epidemic onset times and in the distribution among transmission groups. Lengthening doubling times are generally observed whenever the epidemic in the population concerned is sufficiently advanced for such a trend to be detectable. Although there are indications that these trends are probably continuing, half-yearly (adjusted) incidence continues to increase in most populations. Exceptions have been noted, however, in Norway, Sweden and Belgium, for which observed decreases in incidence for the last two half-years persist even after adjustment for reporting delay (for Belgium, where the epidemic pattern has been much influenced by contacts with Africa, this decrease remains when cases among residents only are considered). In The Netherlands and FR Germany, adjusted incidence has remained almost constant over the last 3 half-years, as had previously been noted for Sweden.

The extent to which the exponential model fits the data over the last three years is quite variable. In some cases it is clearly no longer satisfactory, while in others the coefficient of determination (R^2) remains high. Latest estimated doubling times for all populations with at least 50 reported cases and for which $R^2 > 0.80$ are given in Table 4 and Fig. 6. Those countries in which overall doubling times (1986 - 1988) are shortest (8.2 - 12.4 months) are those in which either the epidemic is at a relatively early stage (Ireland, Yugoslavia, Portugal, Greece) or the predominant mode of

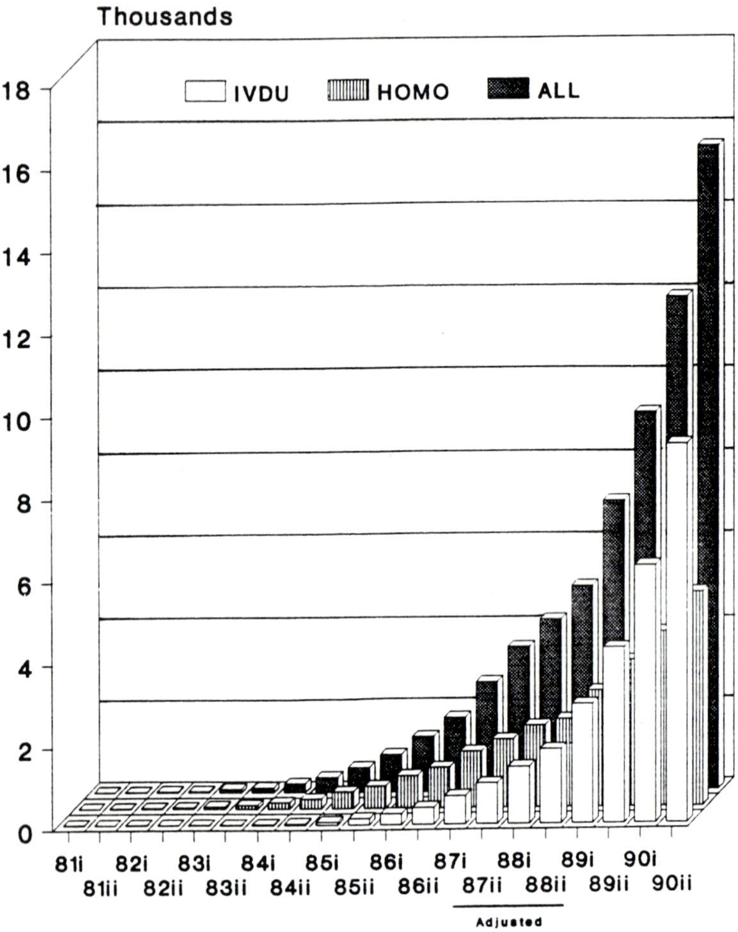

Fig. 5. The AIDS epidemic in the European Community: observed half-yearly incidence of AIDS cases, adjusted for reporting delays, to December 1988 and projections, based on doubling times estimated over 1986 - 1988 (Fig. 4), to December 1990 (see text). Projected cumulative cases to December 1990 are 64,600 (ALL), 26,100 (HOMO) and 28,400 (IVDU). HOMO: homo-/bisexuals; IVDU: IV drug users; ALL: all transmission groups combined

transmission is through IV drug use (Italy, Spain). Both Ireland and Yugoslavia have a rather high proportion of IV drug users among a small total number of cases (21/74 and 21/65 respectively). Data from Austria were not available for analysis, but the rather short doubling time of 10.9 months estimated from data reported up to 30th June 1988 may also be related to the rather high (25%) proportion of cases among IV drug users. Doubling times are longest (20.4 - 23.2 months) in The Netherlands, The United Kingdom, FR Germany and Denmark, in all of which the homo-/bisexual transmission group is predominant (>70% cases). France (15.6 months; 15% IVDU)

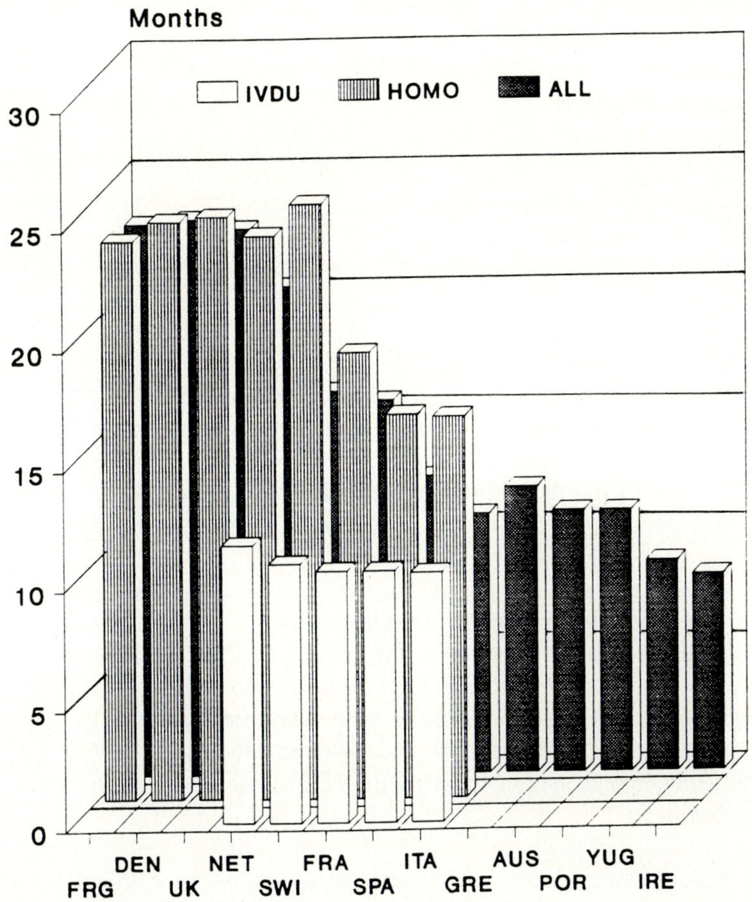

Fig. 6. Estimated average doubling times, in months, of diagnosed AIDS cases over the three year period from January 1986 to December 1988, by country of diagnosis and transmission group, for groups with at least 48 reported cases. No estimation was possible for Norway, Sweden, Belgium, Israel and IVDU in FR Germany (see text). HOMO: homo-/bisexuals; IVDU: IV drug users; ALL: all transmission groups combined

and Switzerland (16.0 months; 28% IVDU) occupy intermediate positions. Due to lack of fit of the model, it was not possible to estimate doubling times in Norway (where incidence has decreased), Sweden (incidence stable), Belgium and Israel.

Estimated doubling times among IV drug users are remarkably similar (10.4 - 11.6 months) in five of the six countries with at least 45 reported cases (Italy, France, Spain, Switzerland, The Netherlands). In FR Germany, adjusted incidence in this group has decreased since December 1987 and no estimation was possible. Short doubling times in cases attributed to heterosexual transmission are noted in Italy (7.3 months), Spain (9.7 months) and Switzerland (8.2 months), although the latter estimate is based on only 63 reported cases. It is understood that the majority of these cases have occurred in partners of IV drug users.

4. HIV seroprevalence data

Data on the prevalence of HIV infection are much less comprehensive and much more difficult to interpret than data on cases of AIDS.

In a number of countries, results of HIV antibody tests are reported routinely by laboratories, alternate testing sites and/or sentinel physicians. These data can be of considerable value in helping to measure the effects of information campaigns and in determining the characteristics of those known to be infected. They are, however, of very limited value in the assessment of seroprevalence, reflecting as they do merely rates among those who, for one reason or another, choose to be tested.

Numerous surveys and studies which include HIV testing have been carried out in both high and low risk populations. Many of these studies were not specifically designed for the assessment of seroprevalence in the population concerned. Protocols differ considerably and practically all studies are subject to some degree of self-selection bias, while demographic and socio-behavioural information necessary for the interpretation of the results is often missing. Despite these limitations, it nevertheless seemed worthwhile to attempt to gather together the considerable amount of such data now existing in Europe.

As a first step, national AIDS surveillance organisations were asked to supply, on standardized forms, basic details and results of both published and unpublished surveys/studies known to have been carried out within their countries since 1984. Details to be supplied included dates of the study, characteristics of study group, study site, sampling method, number tested, number positive and source of the data, with reference where available. Data relating to over 380 studies were reported from 28 countries. The breakdown of these studies by population group and starting date of the study is given in Table 5. After careful validation, these data will form the basis of a European data base on HIV seroprevalence.

While bearing in mind the difficulties of interpretation mentioned above and the fact that the data base is as yet far from complete, some preliminary observations can nevertheless be made.

Table 5. Numbers of European seroprevalence studies entered in the Paris data base at 30 April 1989, by population group and starting date of the study

Group	Starting date:						
	<84	84	85	86	87	88	Total
Blood donations/donors	0	0	17	8	29	9	63
General population	0	0	3	7	7	2	19
Haemophilic etc.	0	2	8	8	5	3	26
Health care workers	0	0	2	2	1	0	5
Heterosexuals	0	1	4	5	5	3	18
Homo-/bisexuals	6	6	13	8	8	4	45
Hospital patients	0	2	1	1	2	1	7
IV drug users	7	11	23	9	18	13	81
Military	0	0	3	0	1	0	4
Pregnant women	0	0	3	6	11	2	22
Prisoners	0	0	2	0	2	2	6
Prostitutes	0	1	9	5	4	3	22
STD patients	1	0	4	9	7	6	27
Transfusion	0	0	4	1	1	2	8
Others	0	1	14	7	6	7	35
Total	14	24	110	76	107	57	388

HIV prevalence among populations assumed to be at high risk

Over the period 1984 to 1988, prevalence rates of up to 40% were reported among groups of homosexual and/or bisexual men. The highest rates (25% - 40%) have been observed in major cities of the northern part of Europe (Table 6), with slightly lower rates (15% - 25%) reported from unpublished studies in Madrid, Berlin and Portugal. Seroprevalence among homosexuals attending sexually transmitted disease (STD) clinics in London in 1987 was also estimated (Department of Health Working Group, 1988) to be in the range 15% to 25%, but the estimated prevalence among other homosexuals in London and those outside London was much lower (around 5%). The few studies which have been conducted outside large cities also report much lower rates (<10%). Extensive testing, up to and including 1988, of homosexual men attending STD clinics in several countries of eastern Europe revealed rates of not more than 6%.

Most of the studies among IV drug users have been conducted either in treatment centres or in prisons. Particularly high seroprevalence rates (40% - 70%) have been reported from France, Italy, Spain, Switzerland and the UK (Edinburgh only). Reported rates are intermediate (15% - 35%) in parts of Austria, Denmark, FR Germany, Ireland and Yugoslavia, and lower (<15%) in twelve other countries (Belgium, Bulgaria, Czechoslovakia, Finland, Greece, Iceland, The Netherlands, Norway, Poland, Portugal, San Marino, Sweden).

Table 6. Highest reported seroprevalence rates among homo-/bisexual men in a number of European cities

Date	City	Site	N	% HIV+	Source/reference
1984	Copenhagen	mail	134	26	Melbye et al., 1986
1984-85	Copenhagen	ATS	662	27	Kolby et al., 1986
1984-87	Stockholm	-	166	37	Sandström et al.,*
1984-87	Amsterdam	STD	746	39	Van Griensven et al., 1989
1986	Paris	mail	267	33	Pollak et al., 1987
1986	London	STD	420	25	Carne et al., 1987
1986	London	STD	212	25	Evans et al., 1989
1987	London	STD	213	21	Evans et al., 1989

ATS: Alternate test site; STD: Sexually transmitted disease clinic
* Abstract: National Meeting of Swedish Physicians, 1987

Among haemophiliacs, seroprevalence appears to be highest (around 50% in 1986) in France (Allain, 1986). Within France, observed prevalence rates varied considerably between regions (from 16% to 72%). Studies carried out at various dates between 1984 and 1988 found rates of between 25% and 45% in Denmark, FR Germany, Greece, Italy, United Kingdom and Yugoslavia, and between 5% and 20% in Belgium, Ireland and Norway. Rates below 5% have been reported from four countries of eastern Europe (Bulgaria, Czechoslovakia, Hungary, Poland).

Prostitutes form a very heterogeneous group. Their motivation for participation in studies is generally low and it is difficult to obtain representative samples. In some countries, information has been obtained from registered prostitutes. Some studies have been undertaken on the street or in bars etc. Information has also been obtained from prostitutes attending STD clinics. The studies which have been carried out suggest that prevalence remains low (<2%) among non IV drug using prostitutes in Europe. However, in a study in Amsterdam (Van den Hoek et al., 1988), 83% of 166 female drug users reported prostitution and prevalence rates among groups such as this reflect rates among IV drug users.

Seropositivity rates among heterosexual partners of infected persons vary considerably according to the risk group of the index case and other characteristics of the couple. Two ongoing studies (Johnson et al., 1988; European Study Group, 1989) in which a majority of the index cases were either IV drug users or bisexual men have reported male to female transmission rates of 17% (N=60) (Johnson and Laga, 1988) and 27% (N=155) respectively. Higher rates (40% - 58%) have been reported in groups with significant African connections (Staszewski et al., 1988; Laga et al., 1988). Comparatively low rates of transmission, 7% in France (Allain, 1986) and 10% in FR Germany (Kamradt et al., 1988), have been reported from haemophiliacs. These observations are consistent with the results of other studies conducted outside Europe (see Johnson and Laga, 1988; Anderson and May, 1988). The observed differences in transmission rates between different groups may however be considerably less when risk factors are taken into account (European Study Group, 1989).

Few studies have been reported on HIV seropositivity rates in non IV-drug using heterosexuals attending STD clinics. In most cases, the extent to which homo-/bisexual men and IV drug users have been excluded is unclear. Studies carried out in the UK suggest that the level of seroprevalence probably lies between 0.1% and 0.5%, with higher rates in the London area than elsewhere (Department of Health Working Group, 1988). Rates in this range are reported from Belgium, Finland and Sweden, with rather higher rates (up to 3%) reported from limited studies in Denmark, France and The Netherlands. Lower rates are reported from Norway and from countries of eastern Europe. This population represents one of a number of potential bridges between the established high risk groups and the general heterosexual population and careful monitoring could provide a sensitive indicator of the spread of HIV.

HIV prevalence among selected groups of the general population assumed to be at low risk

Blood donations are tested routinely in all European countries. Among donations (as opposed to donors) screened in 1987, HIV positivity rates were highest (0.03%) in Spain, France and Portugal, followed by Italy (0.02%), Switzerland (0.01%) and Greece (0.01%) (WHO Collaborating Centre on AIDS, Paris, 1988). Elsewhere, rates did not exceed 0.005%. Direct comparisons between countries are however not very meaningful due to differences in methods of organization of national blood donation systems and to differences in the extent of the provision of alternate test sites. Most countries reported lower rates than in 1986, but this result is also difficult to interpret as it is related to better selection of donors and to improved self-deferral of high risk donors. The screening of blood donors is carried out in order to protect the blood supply and is not designed for the assessment of seroprevalence in the general population. Blood donors are not representative of the general heterosexual population in a country, nor do they form a stable population over time, and neither prevalence rates nor their changes with time are easily interpreted.

Results from the screening of pregnant women have been reported by 13 countries. Most results relate to 1987 and/or 1988, although a few studies were undertaken in 1985/86. Screening was in most cases by consent (two surveys incorporating unlinked anonymous testing were carried out in London). Refusal rates were stated for six studies only and were between 0.4% and 8% in five of these, the refusal rate in the remaining study being as high as 18%. Even low refusal rates can crucially affect the outcome of screening programmes intended to assess seroprevalence rates in low risk populations. In only three countries (Bulgaria, Norway, Sweden) can the studies be regarded as representative at a national level, other studies being mostly confined to particular cities or regions. Reported prevalence rates are lowest (<0.005%) in

Bulgaria, Finland, Iceland, Norway, San Marino and the USSR, intermediate in Sweden and Greece, and higher (0.1% - 0.7%) in certain regions of France, FR Germany, The Netherlands, Switzerland and The United Kingdom. The highest rate (0.7%) was observed in a study carried out in the Paris area during 1987-88 (Brossard et al., 1988). Of 28,715 women tested (refusal rate 2%) over a 17 month period, 218 confirmed positive results were obtained (pers. comm.). Among these, 165 women were already known to be HIV positive, and many of these had been referred to the hospitals in the study for this reason. The seropositivity rate among previously unscreened women was thus 0.2%. Most of these (53) women reported at least one known risk factor for HIV infection. This study thus concluded that heterosexual transmission in the absence of other recognized risk factors remained rare in Paris in 1987.

Results of screening of military recruits and/or military personnel are available from only four countries. Reported seroprevalence rates range from 0% to 0.05%.

Prevalence of HIV-2 infection

Infection with HIV-2 is a problem of particular concern in Portugal, where HIV-2 seroprevalence rates similar to or greater than those for HIV-1 were observed in a 1987 study of prostitutes attending an STD clinic in Lisbon, in the screening of pregnant women with risk factors (1987/88), in Africans requesting testing (1987) and in heterosexual contacts of infected persons (1986-88). Infection among homosexual and bisexual men and among IV drug users is, on the other hand, almost exclusively with HIV-1.

Very little data is available from other European countries. However, a study carried out in 1987 (Couroucé et al., 1988) suggests that HIV-2 infection in France remains uncommon. Among a sample of 100,114 blood donors, 30 of whom tested positive for HIV-1, no sample was confirmed as positive for HIV-2. Among a total of 10,004 persons requesting HIV testing, 713 (7.1%) were HIV-1 positive, while 9 (0.09%) were confirmed as positive for HIV-2 (eight of these cases were directly or indirectly connected with West Africa, the other being a transfusion recipient). It thus seems probable that, Portugal excepted, HIV-2 infection rates remain very low throughout Europe.

Incidence of HIV infection

Several recent studies, in particular in the UK (Carne et al., 1987; Evans et al., 1989) and in The Netherlands (Van Griensven et al., 1989), suggest that incidence among homosexual men has been falling since at least 1985. A similar evolution, due largely to changes in behaviour, is believed to be occurring in many other countries.

In general, however, incidence, as opposed to prevalence, rates of HIV infection in specific population groups are extremely difficult to assess, particularly in low prevalence populations, and most of the available data are inadequate for this purpose. Many of the data were collected with other purposes in mind (e.g. protection of the blood supply, assessment of risk factors) and, although, in some countries, reported prevalence rates in certain groups are reported to have declined over time, probable unquantified changes in the nature of the (often self-selected) samples studied make interpretation hazardous.

Monitoring the future spread of HIV infection, particularly in the low prevalence sectors of the population, will require carefully designed, large scale surveys sustained over several years. Unlinked anonymous screening (UAS) provides the possibility of removing self-selection biases, thus improving the accuracy of estimation of incidence rates in the selected populations. Surveys which continue to rely on named testing of volunteer subjects will almost certainly be flawed by changing attitudes of both subjects and professionals in consenting to the test.

References

Allain, J.-P. (1986). Prevalence of HTLV-III/LAV antibodies in patients with haemophilia and in their sexual partners in France. New England Journal of Medicine 315, 517-518.

Ancelle-Park, R., Brunet, J.-B., and Downs, A.M. (1987). AIDS and drug addicts in Europe. Lancet ii, 626-627.

Ancelle-Park, R. and De Vincenzi, I. (1988). Heterosexual transmission of HIV. In: AIDS and obstetrics and gynaecology. Proceedings of the 19th study group of the Royal College of Obstetricians and Gynaecologists (eds. C.N. Hudson and F. Sharp). 39-47.

Anderson, R.A. and May, R.M. (1988). Epidemiological parameters of HIV transmission. Nature 333, 514-519.

Brossard, Y., Goudeau, A., Larsen, M., Muchet, J., Barin, F., Henrion, R., Barret, J., Chavinie, J., Dupay, A., Engelmann, P., Leroy, B., Papiernik, E., Santarelli, J., Sureau, C., Sender, A., Parnet, F., Gross, E., Courtois, F., Soulte, J.C., Petei, J.C., Mayaux, M.J., and Schwartz, D. (1988). A sero-epidemiological study of HIV in 15,465 pregnant women screened in Paris area between Feb. 1987 and Oct. 1987. IV International Conference on AIDS, Stockholm (abstract 4632).

Carne, C.A., Johnson, A.M., Pearce, F., Smith, A., Tedder, R.S., Weller, I.V.D., Loveday, C., Hawkins, A., Williams, P., and Adler, M.W. (1987). Prevalence of antibodies to human immunodeficiency virus, gonorrhoea rates, and changed sexual behaviour in homosexual men in London. Lancet i, 656-658.

Centers for Disease Control (1989). AIDS weekly surveillance report. January 2, 1989.

Couroućé, A.-M. and the 'Retrovirus' study group of the French Society of Blood Transfusion (1988). A prospective study of HIV-2 prevalence in France. AIDS 2, 261-265.

Department of Health Working Group (1988). Short term predictions of HIV infection and AIDS in England and Wales. HMSO, London.

Downs, A.M., Ancelle, R.A., Jager, J.C., and Brunet, J.-B. (1987). AIDS in Europe: current trends and short-term predictions estimated from surveillance data, January 1981 - June 1986. AIDS 1, 53-57.

Downs, A.M., Ancelle, R.A., Jager, J.C., Heisterkamp, S.H., van Druten, J.A.M., Ruitenberg, E.J., and Brunet, J.-B. (1988). The statistical estimation, from routine surveillance data, of past, present and future trends in AIDS incidence in Europe. In: Statistical analysis and mathematical modelling of AIDS (eds. J.C. Jager and E.J. Ruitenberg). Oxford University Press, Oxford.

European Study Group (1989). Risk factors for male to female transmission of HIV. British Medical Journal 298, 411-415.

Evans, B.A., McLean, K.A., Dawson, S.G., Teece, S.A., Bond, R.A., MacRae, K.D., and Thorp, R.W. (1989). Trends in sexual behaviour and risk factors for HIV infection among homosexual men, 1984-7. British Medical Journal 298, 215-218.

Heisterkamp, S.H., Jager, J.C., Downs, A.M., van Druten, J.A.M., and Ruitenberg, E.J. (1988). Statistical estimation of AIDS incidence from surveillance data and the link with the modelling of trends. In: Statistical analysis and mathematical modelling of AIDS (eds. J.C. Jager and E.J. Ruitenberg). Oxford University Press, Oxford.

Heisterkamp, S.H., Jager, J.C., Ruitenberg, E.J., van Druten, J.A.M., and Downs, A.M. (1989). Correcting reported AIDS incidence: a statistical approach. Statistics in Medicine 8, 963-976.

Johnson, A.M., Petherick, A., Davidson, S., Howard, L., Osborne, L., Sonnex, C., Robertson, R., Tchamouroff, S., Hooker, M., McLean, K., Brettle, R., and Adler, M.W. (1988). Transmission of HIV to heterosexual partners of infected men and women. IV International Conference on AIDS, Stockholm (abstract 4058).

Johnson, A.M. and Laga, M. (1988). Heterosexual transmission of HIV. AIDS 2/supp.1, S49-S56.

Kamradt, T.G.A., Niese, D., Schneweis, K.E., Breckmann, H.H., and Kamps, B.S. (1988). Heterosexual transmission of HIV in haemophiliacs. IV International Conference on AIDS, Stockholm (abstract 4008).

Kolby, P., Pedersen, C., Sindrup, J.H., Gaub, J., Arendrup, M., and Gerstoft, J. (1986). The LAV/HTLV-III screening in Copenhagen. Epidemiological results from four clinics over the period 1 July 1984 to 1 April 1985. Danish Medical Bulletin 33, 268-270.

Laga, M., Taelman, H., Bonneux, L., Cornet, P., Verkauteren, G., and Piot, P. (1988). Risk factors for HIV infection in heterosexual partners of HIV infected Africans and Europeans. IV International Conference on AIDS, Stockholm (abstract 4004).

Melbye, M., Biggar, R.J., Ebbesen, P., Neuland, C., Goedert, J.J., Faber, V., Lorenzen, I., Skinh:j, P., Gallo, R.C., and Blattner, W.A. (1986). Long-term seropositivity for human T-lymphotrophic virus type III in homosexual men without the acquired immunodeficiency syndrome: development of immunologic and clinical abnormalities. A longitudinal study. Annals of Internal Medicine 104, 496-500.

Pollak,M., Schiltz, M.-A., and Lejeune, B. (1987). Premiers résultats de l'enquête 1986: les homosexuels face au SIDA. Bulletin Epidemiologique Hebdomadaire (7), 27.

Staszewski, S., Rehmet, S., Hofmeister, W.D., Helm, E.B., Stille, W., Werner, A., and Doerr, H.W. (1988). Analysis of transmission risks in heterosexual transmitted HIV infection. IV International Conference on AIDS, Stockholm (abstract 4068).

Van den Hoek, J.A.R., Coutinho, R.A., van Haastrecht, H.J.A., van Zadelhoff, A.W., and Goudsmit, J. (1988). Prevalence and risk factors of HIV infections among drug users and drug-using prostitutes in Amsterdam. AIDS 2, 55-60.

Van Griensven, G.J.P., De Vroome, E.M.M., Goudsmit, J., and Coutinho, R.A.(1989). Changes in sexual behaviour and the fall in incidence of HIV infection among homosexual men. British Medical Journal 298, 218-221.

WHO Collaborating Centre on AIDS, Paris (1988). AIDS surveillance in Europe: quarterly report no. 20, Paris.

Demographic Impact of Mortality from AIDS in France: Projection for 1991

M. Guiguet, A.J. Valleron

At present AIDS is still a minor cause of death in France, despite the fact that it is the second country in the world in terms of numbers of cases notified. However, in the next few years, its impact on demography may well be of importance because of two obvious reasons: First, the number of cases has gradually increased and, before the discovery of an efficient treatment, the number of deaths will follow the same trend. Secondly, AIDS is a cause of death which, like motor vehicle crashes, kills selectively young people: only 19% of the 4,887 cases of AIDS in men which were notified by December 31, 1988 to the General Department of Health (Direction Générale de la Santé) in France were over 45, while the figures were 95.6% for cancer, 97.3% for cardiovascular diseases, 59% for suicide.

Quantitative estimates of the likely AIDS impact in France on two demographic indicators, loss of life expectancy (LLE) and potential years of life lost (PYLL) in men, were provided in 1987 for the 1988-1990 period, assuming that the number of cases would continue to increase exponentially (Flandre and Valleron, 1988). There is now evidence that the annual incidence is slowing down and this paper will provide new estimates for the 1989-1991 period which will be compared to the corresponding values presently observed in six causes of death: cancers, diseases of the circulatory system, infectious diseases, alcoholic psychosis, suicides, motor vehicle crashes.

Material and methods

The causes of death which are considered in this paper are: AIDS, cancer (International Classification of Disease numbers (ICD), 9th revision, ranging between 140 and 208), diseases of the circulatory system (ICD 390 to 459), infectious diseases (ICD 1 to 139), alcoholic psychosis (ICD 291-303), suicide (ICD 950-958), motor vehicle crashes (ICD 810-819, 826-829).

The computation of the loss of life expectancy due to a cause of death requires the age distribution of the population and the number of deaths by age for all causes and for the considered cause. The computation of the potential years of life lost requires only the latter. The age distribution of the male French population which is used in this paper is that of 1985 as provided by the Institut National de la Statistique et des Etudes Economiques (INSEE).

The year by year estimation of the number of deaths by AIDS in each age class has required several steps. Indeed, we need this information for the years 1989 to 1991. However, the 1989 values are not available and projections are necessary to forecast the 1989, 1990 and 1991 figures. The first step of the estimation used the incidence data published by the French General Health Department from June 1, 1984 to December 31, 1988. In the second step we computed corrected incidences taking into account the delay of notification of the cases according to the method provided by Downs et al. (1987). At this point, we had estimates of the incidence till the end of 1988. To get estimates of the incidence till 1991, we performed a linear-logistic regression. The estimated annual incidence for the years 1989 to 1991 are presented in Table 1. Finally, the predicted distribution of the number of male cases in each age class was obtained by applying the sex and age distribution observed by December 31, 1988 (Direction Générale de la Santé, 1989) to these annual incidences.

In the third step, we deduced from these values the expected number of deaths in the next years. To describe the duration of the disease, we apply an exponential distribution of mean 1.14 year supplemented by a 8% probability of zero survival time (Reeves, 1988).

The computation of the loss of life expectancy due to a given cause (e.g. AIDS) was done by the standard techniques of life table and mortality analysis (Chiang, 1978) where mortality statistics were those published by the Institut National de la Santé et de la Recherche Médicale (INSERM) for the year 1985. The loss of life expectancy due to a cause is defined as the difference between the observed expectation of life at birth and the one that is expected under the assumption that the disease has been eliminated as a risk of death. Independence between causes of deaths is assumed. For each cause of death, the number of Potential Years of Life Lost (PYLL) is computed (Romeder and McWhinnie, 1978) modifying each death at a given age (older than 1) by the difference between 65 and this age. The percentage of potential years of life lost associated with a cause is computed by dividing the total numbers of PYLL due to this cause by the total number of PYLL due to all causes.

Table 1. Estimated annual incidences and confidence intervals (C.I.)

Year	1989	1990	1991
Incidence	4295	5245	6035
C.I.	(3205-5384)	(3797-6693)	(4108-7962)

Results

Assuming a constant sex-ratio, the linear-logistic model provides estimates of annual AIDS incidence in men of 3,650 in 1989, 4,460 in 1990, 5,130 in 1991. The expected numbers of deaths by AIDS are 2,727 in 1989, 3,610 in 1990, 4,385 in 1991. The loss of life expectancy and the percentage of potential years of life lost associated with AIDS in 1989 and 1991 together with their corresponding values for the other causes of death (1985) which we have considered are presented in Table 2.

Whatever the indicator used, AIDS represents a cause of death whose demographic impact is smaller that the one associated with cancer, motor vehicle crashes, diseases of the circulatory system or suicide. But even for 1989, AIDS is a greater cause of mortality than all the infectious diseases. Projections for 1991 emphasize this tendency; at that time AIDS could have an impact of the same order of magnitude as the one associated with suicide.

Discussion

The two demographic indicators we have used in this paper are and have been widely used to assess the impact of various causes of death on the population. The Centers for Disease Control (CDC) - for instance - regularly provides estimates of PYLL in its Morbidity and Mortality Weekly Report (MMWR). The results we present here are based on estimated values of the numbers of AIDS cases and numbers of deaths. The security of our estimations relies on the fact that we make short term predictions. The

Table 2. Demographic impact of AIDS compared to six other causes of death (France, male population). For AIDS, number in parentheses indicate the 95% confidence interval of the estimates. LLE stands for loss of life expectancy and PYLL stands for potential years of life lost. For all causes (except AIDS) LLE and PYLL are based on the 1985 vital statistics

Cause of deaths	ICD No.	LLE (years)	PYLL (%)
AIDS : 1989		0.24 (0.16-0.32)	5.5 (3.8-7.3)
AIDS : 1991		0.39 (0.27-0.5)	8.9 (6.3-11.5)
Suicide	950-958	0.61	11.0
Motor vehicle crashes	810-819 826-829	0.65	15.0
Cancer	140-208	3.84	21.9
Diseases of the circulatory system	390-459	4.11	13.1
Infectious diseases	1-139	0.16	1.2
Alcoholic psychosis	291-303	0.14	1.7

curve for empirical forecasting chosen is the linear-logistic. Predictions made under this model are optimistic, relative to other types of mathematical curves (Department of Health Working Group, 1988). In the initial stages of the epidemic, future cases were predicted by using an exponential model. The demographic impact of mortality by AIDS based on these estimates was therefore greater (Flandre and Valleron, 1988). Even with the present extrapolations, AIDS impact in France between 1989 and 1991 on the two demographic indicators studied in men is considerable. While there may be a certain amount of imprecision in the figures we present - and this is documented by the confidence intervals provided in Table 2 the general tendencies we found will very likely be observed.

Conclusion

Because AIDS kills selectively the young people, its demographic impact is not negligible even in 1989 when it is compared to causes of death like infectious diseases or alcoholic psychosis. In 1991, AIDS will likely have a demographic impact in terms of loss of life expectancy and of potential years of life lost close to those of suicide and motor vehicle crashes.

AIDS is becoming a cause of death which lowers the life expectancy, a criteria whose continuous increase in most countries bears witness to improved health programmes, and is responsible for a significant percentage of potential years of life lost between 1 and 65 years.

References

Flandre, P. and Valleron, A.J. (1988). Impact démographique de la mortalité par SIDA en France en 1990: le SIDA devant le suicide est proche des accidents de la circulation. Rev. Epidem. et Santé Publ. 36, 196-201.

Downs, A.M., Ancelle, R.A., Jager, H.C., and Brunet, J.B. (1987). AIDS in Europe: current trends and short term predictions estimated from surveillance data, January 1981 - June 1986. AIDS 1, 53-57.

Reeves, G.R. (1988). The overall distribution of survival time for UK AIDS patients. In: Short-term prediction of HIV infection and AIDS in England or Wales. Department of Health, HMSO, London, 80-81.

Direction Génerale de la Santé (1989). Situation du SIDA en France au Décembre 1988. B.E.H. 4, 13-14.

Chiang, C.M. (1978). Life table and mortality analysis. World Health Organization, Geneve.

Romeder, J.M. and McWhinnie, J.R. (1978). Le développement des années potentielles de vie perdues comme indicateur de mortalité prématurée. Rev. Epidem. et Santé Publ. 26, 97-115.

Centers for Disease Control (1987). Premature mortality. Morbidity and Mortality Weekly Report (MMWR) 36, 56-57.

Department of Health Working Group (ed.) (1988). Short term predictions of HIV infection and AIDS in England and Wales. HMS0, London.

Social and Political Aspects of AIDS

J. Santos Lucas

The AIDS epidemic is an evolving phenomenon. Instead of one epidemic, we ended up with a set of epidemics: the HIV epidemic, the AIDS epidemic, and the epidemic of fear. It started as a medical problem and was converted into a multidimensional process. Ethical, political, social, managerial, and economic issues emerged in connection with it.

Rational decision making has been confronted with a large variety of value implications. Clinical reasonings, as well as planning the allocation of resources, have to deal with different perceptions, conflicting demands, and pressure group politics.

In this paper we try to stimulate health planners, health economists and health policy makers to go through different matters and assess their social and economic aspects.

AIDS and the HIV infection in the policy agendas

At the begining of this decade there was some resistance, even in WHO, to accept that a new epidemic was emerging. It took some time for the WHO to adopt specific policies with regard to the HIV epidemic and to take action.

Governments gave, and some are still giving, a halfhearted response to the epidemic. They were unwilling to go ahead with any kind of political decisions. This attitude might be associated with several factors, among them with the perceptions of the policy actors. In the developed world, AIDS was initially perceived and conceptualized as a disease resulting from abuse of sex and sex deviance, as a result of casual sex and homosexuality. As the disease used to be regarded as specific to marginalized groups, it was perceived as not posing a threat to the whole population. Therefore, AIDS issues got little attention and were introduced very slowly into the policy agendas.

In the meantime, some changes occurred within the AIDS policy community. New policy actors were involved in promoting, formulating, and implementing AIDS policies. Gay leaders may be singled out as the first "intruders". In the USA, the Centers for Disease Control Task Force initiated and maintained constant consultation with gay groups. In most European countries, Canada and Australia, the gay movement was officially recognized in government dealings with AIDS matters. Haemophiliac's associations were very active, putting pressure on governmental decision-making related to blood quality control.

To the extent that the epidemic crosses sexual boundaries and becomes more and more prevalent among heterosexuals and children, and among every segment of the productive society, it is likely that other social leaders will commit themselves to the AIDS struggle and get involved in policy making. We are already seeing family associations, community leaders, medical and other health professional's associations, unions and employer's associations debating the implications of AIDS for their own lives and organisations.

The integration of representatives of infected people, AIDS patients, and those social groupings just referred to, in National Committees on AIDS is likely to improve their effectiveness. It is expected that very shortly every country in Europe will have an explicit and consistent set of AIDS policies, with clear objectives, principles, measures, programmes and activities.

Conflicting demands

The AIDS epidemic puts many demands in conflict, such as prevention versus treatment, general or segmented approaches, priority groups, dominance of the medical profession or combination of volunteer and community care.

To give an example, in USA and in many countries of Europe, it is anticipated that drug use will become, in the coming years, the principal route by which the HI virus will be transmitted. Which priority should be given to drug rehabilitation programmes as a consequence of that fact is a matter of policy choice.

Private and public expenditures in caring for AIDS patients are rising. Alternative models of caring for AIDS patients may produce different outcomes and generate different cost estimates. If there is not sufficient empirical evidence to support different options, personal judgement is likely to be called upon. This happened to me, sometime ago, when I had a meeting with some doctors in order to discuss a project to support AIDS patients that were excluded from their families. Within this project alternative housing, emotional and practical support and transportation to and from the hospital would be provided. Some of the participants, however, claimed that a special hospital would do a better job for these patients. The weakness of the discussion rested with the fact that both solutions were based on different belief systems more than in sound evaluation.

Whether AIDS prevention should be considered a public good, is a matter of dispute. If so, one could advocate preventive programmes to be fully financed by governments. Yet, could we hold that condoms should be provided free? What would be the expected social costs and benefits, and the economic costs of this option at national or regional level?

Screening

Screening is not a consensus issue but one that prompts a lot of controversy. A couple of years ago, mass screening was mentioned but very quickly rejected. In these days no one believes in the usefulness and economic feasibility of regulary screening the general population with regard to the HIV antibody. However, some specific forms of universal screening could be defensible, such as universal premarital screening. Should it be enforced? What are the expected costs and benefits of such a decision? The same questions could be raised with reference to mothers-to-be and their newborns.

There are special situations and special groups that could be submitted to mandatory screening. It is well accepted that blood donors must be tested at the point of entry. However, should specific workers, such as health professionals, pilots or bus drivers, be screened periodically? What are the advantages and disadvantages? Many admit that it should be enforced that prostitutes be screened periodically. How effective this programme could be remains to be seen, too.

Informed consent and mandatory counselling

Although informed consent is already a common practice in many places where mandatory screening and testing are performed, it is not yet universal. Should informed consent be mandatory whenever individuals are tested? Should policies regarding informed consent be adopted in blood institutes, health centres, clinics and hospitals before testing?

Disclosure of a test result has many implications, particularly at psychological level. Therefore it may be pondered whether pre- and post-test counselling be mandatory as a prerequisite for testing. If so, costs of testing should take account of the adoption of a mandatory counselling policy and its expenses. In some cases, counselling will be provided by psychologists or social workers, in others by volunteers. More frequently GPs have this responsibility. Different models of counselling provision have different cost implications to be taken into account.

Confidentiality

The individual right to privacy prevents disclosure of any kind of information about test results. However, public health values conflict with the right to privacy whenever someone puts others at direct risk. Accordingly, Daniel Koshland has challenged the idea of keeping the information of seropositivity secret. "Should confidentiality be preserved at any cost?", he asks. "What is the responsibility of a physician in informing spouses and children, to say nothing of others who might become infected?"

If confidentiality is to be broken, counselling should be provided to support the person in revealing his or her health status. Yet, he or she may refuse or avoid it.

Infected prostitutes may be an even worse case for concern. Similarly, infected drug addicts who involve themselves in transmitting the virus deliberately, may give grounds for disclosure of their condition. What kind of policies and programmes should be adopted and implemented regarding these two groups of the infected population? What are the alternatives and at what cost?

Connected with the disclosure of the seropositivity status is contact tracing. Through this measure anyone potentially at risk is contacted in order to reduce his or her probability of (re)infection and to contain the spread of the disease. Again, the acceptability of mandatory contact tracing for infected people is a matter of debate.

Discrimination

Confidentiality mingles with discrimination issues. Should a doctor reveal test results to an insurance company? Concurrently, should society allow an insurance company to discriminate and refuse an HIV infected person to subscribe to an health insurance policy? The financial consequences of such decisions are obviously very important for the individual as well as for the whole society.

Discrimination at the work place is another complex issue, with great implications for both the employees and the management of companies. Firing HIV infected people is less likely than firing AIDS patients. Some countries have already started to oppose this behaviour. In the USA, the Rehabilitation Act is now protecting AIDS victims and seropositives. A policy statement was issued by the US President requiring federal employees to treat HIV infected employees on a case-by-case basis in evaluating job performance, health and safety factors, just like any other employee for other purposes.

How much protection from the law does any infected person have in order to rule out discrimination in hiring procedures? If the epidemic grows more serious, as is expected, what may the impact on the economy as a whole and on the financial stability of some companies be?

Discrimination in the education system has been observed. Seropositive children are facing enormous difficulties in many places to pursue their studies. These vulnerable children from vulnerable families are getting into even more precarious situations. The result is not only human suffering but a new burden to society. Landlords and neighbours are also a source of discrimination. Cases of eviction have been reported.

Discrimination also takes place in health care systems. Some doctors avoid performing surgery in infected patients. Some nurses avoid direct contact with them and quit jobs in hospitals that treat AIDS patients. How to reverse this trend? What kind of incentives to put at work?

AIDS is still a stigmatized disease. Education and counselling of those involved in discriminative behaviour would stimulate a change in attitudes and behaviours, but at a certain cost.

Social implications

Seropositives and AIDS patients go through a course of disruptive events. On top of their infection or disease, some will experience light or severe psychological imbalances, isolate themselves or be excluded from their social networks. Their family structures or stable sexual relations are likely to be ruined. They will have to rebuild their sexual networks at a time of low morale. They would benefit from being involved in leisure activities which could help them in buffering stress factors. This can also be costly. Yet, they are more likely to be absent from work, to be fired, not to be hired, to see a reduction of earnings, to have more medical and pharmaceutical bills to pay. As a result of separation many will need a new place to live, without having very much money available to pay for it. Financial insolvency is expected.

Community-based groups have been at the forefront of the fight against AIDS. Should or should not funding be provided to community-based groups to care for infected people and AIDS patients, to provide counselling, emotional and practical support, and to provide housing? Should or should not funding be provided to community-based groups to train counsellors, educators, and home helpers? Should or should not volunteer work be strengthened? Should professional work replace volunteer work in AIDS prevention? Will professional work be sufficient to face the needs?

Concluding remarks

These are just a few of many social and policy issues that we are now facing while coping with this deadly disease. It is important to have economic measures of each alternative, related to each type of action, either to preventive care or palliative cure. Nevertheless, decisions are marginally determined by those quantifications. To be effective, planners and economists should work with policy actors, inside and outside government. Their contribution is likely to be of great importance in winning the war against AIDS.

References

Institute of Medicine (1986). Confronting AIDS. Directions for public health, health care and research. National Academy Press, Washington, DC.

Koshland (Jr.), D. (1988). The AIDS issue. Science 5, February.

Economic Aspects of AIDS

J. Rovira

Introduction

This paper tries to set up a conceptual framework which would allow us to place the different possible economic approaches to AIDS and HIV infection into a broad perspective and to discuss the potential usefulness and limitations of these approaches.

"Economic aspects" and "economic approaches" are very loose expressions, which may have different meanings to different people. Therefore, for the purpose of this paper it seems advisable to start by trying to define their content and boundaries. An enlightening starting point to this discussion is the distinction made by Williams between a topic - i.e. area of study - and a discipline - i.e. mode of thinking (Williams, 1979).

Economic analysis is a discipline which can be applied to the study of the economy - i.e. the economic system -, a topic whose boundaries are conventionally defined as embracing those phenomena of society that are related to resources, wealth, consumption, production, distribution, and so on; but the tools of economic analysis can and have been applied to other topics, which fall clearly outside what people usually include in the substantive meaning of "the economy": criminal behaviour, marriage or health are examples of topics which have also been the focus of economic analysis.

Health Economics can be defined as the application of the discipline "economics" to the topics "health" and "the health system". In the same line of reasoning, the economic effects of AIDS and HIV infection can be thought of as the application of "economics" to these specific sub-areas within the broader area of "health".

The rest of this paper is divided into two parts:
The first part will focus on substantive aspects, i.e. on the areas of study which should be considered in applying economic analysis to AIDS and HIV infection. The second part will consider the analytical tools of economics which can be applied to the study of AIDS and HIV infection and their impact on the economy and the society as a whole.

Areas of study in the economic analysis of AIDS and HIV infection

The effects of AIDS and HIV are not limited to health and to the health sector, but spread out through most aspects of the economy and the social system, which therefore need to be taken into account in the analysis. Well-being, however broadly or narrowly it may be defined, is another topic to be considered, for it has traditionally been one of the basic concerns of economic analysis, especially in normative, but also in positive analysis. Within positive economics, human behaviour is usually explained by supposing that people are always trying to attain a maximum level of well-being. In normative economics, the maximization of well-being is explicitly the final objective that justifies the conclusions drawn from the analysis.

Our review will therefore proceed from the six-area scheme outlined in Fig. 1, accepting the relative arbitrariness of the resulting framework[1)]. AIDS can affect and be affected directly and indirectly by factors pertaining to any of the five remaining areas. The resulting set of relationship will be taken as the classification criterion.

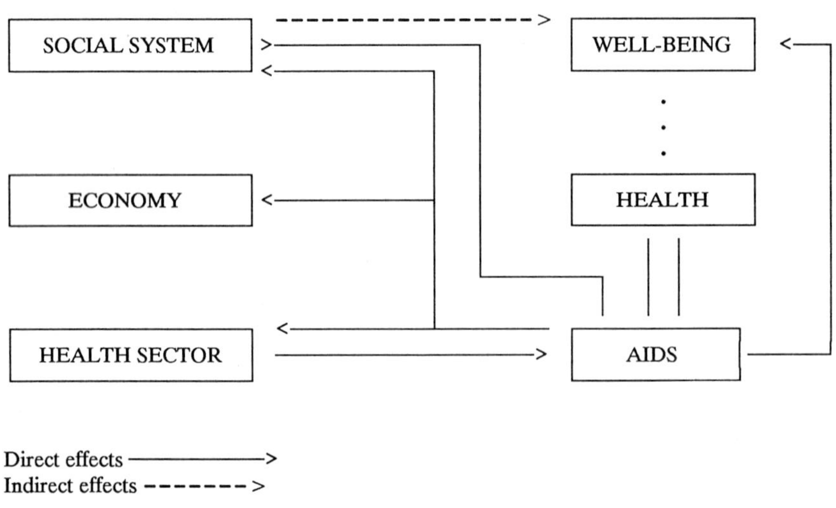

Fig. 1. The economic aspects of AIDS: main areas of study

1) AIDS may alternatively be included in the area of health and health in that of well-being. Similarly, the health sector is part of the economy, which in turn is part of the social system. In the proposed scheme, the social system is assumed to exclude the economy, and the economy to exclude the health sector; moreover, AIDS, health and well-being are conceptualised as separate entities.

Effects of AIDS on health

With AIDS being a disease, it is obvious that its existence and spread mean a reduction in health in the form of reduced life expectancy and quality of life to those suffering from the disease. The high mortality rate associated with AIDS as well as the irreversibility and severity of the disease have a significant demographic impact, especially among the high risk groups, which in turn will have indirect effects on the health sector and on the economy as a whole, e.g., changes in the utilization of health services and in productivity.

However, indirect positive effects of AIDS on health are also likely, measures aimed at preventing AIDS transmission will probably reduce the incidence of other transmissible diseases like Hepatitis B or STD (Sexually Transmitted Diseases). Likewise, the high incidence of AIDS among IVD (intravenous drug) users, coupled with the low survival rates of those contracting the disease, may result in the reduction of drug addiction as a public health problem.

These kinds of benefits are usually neglected when estimating the costs of AIDS.

Effects of health on AIDS

A high prevalence of IVD addiction is a factor enhancing the spread of the AIDS epidemic. At the individual level, the presence of some STD seem to increase the risk of sexual transmission of the HIV.

Effects of AIDS on well-being

AIDS, like any other disease, is a source of pain and distress not only for the patients but also for their relatives and friends. The loss of well-being is a result not only of the physiological but also of the psychological and social consequences of AIDS, such as the stigma and discrimination associated with the disease.

Loss of well-being also reaches healthy individuals who fear the likelihood of contagion and are induced to restrict their behaviour, especially, their sexual behaviour.

Societal well-being is also indirectly affected by a reduction of resources which, because they need to be diverted to AIDS, are no longer available for other ends.

Effects of AIDS on the health sector

AIDS increases the requirements of health care resources. These resources must be detracted from other uses within the health sector, or obtained from outside it, in order to be allocated to the personal care of AIDS, ARC and HIV patients. Preventive measures not directly involved in treating AIDS patients, include the screening of blood donations, the generalization of the use of rubber gloves by health personnel, and general preventive activities undertaken by the health sector such as information, health education, etc.

The premature death of most AIDS patients means a reduction in their future general health care consumption. Moreover, there seem to be other effects on health-care resource availability: some people are less willing to consume blood products, while the number of blood donations may rise as a result of the added inducement, to some individuals, of a free HIV test. (However other people may be reluctant to donate blood out of an irrational fear of contracting AIDS.) Autologous transfusion may rise because of people trying to avoid any possibility of transmission by blood transfusion.

AIDS may also change the attitudes and behaviour of health personnel, who may refuse to treat AIDS and HIV patients or even risk groups, or at least may ask for safer working conditions or higher salaries.

AIDS can affect the behaviour of health care insurers, especially private insurers, who may refuse to insure AIDS treatment costs. The unwillingness of private insurers to cover these risks may induce the public system to take up the coverage of AIDS treatment. The final outcome could be a change in the public-private mix, maybe with far-reaching consequences.

The high cost of AIDS treatment can induce the setting up of new cost control mechanisms, which may later be applied to other activities. This seems to have been the case of zidovudine prescription control in Spain, which may be extended to other drugs in the future.

Effects of the health sector on AIDS

The amount of resources devoted to AIDS will depend in part upon the ability of the health sector to attract new resources or redeploy the existing ones.

Although the interventions of the health sector have had, up to now, only a limited impact on the natural course of the disease at individual level once the virus is transmitted, there is a wide scope for influencing the spread of the epidemic by means of preventive measures, as well as for mitigating the effects of AIDS on the patients' well-being.

The effects of AIDS on the economy

Insofar as the resources devoted to AIDS are not diverted from other health activities, the result will be a reduction either of public or private expenditure, or both, for other activities.

However, some industries providing medical and paramedical goods (pharmaceutical industry, condom production) will increase their output, investment and research activities.

The mortality and morbidity of AIDS will cause productivity losses, which may be relatively high in comparison to other diseases because of the relatively low age of the individuals affected. This effect may be counter-acted by the probably low activity rate of some of the main risk groups, e.g., IVD users.

AIDS will pose important resource requirements on the public and voluntary welfare services - especially personal social services - and on income maintenance programmes, such as sickness subsidies. However, as in the case of health services, some future expenditures (e.g., pensions) will decrease due to early mortality.

Life insurance is one of the economic activities that may experience the biggest impact. The insurers will undergo unexpected losses and may try to discriminate against HIV carriers and even against high risk groups, by denying them insurance or by setting up high premiums which may be impossible for many individuals to afford, thus leaving them without coverage. Here again, a response by the public sector may come up to compensate for the withdrawal of the private sector.

Tourism to areas with a high prevalence of AIDS may go down; where tourism is a relatively dominant activity, this can generate acute economic problems for whole areas.

Prostitution will probably decrease as long as it is perceived to be a high risk activity. A similar trend may occur in the illegal IVD market, as a result both of changes in behaviour and of reduction in the population involved in this market due to mortality.

Effects of the economy on AIDS

The main effects under this heading probably follow an indirect path, on the one hand via the amount of resources which can be allocated to the health sector and, in general, to preventive actions and, on the other, via lifestyles, educational levels and attitudes associated with income and wealth.

Effects of AIDS on the social system

It is apparent that AIDS is changing social values and attitudes towards some types of behaviour, patients and risk groups. The degree of acceptability of homosexuality and drug addiction, sexual freedom, intimacy and individual rights may be some of the areas where AIDS can produce far-reaching changes.

Effects of the social system on AIDS

The extension of some types of sexual behaviour is probably the prime factor influencing the spread of AIDS. Moreover, the attitudes of society towards the sick and the risk groups will influence societal responses, such us a commitment to preventing AIDS, acceptance or discrimination of those affected, which will have a clear effect on the development and consequences of AIDS.

Economic approaches to AIDS

One article in this volume presents an overall view of a worldwide literature survey and a European project survey on the economics of AIDS undertaken by the MEDIS Institute, which allows us to draw some conclusions as to the pattern of research activities in this field (Schwefel, this volume):

1. The cost of AIDS is the topic that seems to attract most attention. However, most studies deal only with hospital cost. The financing of expenditure on AIDS has attracted some attention in the USA where, given the limited public coverage, the financial consequences of AIDS can be very disruptive for patients and their families.
2. A lot of work has also been done in the area of projecting the future development of AIDS, but so far these studies have had limited or no economic content.
3. There are few "truly" economic studies, like cost-benefit or cost-effectiveness analyses, or other types of approaches focusing on efficiency or resource allocation problems related to AIDS.

To evaluate the relevance and priorities to be attached to the different topics and methodologies which have been or can be applied in the economic studies of AIDS, it is important to consider their usefulness and the objectives they try to attain. These objectives are rarely explicit, and many studies seem to have been carried out mainly to show the magnitude of the burden of AIDS on society, which can provide a justification - however fallacious - of the need to devote more resources to the different activities - prevention, treatment, or research - related to AIDS. Of course, these activities should be advocated on the basis of their ability to reduce that burden or to attain health policy objectives. The proper economic approach to assist decision making in these matters is the economic evaluation of the programmes or alternatives designed to reduce the disease, not the total burden of the disease.

Cost studies can be seen as a first step towards evaluative or projective studies, which can be useful tools in planning and decision making. Cost studies can also be carried out with the objective of setting up reimbursement fees for health care providers or to more specific ends. But if they are to serve these purposes, the costs computed should refer to individual patients and, optimally, to the lifelong flow of costs generated by an HIV or AIDS patient. Aggregated costs at the level of institution or region do not provide any useful starting point for evaluative or projective studies.

Another important issue to consider is the range of costs which are relevant for decision making. Economists have tended to develop their own rules and procedures for defining, measuring and valuing costs. The net social cost - or opportunity cost - is probably the most favoured cost concept among economists, because of its foundation on welfare theory, but it may not be the prime concern of decision makers and planners. Intangible effects which are often quoted but seldom estimated in economic analyses may well play a major role in the case of AIDS decision making.

Productivity losses, an increasingly criticized but still the most usual way of quantifying indirect costs, may be especially unsuited to the evaluation of AIDS policies, as there is a varying but, in some countries, large number of AIDS patients who are not labour-active.

One example can illustrate the lack of tuning between economic analysis and decision making. A study on the cost-benefit aspects of AIDS prevention (Ochi et al., 1987) concluded that systematic screening of blood donors for HIV was not justified in Japan on economic grounds. Shortly after its publication, the measure was enforced (Lee and Moss, 1987).

Conclusions

The main contributions of economic analysis to decision making in the field of AIDS can probably be found in one of the following areas:

1. Projecting future needs or resource requirements within and outside the health sector.
2. Foreseen changes in specific markets or sectors - e.g. life and health care insurance, labour markets, etc.
3. Evaluating alternative courses of action within and outside the health sector in order to prevent, treat and reduce the negative effects of AIDS on the welfare of society.

To attain a higher credibility and, hence, effectiveness economic analysis should probably:

1. Adopt broader approaches, which does not mean to give up the traditional ones, but to enlarge them with new dimensions and perspectives which are felt to be relevant by society and decision makers.

2. Collaborate closely with other disciplines - health and social sciences - to take advantage of the complementarity of their different points of view and methodologies.

References

Lee, P.R. and Moss, A.R. (1987). AIDS prevention: is cost-benefit analysis appropriate?. Health Policy 8, 193-196.

Ochi, G. et al. (1987). AIDS prevention in Japan and its cost-benefit aspects. Health Policy 8, 17-27.

Schwefel, D. (1989). Social Sciences, Economics and AIDS. Paper presented at the EC-COMAC Conference on the "Economic Aspects of AIDS and HIV-Infection" (In this volume).

Williams, A. (1979). One economist's view of social medicine. Epidemiology and Community Health 33, 3-7.

Patterns of Health Care and Social Support Systems

The US Hospital AIDS Survey: Structure and Substance

D.P. Andrulis

The U.S. hospital AIDS survey: structure and substance

Acquired Immune Deficiency Syndrome (AIDS) throughout the 1980s has evolved into a formidable challenge for the health care systems of the affected countries. While the spectrum of health care providers are or will be involved with treating the individuals afflicted with this condition, it is the hospital sector that represents the primary if not only source of treatment for so many people with AIDS.

In 1986 and again in 1988, the National Public Health and Hospital Institute (NPHHI) developed and disseminated national surveys on hospital care for patients afflicted with AIDS in the United States. The first survey requested 1985 calendar year information from 4.65 members of two hospital associations: the National Association of Public Hospitals, which represents primarily large city, publicly owned or publicly subsidized institutions, and the Association of American Medical Colleges' Council of Teaching Hospitals, which represents major public and private teaching institutions. The 1988 version requested similar 1987 information from members of these two associations as well as institutions represented by the National Association of Children's Hospitals and Related Institutions and the National Council of Community Hospitals, bringing the total number of participating facilities to 623. Results from these two surveys currently represent one of the most comprehensive examinations of hospital care for people with AIDS (PWAs). (A 1989 version of the survey has been disseminated to members of these four organizations as well as the 600 hospitals belonging to the Catholic Health Association.)

This report discusses how the surveys were developed. It does not review survey methodology in general. Instead, it describes the methodology behind the study and presents the procedure conducted for its execution, identifying strengths and limitations. A final section considers the feasibility of replicating such a study in European Community countries.

Scope of the study

Constructing the Hospital Study Universe. Selection of the hospitals for study is obviously critical to the value of the research. It affects generalizability, validity and ability to monitor AIDS care over time.

Determining which hospitals should be included in an AIDS survey, if all hospitals are not to be contacted, is dependent on the questions under study. What proportion of patients and characteristics of patients served by study hospitals would be sufficient to represent the nation's AIDS population? Should the study focus on hospitals treating the highest proportion of AIDS patients? Is the study attempting to document treatment characteristics in an "average" hospital? Is there a specific target population of particular interest? Implied in these questions are the research and policy needs the study is intended to address: identifying AIDS resource and financing decisions at the national regional, city or hospital levels; identifying the burden of care distribution; assessing the effect of alternative treatment programs; monitoring changes in hospital use and costs. Determining these and other primary study needs should provide substantial direction for answering the key questions regarding scope of the project.

Lessons from the U.S. Hospital AIDS Survey have indicated that two key factors set the stage for any analyses that follow. AIDS has most frequently affected individuals residing in large U.S. cities. Even as it spreads throughout the country rather than being concentrated on the east and west coasts, the epidemic continues to be found most often in urban areas.

The composition of the AIDS population also affects the type of hospitals most likely to provide treatment. For example, in the U.S., PWAs who are insured, employed and who have more than a subsistence income are likely to be treated in private hospitals. Conversely, unemployed and/or uninsured patients with few personal resources will come to rely on public hospitals and a relatively few private institutions for their care. PWAs who happen to be homeless, IV drug users and prostitutes are also likely to be treated in public hospitals.

Successfully soliciting the active cooperation of associations representing hospitals to be surveyed was an essential component of the U.S. study. Perceived by their memberships as advocates, their hospitals are more likely to respond positively to association requests for information than outside organizations or governmental agencies that may be seen as antagonistic to the goals of many institutions. Moreover, the success in building coalitions among various groups is a valuable method of collecting important information.

Selection of survey questions. Once the parameters and limits of the U.S. study were set, we identified the survey topics and specific items that would address our concerns. In both 1985 and 1987, we developed questions around five issue areas: hospital utilization; patient demographic/risk group/residence characteristics; hospital organization, staffing and community relationships; outpatient care; and financing and sources of support. In 1987 we added a section on Zidovudine and other specific treatments. Where appropriate, definitions of terms were provided (e.g. the CDC definition of AIDS, identifying what constitutes an outpatient visit). Where we were unable to devise a universally acceptable description (e.g., other HIV infections, case management), we asked responding institutions to define the term.

Critical to the value of the survey was the inclusion of questions to validate responses. For example, the number of inpatient days should equal the sum of acute and special care days. The number of patients should not exceed the number of discharges. Cross-checking responses to these items allowed us to assess data quality and difficulties in survey completion. Finally, we contacted all participating hospital associations, asking them to pilot the instrument to one or two of their members. We also obtained assurances from each association that they would actively assist in encouraging their respective memberships to respond to the survey.

Conducting the survey

Obtaining successful information is contingent on providing detailed instructions for survey completion and describing how the survey information will be used. We stressed that results of the study would assist in developing policy at national and state levels. We also strongly guaranteed confidentiality of hospital information. No individual hospitals would be reported nor would hospital specific data be identified.

While some guidance can be incorporated into the instrument, the cover letter is the vehicle for providing overall direction. The U.S. Hospital AIDS Survey cover letter, which was addressed to the hospital chief executive officer or administrator, included suggestions for three specific areas:

- <u>Survey coordination.</u> Since completing the survey required the participation of several departments within the hospital (e.g., infectious disease, pediatrics, finance, outpatient), we recommended that an individual be designated to coordinate all responses. Hospitals were also asked to designate a contact person and telephone number for follow-up.
- <u>Obtaining financial information.</u> Completion of financial information on AIDS hospital treatment, while important, should not deter potential respondents from returning the survey. Still, we advised hospitals to supply as much of the requested cost and revenue data as possible, preferably by finance office staff.
- <u>Returning the survey.</u> Since it was our intention to obtain responses from as many hospitals as possible, we advised all hospitals treating any number of AIDS patients or no AIDS patients at all to return the survey. As with the financial information, we also suggested that the inability to complete one section of the survey should not preclude responding or result in inordinate delays.

The cover letter also allowed a turnaround time of two months for hospitals to fill out and return the survey. A second mailing followed approximately two weeks after the first closing date. Since feedback to participating institutions was regarded as critical to current and future response, we also noted that all hospitals would receive copies of reports based on the survey results.

As hospitals replied, all answers were reviewed before computer entry. As necessary, hospitals were called to clarify information. We identified, in particular, key questions that were not being answered (e.g., financial information) and sought additional responses.

Survey results and survey analysis

The response to the 1987 U.S. Hospital AIDS Survey was very positive. In all, 341 hospitals responded, and 59% of the universe that formed the analytical base. Two hundred and seventy-six hospitals provided information on 14,145 AIDS patients treated during 1987, representing 52% of the estimated number of patients alive at any one time in that year, according to the U.S. Centers for Disease Control.

For the purposes of the U.S. analysis, we examined the hospital survey responses according to two primary characteristics: hospital ownership (i.e. public or private); and region of the country (i.e., census regions: northeast, midwest, south, and west) (Andrulis, Weslowski and Gage, in press). Subsequent analysis compared major cities in the U.S. (i.e., Los Angeles, San Francisco, Chicago, Houston, Washington, New York/Newark) according to changes in utilization, patient mix and financing for 1985 and 1987 (Andrulis and Weslowski, 1989). Other published reports have examined ambulatory care (Andrulis and Beers, 1988), long term care issues (Andrulis, 1989), the effect of AIDS on public hospitals specifically (Andrulis, in press), the role of Medicaid (Andrulis, Beers, Bentley and Gage, 1987), and the characteristics of pediatric AIDS in this country (Andrulis, Weslowski, Brady, Hintz and Parrott, 1987).

Strengths and limitations of a hospital based AIDS research methodology

Accurately monitoring and assessing the effect of the AIDS epidemic on hospitals nationally cannot be accomplished through one approach. However, a survey based methodology can provide a useful perspective which, in conjunction with local, state or regional studies, can examine a broad spectrum of issues.

The U.S. Hospital AIDS Survey has a number of potentially valuable strengths. It can capture a large amount of information on AIDS related issues from many hospitals. It is sufficiently flexible to allow a nation to include all hospitals, to survey hospitals in certain cities or regions, or to target institutions with specific mixes of patients or other characteristics of concern. Since interest in institutional effect is likely to remain high, objective presentation of findings may also be appropriate for journal publication. For example, and as noted above, different parts of the 1985 and 1987 U.S. Hospital AIDS Survey results have been reported in a number of journals and books.

Critical to a successful response is the guarantee of institutional confidentiality. The survey enables confidentiality to be incorporated effectively into the study protocol. Hospitals are promised that, without their permission, provider-specific information will not be released to anyone or any organization under any circumstances. Only aggregated hospital information will be released. The analysis can be conducted in the study country by an objective organization, perhaps in conjunction with other interested parties (e.g., hospital associations). Another option would allow a research institute from another nation to analyze available data.

Its relative methodological simplicity may make the survey easier to undertake, since it relies on information many hospitals capture or can obtain. Such an approach can be relatively easily modified from year to year to adapt to changes in treatment or service delivery technology, and to allow for monitoring of trends. This methodology may also assist in monitoring other measurements of the AIDS epidemic. For example, the Centers for Disease Control is providing support to validate pediatric HIV responses to the U.S. Hospital AIDS Survey which, when completed, will represent a reference point for comparing information on this affected population. Finally, the relative universality of many terms in the instrument (e.g., average length of stay, number of hospital days, number of deaths, demographic and risk group characteristics) would facilitate international comparisons for a period of time and over several years.

While the survey-based technique for AIDS hospital research represents a number of potential strengths, its composition also includes uncertainties and limitations. These factors must be weighed before using this approach and must be monitored if the survey is undertaken.

Most importantly, the survey information is only as good as the data provided by the hospitals. If the hospitals find some of the information too difficult to supply, responses are less likely to represent an accurate portrayal of the AIDS situation. Such encumbrances may also decrease responses and decrease the likelihood that non-inpatient information can be reported.

Conflicting political agendas (e.g., a hospital association antagonistic to an entity financing the research) may further becloud reporting of accurate information if allowed to enter into the data collection process.

While the structure of the survey is relatively straightforward, responses will require hospital staff to devote a substantial amount of time completing it. This is especially likely if they treat large numbers of AIDS cases.

While the survey is adaptable, major changes in the instrument or in the composition of hospital response groups from year to year may encumber comparisons over time. For example, if key questions are modified or if new hospitals are added between two study years, the information reported by the institutional group in the second year may represent something quite different from the first study year results.

Because the institution is the unit of analysis, the survey cannot capture patient-specific information. Thus this approach cannot determine the extent to which an AIDS patient has used more than one hospital for treatment. It also cannot provide data on multiple characteristics of patients (e.g., comparing length of stay for IV drug users with homosexuals' length of stay), unless it uses a hospital breakdown that may not provide accurate information (e.g., examine the length of stay in hospitals treating the highest proportion of IV drug users with hospitals treating the highest proportion of homosexuals).

Considerations for study replication in other countries

The survey based approach to measuring the effect of AIDS on hospitals may represent a useful tool for other countries to consider. However, before electing this methodology, there are a number of key issues that should be addressed.

Hospital concern regarding AIDS. It is important to assess the level of concern for AIDS and its impact on hospitals. If concern is high (but not necessarily a high AIDS case-load), cooperation could be increased as well. Conversely, if only a few hospitals perceive the need to monitor the epidemic's institutional effects closely, a survey that extends much beyond that group may not yield much useful information.

Hospital data base sophistication. While many of the questions in the survey may seem basic, it is important to determine if hospitals can actually provide such information. Working with representative associations and piloting the instrument would answer this question. If institutions cannot respond or can supply requested data only with great difficulty, another approach may be necessary (e.g., special studies in a few hospitals).

Hospital association support. While not essential, gaining the cooperation and endorsement of associations representing study group hospitals will work to insure a successful study. These organizations can also be recruited to assist in obtaining accurate information from as many facilities as possible.

Participation by major providers of AIDS treatment. While broad based participation is important, the involvement of the major providers of care to AIDS patients is essential if the study is to ascertain accurately the effect of the epidemic for the most heavily involved institutions. Also, including these hospitals is likely to capture a large segment of the AIDS population.

Uniform definition of AIDS. It is imperative that the hospitals under study use the same definition of AIDS in completing the survey. Without this uniformity, reported results will be virtually uninterpretable. Whatever definition is used, it should be included with the survey when it is disseminated. Acceptance of a more widely used definition (e.g. the Centers for Disease Control definition) may facilitate cross country comparisons.

Conclusion

The U.S. Hospital AIDS survey may be a useful tool for many countries concerned with the current and future effects of the epidemic on their primary health care providers. Its capacity to yield a broad-based representation of utilization, patient characteristics and financing among key providers, when incorporated with more patient- or institution-specific studies, can result in an effective method of monitoring the course of AIDS services. It could also assist governmental and other organizations in identifying service needs, problems in health care delivery, the effect of new interventions, changing characteristics of AIDS care and in setting health care program objectives.

As this epidemic continues through the 1990s, it will be important to compare its health care impact internationally as well. In this context, such an approach could assist in furthering efforts to direct the development of an international health care policy to combat this tragic illness.

References

Andrulis, D. (1989). Hospital medical treatment for people with AIDS and the need for a long term care strategy. In: AIDS and long-term care: a new dimension (eds. R. Southby and D. Infeld). National Health Publishing, Spring.

Andrulis, D. (in press). AIDS and our cities' public hospitals: crisis at the frontlines of an epidemic. The Twentieth Century Fund, New York.

Andrulis, D., Beers, V., Bentley, J., and Gage, L. (1987). State medicaid policies and hospital care for AIDS patients. Health Affairs, Winter.

Andrulis, D. and Beers, V. (1988). Coordinating hospital and community-based care for AIDS patients. The Journal of Ambulatory Care Management 11(2).

Andrulis, D. and Weslowski, V. (1989). Hospital trends and the financing of medical care for AIDS patients. Paper presented at a conference sponsored by the National Center for Health Services Research and the Health Care Financing Administration 'New Perspectives on AIDS': Progress in Health Services Research, Miami, Florida, May 17-19, 1989.

Andrulis, D., Weslowski, V., and Gage, L. (in press). The 1987 U.S. Hospital AIDS Survey. Journal of the American Medical Association.

Andrulis, D., Weslowski, V., Brady, M., Hintz, E., and Parrott, R. Pediatric AIDS and hospital care in the United States: 1987. Submitted for publication.

Description and Analysis of Patterns of Outpatient Care for AIDS Patients and HIV Infected Persons

G. Brenner

The number of persons with AIDS in the Federal Republic of Germany is known from the cases reported to the AIDS Centre at the Federal Health Office. On 31 December 1988, 1,823 living people were registered there as suffering from AIDS. No reliable statistics, however, exist with respect to the number of people infected with HIV. Widely differing estimates render it impossible to make any statements on the rate of infection.
Similarly, there is also little information available on the extent to which physicians in private practice are involved in providing outpatient care for AIDS patients and HIV infected persons, or on any other institutions with which they might be cooperating in this field.

However, such information is urgently required in the interests of health care planning, in particular for preventive actions and for specific support to be directed at doctors providing care. A fairly accurate quantitative basis is also necessary for an assessment of the economic impact of AIDS on outpatient care.

In October 1987 and again in October 1988, the Central Institute conducted a comprehensive survey among all doctors working in outpatient care in the Land of Hesse, where 9.1% of the inhabitants of the Federal Republic of Germany live, and 9.5% of West Germany's office-based physicians work (Fig. 1). Both the structural composition of the population and the regional distribution between urban and rural areas mean that the results from the Hesse survey can be extrapolated to give a fair idea of the situation in the Federal Republic of Germany as a whole.

In the following, some of the results of the survey conducted in October 1988 will be presented. On a questionnaire all 6,000 office-based physicians in Hesse were asked to give the number of HIV positive, LAS/ARC and AIDS cases receiving outpatient treatment or care. The answers were categorised according to sex and high-risk groups. We also asked for information on the number of HIV (ELISA) tests performed or arranged as well as on the type of cooperation with other institutions outside their own practices.
Replies came from 3,318 physicians, representing 56% of all questionnaires sent out. Taking this response rate as a basis, some generalised statements for the Land of Hesse, and even for the Federal Republic of Germany as a whole, are possible.

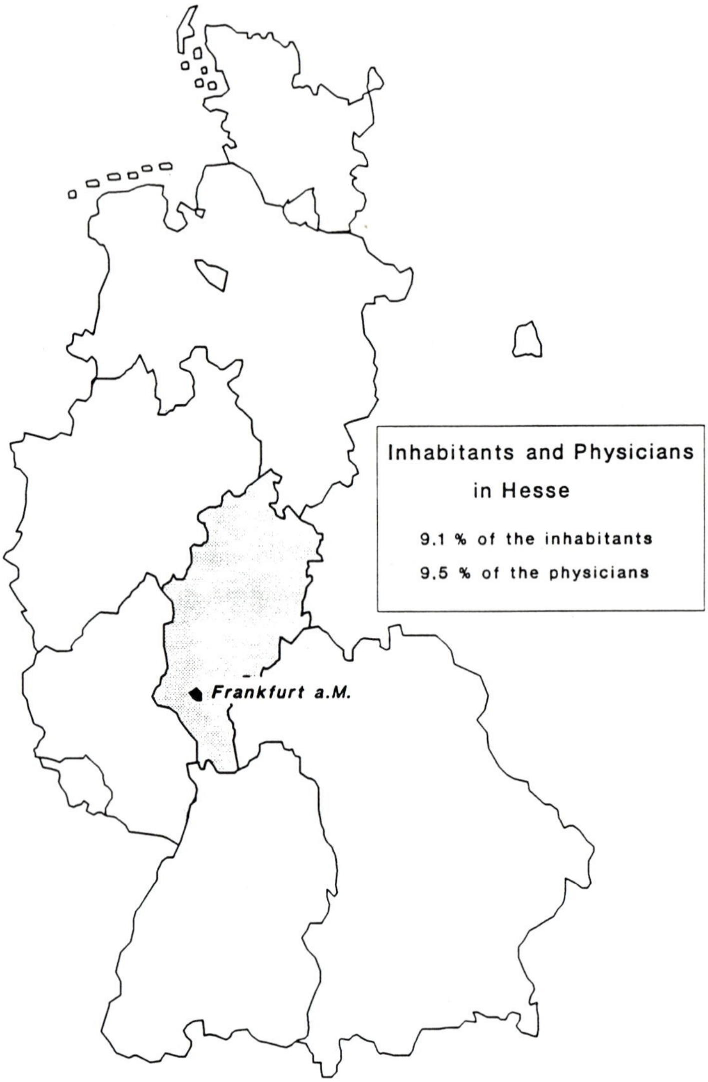

Fig. 1. Land Hesse in the FRG

Fig. 2 shows that, while many types of office-based physicians were involved in the treatment and care of HIV and AIDS patients, 77.2% of all cases concentrated on general practitioners, internists and dermatologists. It is with these doctors that most initial contacts are made. 22.8% of HIV patients and 25.0% of AIDS patients, however,

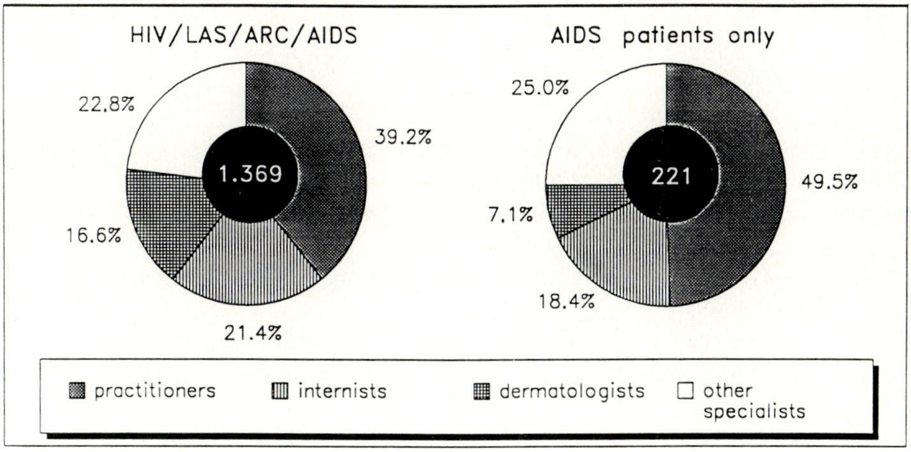

Fig. 2. HIV infected, LAS/ARC and AIDS patients in outpatient care in 3/1988 in Hesse

were treated by other specialists. It can be assumed that most contacts with these were secondary contacts. In order to avoid duplications these contacts are not included in the absolute figure.

Taking account for the rate of participation and the population of Hesse, it is possible to calculate from this basic table that 221 AIDS cases and 1,369 cases of HIV (including LAS/ARC patients) were treated by doctors in private practice. These figures do not contain the contacts with specialists.

The possibility of biases cannot be totally excluded. The extrapolated figures are calculated under the condition that those 56% of the physicians who answered the questionnaire, are representative for all physicians in Hesse. If one assumes that all physicians in Hesse who are involved in the treatment and care of HIV and AIDS patients, had in fact answered the questionnaire and none of the non-respondents had any HIV or AIDS patients, then the absolute figures mentioned above would have to be lower; under this assumption, 767 HIV and 124 AIDS persons would be the minimum figure.

A comparison of the clinical picture obtained from the results of the Hesse survey with the number of AIDS cases registered at the Federal Health Office, reveals a good degree of correspondence. Based on Hesse's 221 AIDS cases we would arrive at the extrapolated figure of 1,841 people suffering from AIDS and receiving outpatient care in the Federal Republic of Germany. As mentioned before, on 31 December 1988 in fact 1,823 AIDS cases were registered at the Federal Health Office.

Given the close degree of congruence between the figures extrapolated from the Hesse survey and the actual figures for the Federal Republic of Germany, it is possible to conclude the following:

1. The number of AIDS cases reported in the Federal Health Office's AIDS register is identical with the number of AIDS cases receiving outpatient medical treatment. In other words, all known AIDS patients are also known to the ambulatory care sector.
2. Cases that are not known in the outpatient sector are not receiving hospital treatment either.
3. If there was a significant number of initial contacts that receive hospital treatment only, the actual number of AIDS cases registered at the Federal Health Office would be too low.

I tend to agree with the first two assumptions, as the outpatient sector is usually the first point of contact for all diseased people, with hospital treatment only following at a later stage. If one considers this argument a plausible one, then the results of the Hesse survey can be generalized.

An important conclusion to be drawn from the study appears to be that the ratio between the number of AIDS cases treated and the number of HIV positive patients (including LAS/ARC patients) receiving treatment is around 1:7. Although this may give us correct information on the number of HIV positive cases treated, it does not help to estimate the actual number of HIV positive persons in the population at large.

For the Federal Republic of Germany as a whole, this would mean that, in addition to the approximately 1,800 registered cases of AIDS, a number of around 12,000 HIV patients (including LAS/ARC patients) received treatment from doctors in private practice.

The computation of the estimates for the Federal Republic is based on the assumption that the situation in Hesse is representative for the country as a whole. As we know, in terms of the structure of population, physicians and even of morbidity Hesse represents well the situation in the Federal Republic. But one can still be in doubt if the AIDS problem, too, follows these general aspects (Fig. 3).

Other estimates put the number of people in the Federal Republic of Germany infected with HIV at between 30,000 and 100,000. If the lower figure of 30,000 is correct, it is possible to say that around 40% of the infected people are currently receiving outpatient medical treatment. In other words, a large proportion of infected people do obviously not yet require any medical treatment.

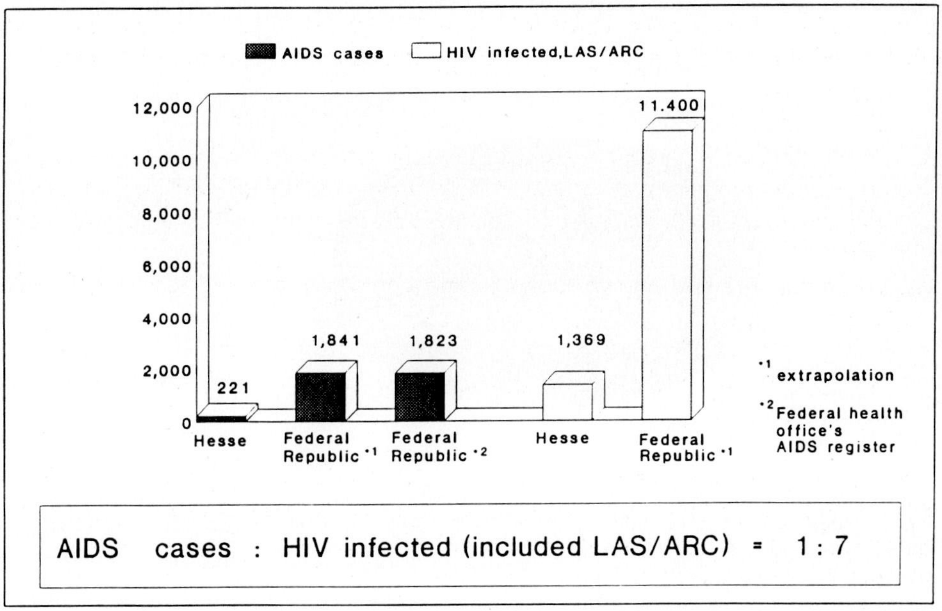

Fig. 3. AIDS cases and HIV infected persons treated in outpatient medical care 1988 in Hesse and in the Federal Republic

The number of positive tests (ELISA) for antibodies to HIV (0.9%) also reveals that the actual number of people infected with HIV is significantly higher than the number of HIV positive cases receiving treatment (Fig. 4).

From the reports submitted by the doctors we must assume that at least 36,000 tests of antibodies to HIV were performed or arranged in Hesse by office-based physicians in the third quarter of 1988 alone. However, the average number of tests charged to health insurance funds in Hesse per quarter of the year was only around 12,500 (Fig. 5). From this I am able to conclude as follows:

1. The number of HIV antibody tests undergone by the general public is three times higher than indicated by the official clearing statistics.
2. People are highly aware of the AIDS issue and prefer to pay for tests privately in order to avoid any record of them being kept.

Consequently, it is possible to estimate that each year 1.2 million HIV antibody tests are performed in the Federal Republic of Germany on an outpatient basis as opposed

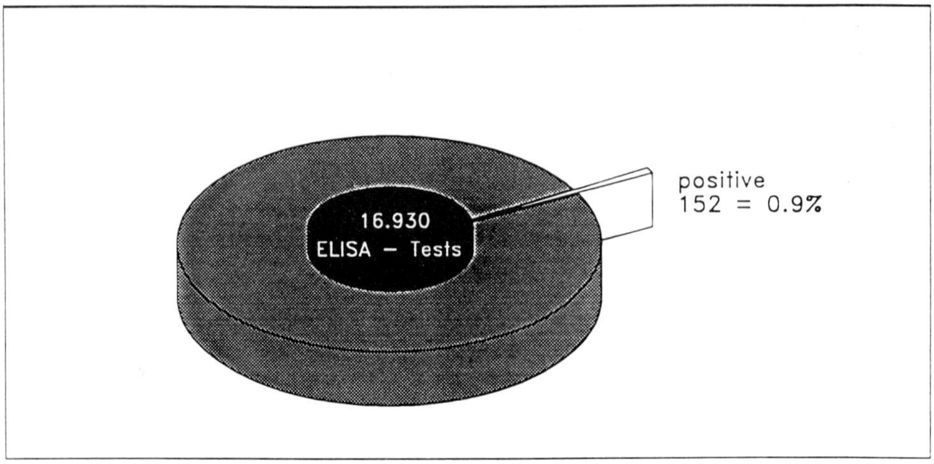

Fig. 4. Calculation of positive results of HIV antibody tests made by laboratories in Hesse in 3/1988

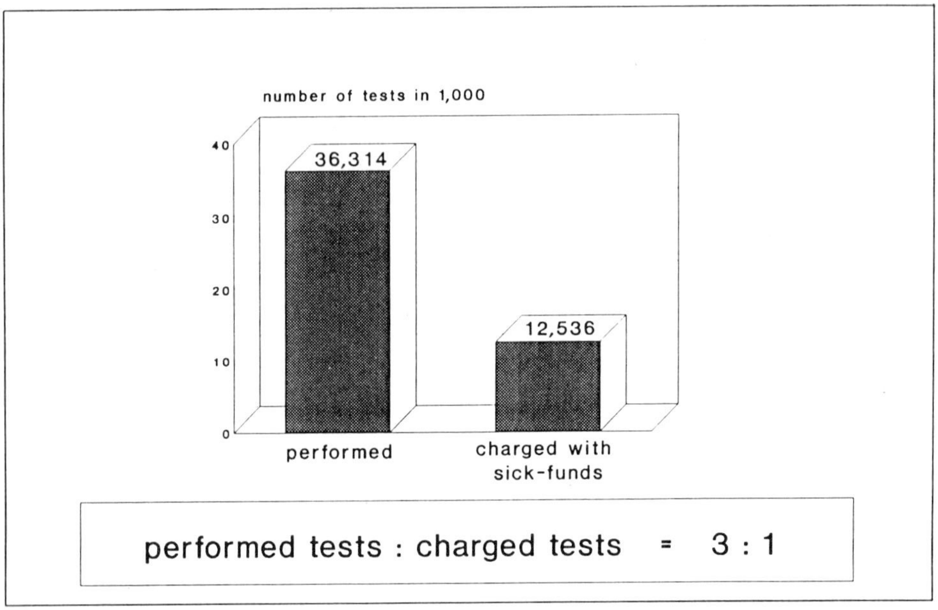

Fig. 5. Performed versus charged HIV antibody tests in 3/1988

to 400,000 charged to the health insurance funds. Assuming that 0.9% of tests prove positive, this would mean that there are around 11,000 new carriers of HIV each year (Fig. 6).

If one converts the results of the study conducted in Hesse to the reference figure of 100,000 inhabitants, it can be shown that, for physicians' practices in the Federal Republic of Germany, the annual figures per 100,000 inhabitants would be 3 AIDS patients and 19 HIV positive patients (including LAS/ARC) who receive treatment, as well as 18 persons who test positive (Table 1).

I should now like to examine briefly the number of doctors involved in the treatment of AIDS patients and people infected with HIV. The study revealed that 84.0% of doctors in private practice did not have any HIV patients under care, 9.2% of them had only 1 such patient, 5.6% were treating between 2 to 5 patients, with 1.2% of doctors having more than 6. In individual cases, doctors had more than 50 HIV patients (Table 2).

The fact, however, that as many as 84.0% of physicians did not treat any AIDS patients or people infected with HIV, should not lead to the conclusion that the problem of AIDS is not an issue in their practices - witness the extremely large number of HIV antibody tests which are either carried out or arranged there.

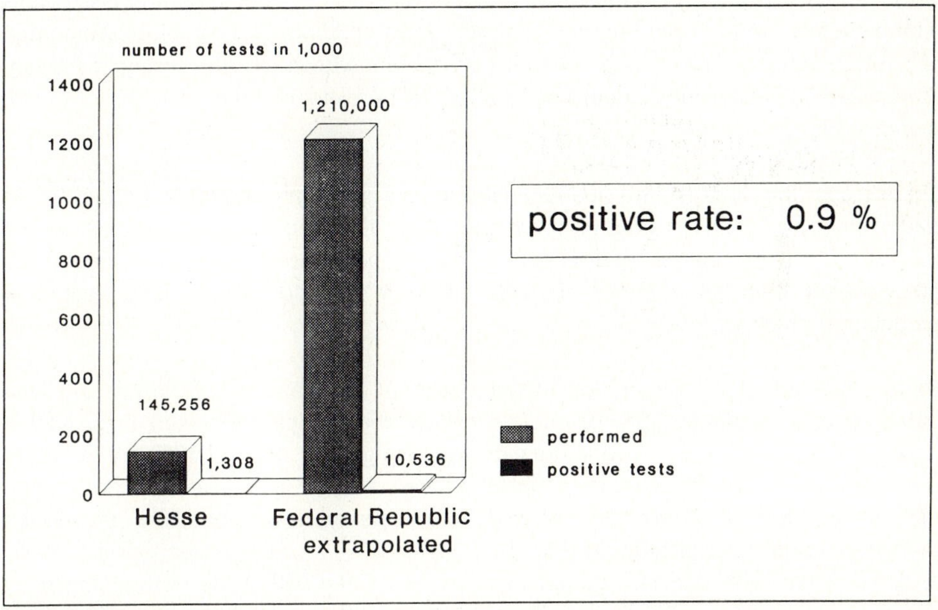

Fig. 6. Performed and positive HIV antibody tests in Hesse and the Federal Republic compared (1988)

Table 1. Cases per 100,000 inhabitants in outpatient medical care in the Federal Republic of Germany

	Hesse	Federal Republic
Treated AIDS patients	4	3
Treated HIV infected, included LAS/ARC	25	19
HIV tests p.a. (ELISA)	2,620	1,980
Positive tests p.a.	24	18

Table 2. Distribution of physicians with HIV, LAS/ARC or AIDS patients in 1988

Number of patients	Proportions of physicians in %
no cases	84.0
1	9.2
2-5	5.6
6-10	0.6
11-50	0.5
51-100	0.1
>100	0.0

Around two thirds of all doctors have arranged for HIV tests to be performed, in other words, the question of AIDS must play a role in diagnostics, treatment, and discussions with patients in at least two thirds of all practices. In addition, one can also assume that at least some of the remaining one third of doctors who have not arranged for any diagnostic AIDS measures, deal with the AIDS problem in their consultations with patients (Fig. 7).

On average, the doctors who had arranged for an HIV antibody test to be performed had arranged 12 tests per quarter of the year. Even the number of patients with whom the AIDS problem had to be discussed in preparation of tests to be arranged, is 22 times higher than the number of AIDS cases or HIV positive patients treated in ambulatory practices.

As to the question of cooperation in the treatment and care of people infected with HIV and AIDS patients, 70% of doctors believe that cooperation with a hospital is necessary, well above 30% cooperate with self-help groups, around 18% are in favour of cooperation with psychologists or social workers, and 12% believe that cooperation with some form of home care services is necessary; less than 10% mentioned theologians and other institutions (Fig. 8).
As to whether AIDS and HIV patients should be treated within the normal course of business of practice, 39% of the doctors questioned regarded the care of people infected with HIV and AIDS patients within the normal course of business of a practice as problematic, while 42% of doctors did not see any problems in such integration.

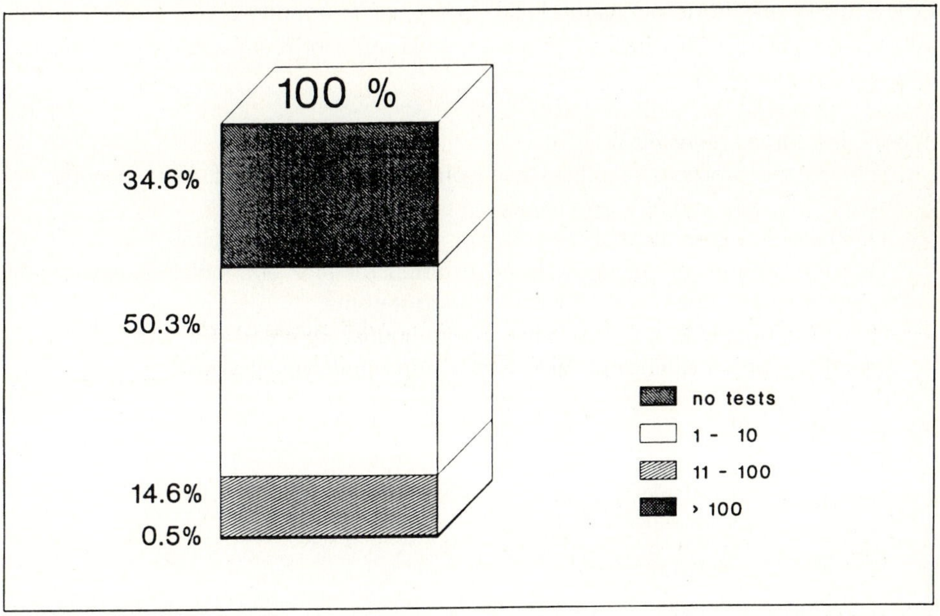

Fig. 7. Distribution of physicians arranging HIV antibody tests in Hesse in 3/1988

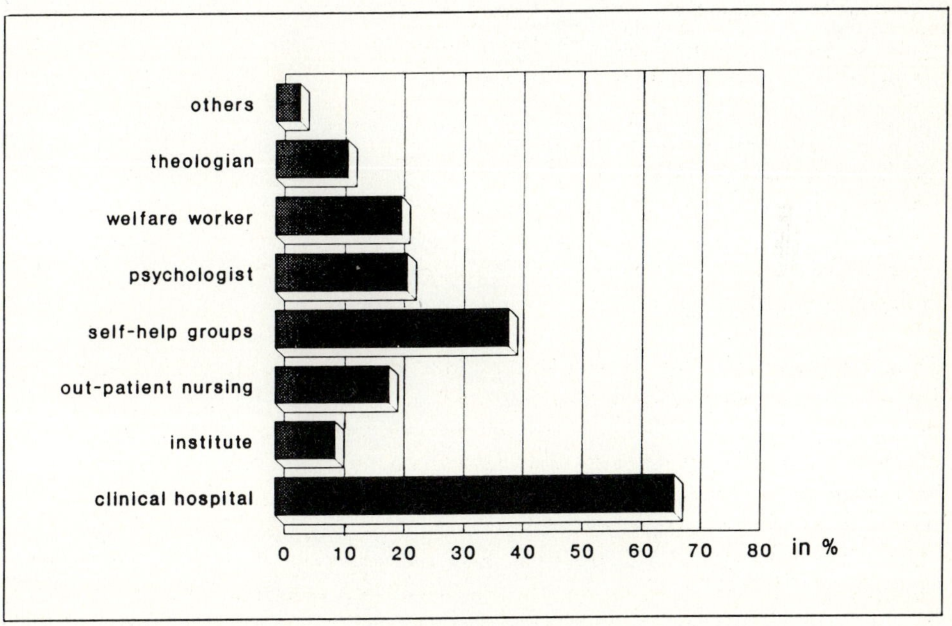

Fig. 8. AIDS related cooperation of office-based physicians with other professions

Only 15% of all physicians were clearly in favour of treating a higher-than-average number of AIDS patients in their practices, while 55% of them were against such an extension of their work.

In brief, the survey revealed

- That, in the practices of office-based physicians, the care of AIDS patients and people infected with HIV takes place on a large scale
- That there is a great deal of cooperation, particularly with hospitals
- That the number of people who were tested for HIV antibodies is considerably higher than indicated by the official clearing statistics
- That it is possible to determine basic figures required for quantifying the prevalence and incidence of AIDS and HIV in physicians' practices.

Association of Office-Based Ambulatory Physicians of Hesse Corporation under Public Law

Central Institute for Office-Based Ambulatory Care in the Federal Republic of Germany

AIDS in Office-Based Ambulatory Care

Questionnaire

1. Do you treat, and take care of, patients with HIV infection, LAS, ARC oder AIDS in your office?

☐ no (go on with question 4) ☐ yes

2. How many cases do you treat or take care of at the moment?

	male	female
HIV positives (asymptomatic)	....	....
LAS/ARC cases	....	....
AIDS cases	....	....

3. How many of these cases are, according to anamnesis, attributable to the individual risk groups?

	male	female
homosexuals	....	....
i.v. drug users	....	....
haemophiliacs, other recipients of blood products	....	....
prostitutes	....	....
foreigners from endemic areas (Central Africa, Haiti, Brazil)	....	....
children of infected mothers	....	....
other risks	....	....
risk group unknown	....	....
no risk	....	....

4. a) How many HIV antibody-tests did you order or perform during the last quarter of the year?

☐ none approx. number ....

b) Where do you have your confirmatory tests (western-blot, immunofluorescence) performed?

☐ lab physician ☐ institute

5. In the treatment and care of AIDS patients, cooperation with other medical or non-medical experts and institutions is sometimes necessary. With whom would you think cooperation is necessary and which cooperation would you initiate?

- ☐ clinic: ....
- ☐ institute: ....
- ☐ home care service
- ☐ self-help group ☐ psychologist
- ☐ social worker ☐ theologian
- ☐ others, i.e.: ....

6. a) Are there any problems in integrating the care for HIV infected and AIDS patients in the every day work of your office?

   ☐ yes ☐ no

   b) If yes, would you agree to primarily treat AIDS patients in your office?

   ☐ yes ☐ no

   c) Would you actively participate in AIDS education (e.g. in schools)?

   ☐ yes ☐ no

Comments:

Are you   Date   Stamp

Office-based physician ☐
with access to hospital beds ☐
Hospital based physician with ambulatory practice ☐
Hospital based physician with out-patient office ☐

Thank you very much for your cooperation.

Association of Office-Based Physicians for Ambulatory Care of Hesse

Central Institute for Office-Based Ambulatory Care in the Federal Republic of Germany

AIDS in Office-Based Ambulatory Care

Questionnaire for lab physicians and laboratory associations

1. How many HIV antibody tests (ELISA) did you perform during the last quarter year?

   number: ....

   ☐ none

2. How many tests were positive?

   number: ....

3. Do you perform the confirmatory tests yourself? If so, please report the number of tests performed during the last quarter.

   ☐ no (please go on with question 5)

   ☐ yes, number of western-blot tests: ....

   number of immunofluorescence tests: ....

4. How many confirmatory tests were positive?

   number of positive tests (western-blot): ....

   number of positive tests (immunofluorescence): ....

5. Do you send serum to other labs for confirmatory tests?

   ☐ yes

   ☐ no

Comments:

Date Stamp

Thank you very much for your cooperation.

Social Support Systems for People Affected by AIDS. Observations from West Germany

W. Satzinger

To deal with the subject of "social support systems" in relation to AIDS, is - from the outset - like entering a scientific jungle. For, as one approaches it, one is faced with a broad array of highly different conceptual frameworks, methodological issues and research designs, which originate from several academic disciplines and have produced a lot of diverse, even contradictory evidence. What can be attempted in this article is only to give a brief overview of

- The definitions and hypotheses surrounding the concept of social support
- General systems of social support and their relationship to provisions of social security and welfare
- The forms and flaws of AIDS specific social support systems in West Germany.

Social support

It was in the mid-1970s that "social support" became the catch-word around which a (not entirely new, but so far fairly neglected) area of sociomedical and epidemiological research was opened up. "Social support began to be examined in the context of the psychosocial dynamics of physical and mental health", and conceptually it was "integrated into the (familiar) stressor-illness model" (Lin et al., 1985, 247).

Since then, research on the forms and roles of social support and, particularly, on the measurement of its effects has had a tremendous boom (House and Kahn, 1983, Table 1), and today the relevant literature fills shelves.
Irrespective of all the differences in purpose, methods and results of those studies, there seems to be some agreement as to the components of the social support construct. Those are the quantity and quality as well as the types and sources of social support, which can be described in the following terms (see Ostfeld and Eaker, 1985, 68,99; Jacobson, 1986, 252):

- Quantity of social support
  - number of social relationships
  - size and density of social networks
  - frequency of social interactions

- Quality of social support
  - accessibility
  - symmetry/reciprocity of supportive actions
  - intimacy of contacts
  - sociodemographic homogeneity of networks
- Types of social support
  - emotional/affective
  - cognitive/informational
  - material/instrumental
- Sources of social support
  - family, relatives
  - friends, colleagues, neighbours
  - significant others

Of course, there exist some variations to this theme:
- Jacobson (1986, 256), for instance, points out that the question of the effectiveness of any social support is not only one of quantity, quality, type and source but also of its timing: that means one should not only ask "Who gives what to whom regarding which problems?", but also when this is done within the process of stress-experiences and situations of need for help;
- Wethington and others (Wethington and Kessler, 1986) claim that perceived (potential) support might well be more important than actually received support in helping somebody to adjust to adverse life events.

But, all in all, scholars today demonstrate a high degree of conformity when it comes to the basic properties of the social support concept. Far less harmony, however, exists, with respect to the assessment of the effects of social support on a person's health. There, opinions and even experiences differ widely, depending on the various frames of reference, theoretical paradigms and practical settings in relation to which specific observations have been made.[1)]

---

1) In the context of this article, it is by no means possible to address this issue adequately. It must suffice to mention some of the research literature involved, e.g.:
Kaplan, B.H. et al. (1977). Social support and health. Medical Care 15, Suppl. 5, 47-58;
Schaefer, C. et al. (1981). The health-related functions of social support. Journal of Behavioral Medicine, 381-405;
Bell, R.A. et al. (1982). Evaluating the mediating effects of social support upon life events and depressive symptoms. Journal of Community Psychology 10, 325-340;
Broadhead, W.E. et al. (1983). The epidemiologic evidence for a relationship between social support and health. American Journal of Epidemiology 117(5), 521-537;
Hammer, M. (1983). "Core" and "extended" social networks in relation to health and illness. Social Science and Medicine 17(7), 405-411;
Asher, C.C. (1984). The impact of social support networks on adult health. Medical Care 22(4), 349-359;
Badura, B. and Waltz, M. (1984). Social support and the quality of life following myocardial infarction. Social Indicators Research 14, 295-311;
Sarason, I.G. and Sarason, B.R. (eds.) (1985). Social support: theory, research and applications. Martinus Nijhoff Publishers, Dordrecht;

Putting all particulars aside, the leading hypotheses in this respect, however, contend that social support may be beneficial to health by performing four functions while playing two basic roles (see Ostfeld and Eaker 1985, 65,84):

First, as regards receiving good health care
social support may
- facilitate the finding of good health care (informational function)
- directly, i.e. through money, transport, etc., assist the obtaining of care (instrumental function);

Secondly, by improving personal behaviour and well-being
social support may
- enhance norms of health-conducive behaviour (cognitive function)
- advance well-being through promoting personal self-esteem (emotional function).

At the most general level, it is proclaimed that social support can act as a "buffer" between an adverse life event and its mental as well as somatic consequences. Over the years, the buffer theory has attracted a lot of attention but has, it seems, not been able to produce conclusive and undisputed evidence.
As one of the prominent scholars in this field stated:

> "Even though the evidence for the buffering effect of social support is equivocal, the idea that social support may serve as a buffer against the potentially harmful effect of life events remains theoretically intriguing and practically inviting" (Lin et al., 1985, 247).

In the context of AIDS, those beneficial buffering effects of social support are obviously taken for granted. Wherever you look, the importance of social support for the care of people affected by AIDS is not questioned at all: it is rather emphasized throughout. Apparently, it is considered - in the absence of effective medical treatment - to be almost the only means of improving the situation of those persons.

Let us take, for example, the "Gay Men's Health Manual for the Age of AIDS", published under the (rather pretentious) title "Strategies for Survival". A large chapter of that volume is dedicated to "social support" which, in turn, is rather loosely defined:

Berkman, L.F. (1986). Social networks, support, and health. American Journal of Epidemiology 123(4), 559-562;

Waltz, M. (1986). Social support and coping with physical illness. Social Indicators Research 18, 71-93;

Patrick, D. et al. (1986). Psychosocial support and change in the health status of physically disabled people. Social Science and Medicine 22(12), 1347-1354;

Friedland, J. and McColl, M. (1987). Social support and psychosocial dysfunction after stroke: buffering effects in a community sample. Archives of Physical and Medical Rehabilitation 68, 475-480.

In a "meta-analysis", results of 55 empirical research studies on the relationships between social support and health were reviewed and found to differ considerably; see Schwarzer, R. and Leppin, A. (1988). Sozialer Rückhalt und Gesundheit. Göttingen, 240 seq.

"social support - friendship, companionship, community, love, whatever we call it..." (Delaney, 1987, 157).
There, social support is associated with intimate friendship, with living in social circles in a give-and-take relationship, with participation in the gay community, and with going public as a homosexual - all that is presented as possibly the best way of becoming able to cope with antibody-testing, the diagnosis of AIDS, with the loss of friends, with the final days of one's own life.

Take - as another example - the Self-care Manual, edited by the AIDS Project Los Angeles. Again, social support plays a crucial role; it should be provided by family members and "significant others", also by specific "support groups", and it is supposed to help promote one's state of health through emotional stabilization.
But then, this manual goes a bit further and entails some paragraphs that deal with "tapping social services" and "benefits counseling". There, a different form of social support for persons-with-AIDS is implied: it is the field of professional as well as public support. And the manual gives a lot of advice as to: what sort of assistance one can get from hospital social workers and local AIDS agencies, and what legal entitlements exist with respect to social security schemes and health or disability insurances (Moffatt, 1987, Section II, VII and passim).

Social support systems

This leads us to a different level of consideration altogether. In our discussion so far, "social support" has mainly been confined to be provided by <u>informal</u> relationships and networks. But as the subject of this article is "social support <u>systems</u>", and although - in a sociological understanding - families or groups of friends or colleagues can well be conceptualized as social "systems", it would not be appropriate to limit the view just to these. Rather, a distinction has to be made between informal, formal and perhaps even semi-formal systems of support, their related sources and the sort of persons who can benefit from them respectively, as is outlined in Fig. 1.

To differentiate between formal and informal support systems is, of course, no novelty in this area of research[2]. Nor is the fact that our description of social support has so far centered so much on informal systems, a mere coincidence: it rather reveals a certain bias - I would call it a U.S. bias.

For, in the United States of America, a lot problems are left to individuals, to their personal capacity of solving them, which in many other countries are dealt with by public institutions[3]. The literature on social support, however, is - as, of course, in

2) As long as 15 years ago, Caplan stated that support systems consist of "formal and informal relationships and groups through which an individual receives the emotional, cognitive, and material supports necessary to master stressful experiences". See Jacobson, 1986, 252.

3) Consider, as just one indicator, the fact that, in 1987, around 37 million U.S. Americans were found not to be covered by any health insurance (see Short, P.F. et al. (1988). Uninsured Americans: a 1987

Category of systems	Source of support supply	Entitlement to support by being
Formal	Social security laws/institutions; insurances; health and welfare professionals;	Member of the society
Semi-formal	Counselling agencies; self-help/ community-based organizations; peer groups	Member of a specific group of people
Informal	Relatives, "significant others"	Individual person

Fig. 1. Social support systems - types, sources and beneficiaries

many other areas of psychological and socioeconomic research - dominantly American in origin. That is why the term "social" in this context is mostly used as indicating the immediate human environment of a person; rarely it is also used (as it would certainly be in West Germany) in the meaning of "societal", relating to the society as a whole, to its official institutions and legal regulations with respect to sickness and social welfare.

This observation only confirms what is well-known in essence, but often forgotten in reality: that even to a fairly global matter such as AIDS, our approach must - to a great extent - be country-specific because:

> "Every society reacts in its own way to infectious diseases, has its own approach to the organization and funding of health care, has its own sociocultural history as far as sexual emancipation is concerned, etc.... All of the social and economic means of reacting to the HIV epidemic, i.e. the regulations for and methods of organizing and funding the health care system, the standards and values with respect to sexuality, etc., will in fact both determine the form of reaction to the HIV epidemic and be influenced and/or changed by the HIV epidemic; they exist in continuous interaction" (STG, 1989, 4-5).

This is particularly true with respect to the facilities a society provides for diseased people. In West Germany for one, quite in contrast to the USA, we have a system of social security whose classical components are:

- Health insurances, covering almost everybody and almost every expenses for medical treatment
- A comprehensive payment scheme for occupational and general invalidity

---

profile. NCHSR paper, Nov., Rockville, MD). If one adds to these all persons who are obviously underinsured, the number of people having no official financial support in the case of illness amounts to some 56 million - more than a fifth of the total population (see Salmon, J.W. (1989). Letter from USA. Dr. med. Mabuse, 59, April/Mai, 56-7).

- An unemployment insurance, mandatory for every worker and employee and covering, to different degrees, a few years of joblessness
- And, as a last resort, a social assistance scheme for all those who are not (any longer) protected by other provisions of the social security network and have no resources left of their own.

All this is principally open to nearly every member of society, including of course people with AIDS (Nees, 1988, 30 et seq.). And this is similar in a number of West European countries (see Table 1), let alone the ones of Eastern Europe. So, a lot of problems for which in many parts of the USA a sort of private "system" of social support has to come up, are here partly or even completely dealt with in the existing framework of what is called the modern welfare state.

This is by no means to say that people with AIDS face no problems for which they would need specific social support. Of course, here too, they need
- Relatives and friends, people who care, for emotional support
- Practical information and sometimes legal advice in order to learn how to "tap" the social services and to materialize their rights to financial benefits
- The political backing of others in order to sustain the pressures and attacks of some sections of the public that are hostile to them as homosexuals, drug-addicts, prostitutes.

This is why, in West Germany too, a considerable number of institutions have been established over the last few years whose specific task is to serve the needs of people affected by AIDS, to provide them with support - informational, practical and emotional. The basis of their support-giving function might be called semi-formal: because it is personal in nature but independent of private bonds someone might or might not have; also because it is official, publicly funded (and therefore free of charge) but anonymously provided and not depending on somebody's insurance status or other forms of legal entitlement.

Table 1. Coverage of social security systems in Western Europe. Average percentage of population covered by social insurances in 13 West European Countries (1975)

Subject	Percentage
Health care	91
Accident/invalidity	81
Unemployment	63
Old-age pension	94

Source: CEC (Commission of the European Communities), 1988; Alber, 1987, 236-239

The institutional setting of these semi-formal social support systems in West Germany includes:
- Community-based organizations (especially Deutsche AIDS-Hilfe)
- General agencies for psychosocial AIDS counselling
- Group-/problem-specific federal programmes (e.g., women/children/drugs and AIDS)
- About 350 AIDS advisors at local offices of public health.

Most prominent among these organizations is the Deutsche AIDS-Hilfe, originally an off spring of self-help initiatives of the gay movement (just like GMHC in New York), but now working on an even broader basis and subsidized with public money, very similar to the San Francisco AIDS Foundation (Deutsche AIDS-Hilfe, 1986, 15). A branch of this organization can today be found in almost every major town of West Germany. Apart from that, we have an equally big number of so-called Psychosocial AIDS Counselling Agencies, usually staffed with a psychologist and one or two social workers and mainly paid for by federal, state or municipal authorities.

In addition, several federal programmes are to be mentioned in this context: including one for "Women and AIDS", one for "Children and AIDS", one for "Drugs and AIDS", one for "Home Care for People with AIDS", and yet another one that provides all public health offices of the country with, at least, one special AIDS advisor.
Up to the year 1991 (which is the designated end of their trial period), the costs of these federal programmes alone - involving about 700 professionals for their field work - will amount to approximately 145 million Deutschmark. There are no comparable figures for the related expenditures of various state and local governments, but it appears safe to assume that they, taken together, will easily match that of the federal government.

However, if all this conveys the impression that everything is fine with respect to psychosocial support for people with AIDS in West Germany and everybody is looked after well, that picture would be far too rosy. Rather, a number of qualifications have to be made:

For one thing, there is of course a difference between official entitlement and practical availability or accessibility. This may vary from region to region and even from town to town, depending on the directions of local AIDS policies and on the attitudes of local authorities. It certainly varies with respect to different groups of people - HIV infected drug users, for fear of being criminalized, surely face more difficulties in using such services than haemophiliacs or even homosexuals do.[4)]

---

4) In general, as we do not know how many people of this country are HIV infected (at present, estimates range from 30,000 to 100,000 out of a population of nearly 60 million), let alone how many may be considered to belong to one of the "high-risk groups", it is impossible to estimate the percentage of those who are actually benefitting from official support programmes. Even their absolute numbers are unknown, as there is no comprehensive record of utilization of support institutions; and if there were one, to make a distinction between persons and cases of contact would

Secondly, the supply of support is not equally adequate to all persons concerned. AIDS counselling, for instance, has got a certain middle class bias in its contents and ways of communication; quite a few people tend to feel excluded from its predominantly psycho-cultural approach.
Also, there is a lot of uncertainty as to the targets of dealing with drug addicts (witness the dispute between AIDS counsellors and drug experts over the methadone issue!), which does not help to attract these people to the support-giving agencies.

Thirdly, community-based organizations, which play such a pivotal role as mediators between their clients and the social security system, are more and more getting under pressure - for at least two reasons:
One is that the numbers of afflicted and even ill persons will soon exceed the numbers of volunteers to support them (already there is a shortage of people who are prepared and capable to look after IV drug users); and there is nobody to replace volunteers once they are "burnt out" or fall ill themselves.[5)]

Another reason is that these agencies, the more they get subsidized, the more they become professionalized and officialized, and by this, they may lose some of their appeal to the very groups of population whose self-help body, advocates and political lobby they used to be. So far they have been able to be a bridge between the different "scenes" and the official care and welfare system, and they won public support (and money) for that function, which they fulfill with special competence and - not to forget! - with a large contribution of donated labour. In future, a gap might arise between them and those they are supposed to represent and support.

These are but a few of the flaws in that seemingly well-equipped system of ours, established for the social support of people affected by AIDS. The number of shortcomings would increase if we proceeded to differentiate more exactly between the different high-risk groups or between persons in different stages of HIV infection and AIDS - each has specific needs, and these vary from place to place and over time: many of these people will not only lose their job, earning and flat in that process, but also their relatives and friends - the very sources of informal support they would then need more than ever before.

What I am trying to point out, is:
If we are to assess the importance, potential supply and possible impact of social support systems with respect to AIDS, we have to look closely at the psychosocial and socioeconomic situation of the persons concerned; and this includes that we take into account that

---

prove to be very difficult statistically.

5) If U.S.-American experiences are anything to go by, voluntary work will remain a vital element in the support of PWA and the fight against AIDS. Its supply, however, might - in the long run - not be sufficient to match the needs unless it receives more assistance, material and immaterial, by public policy than hitherto. See Arno, 1987, 190 seq.

- The type and severity of problems depend, to a high degree, on the specific characteristics of the main groups of affected people and on the psychosocial corollaries of the different phases of the disease's development.
- The way (and the extent to which) these problems can be dealt with largely depends on the norms and institutions that are characteristic of each country's specific social security and welfare system, and of the regional or even local variations of its implementation.

Biologically, the virus may act similarly all over the world; but how people can cope with it, varies considerably. Social support may not save their life but decisively improve its quality. Formal support systems, even where they are fairly comprehensive, can't do everything; they need to be supplemented by informal as well as semi-formal ones. And the latter should be further promoted as a basic and, probably, the best approach to the problem of AIDS - and not only because (this is said as a reverence to the main topic of this book) they are the most cost-effective one.

Acknowledgement. I am very grateful to my colleague Dr. Ursula Härtel for her invaluable assistance in providing me with basic literature and useful comments on the social support concept.

References

Alber, J. (1987). Vom Armenhaus zum Wohlfahrtsstaat. Campus, Frankfurt.

Arno, P.S. (1987). The contributions and limitations of voluntarism. In: AIDS. Public Policy Dimensions (ed. United Hospital Fund). New York.

CEC (Commission of the European Communities) (1988). Comparative tables of the social security schemes in the member states of the European Communities. 14th edition, General Scheme, Luxembourg.

Delaney, M. and Goldblum, P. (1987). Strategies for survival. A gay men's health manual for the age of AIDS. St. Martin's Press, New York.

Deutsche AIDS-Hilfe (ed.) (1986). Eine Stadt lebt mit AIDS. Hilfe und Selbsthilfe in San Francisco. Nishen, Berlin.

House, J.S. and Kahn, R.L. (1983). Measures and concepts of social support. Typoscript, University of Michigan, September.

Jacobson, D.E. (1986). Types and timing of social support. Journal of Health and Social Behavior 27, September, 250-264.

Lin, N., Woelfel, M.W., and Light, S.C. (1985). The buffering effect of social support subsequent to an important life event. Journal of Health and Social Behavior 26, September, 247-263.

Moffatt, B.C. et al. (1987). AIDS: A self-care manual. AIDS Project Los Angeles. IBS Press, Santa Monica.

Nees, A. (1988). Soziale Sicherung der AIDS-Kranken und ihrer Angehörigen. In: AIDS. Brennpunkte Sozialer Arbeit (eds. C. Mühlfeld et al.). Diesterweg, Frankfurt.

Ostfeld, A.M. and Eaker, E.D. (1985). Measuring psychosocial variables in epidemiologic studies of cardiovascular disease. NIH Publication No. 85-2270, U.S. Department of Health and Human Services, Washington, March.

Salmon, J.W. (1989). Letter from USA. Dr. med. Mabuse, 59, April/Mai, 56-7.

STG (Steering Committee on Future Health Scenarios) (1989). Guidelines for the feasibility study on "The Socio-cultural and Economic Impact of AIDS on Society". Typoscript, Rijswijk, Netherlands, January.

Wethington, E. and Kessler, R.C. (1986). Perceived support, received support, and adjustment to stressful live events. Journal of Health and Social Behavior 27, March, 78-89.

Use of Sentinel Systems in the Evaluation of the Impact of AIDS and HIV Infection

G. Thiers, M. Denayer, A. Stroobant

Economists who want to study the economic impact of a certain disease on society are often confronted with the problem of the lack of reliable morbidity data. Although mortality data are often available (cf. European Community Atlas of Avoidable Death) there is still a lot of discussion on their quality and their comparability between countries or parts of countries (Holland, 1988). Morbidity data for the general population are generally lacking while the use of morbidity data from hospitals is difficult since the corresponding population is unknown, the so-called denominator problem.

In recent years sentinel systems have been developed in order to obtain more valid epidemiological information for the general population. Sentinel systems try to collect valid information on a sample of the total population, which is called the "sentinel population".

Sentinel surveillance is based on the principle that information collected under high quality standard conditions in a limited number of places is preferable to information collected haphazardly everywhere. The collected information is more reliable because among other things it is possible to train and to supervise regularly a limited number of data providers (Dondero et al., 1988; National HIV Seroprevalence Survey Centers for Disease Control, 1988).

We are going to describe two different sentinel systems which can presently be used for the study of certain aspects of the impact of AIDS : "Sentinel General Practices" (SGP's) and the use of a sentinel population comprising by STD patients.

1. Sentinel general practices

In several countries SGP's have been established one or two decades ago. It is now generally accepted that they can provide reliable epidemiological information about incidence of diseases or health problems in a population.

It is also for this reason that since July 1988 the COMAC - Health Services Research has been supporting a concerted action called eurosentinel. Its purpose is to coordinate activities in the field of SGP's in the different member states of the

European Community, and to assist starting networks. The ultimate goal is to establish, if possible, a European network of SGP's.

Given the very low incidence of AIDS or HIV infection in the general population up to the present, GP's are not an appropriate tool to study the incidence of the disease. In Belgium, however, we have already studied the demand of patients for a serological HIV test through SGP's. Since May 1988 this item is inducted in the Belgian registration programme.

The objective is to evaluate in which way the GP is confronted in its daily work with the AIDS problem, the epidemiological characteristics of people seeking help and the reasons for demanding an HIV test.

It will be possible to repeat this type of registration at intervals in the future in order to evaluate changes in incidence or epidemiological characteristics. All demands for a test are registered, whether the GP decides to do the test or not.

1.1 Frequency of the demand

Between 2nd May 1988 and 1st January 1989, 668 requests for an HIV test were registered through a network of 172 SGP's in Belgium. This covers a sentinel population estimated at 160,000 persons. Presently there is less than one (0.5) request per month and per doctor. Fig. 1 shows that the largest group of patients who present themselves to the GP with a demand for an HIV test is between 25 and 29 years (Institute of Hygiene and Epidemiology, 1989b).

In 586 of these 668 patients (= 87.5%), the GP ordered a laboratory test. By extrapolation it can be estimated that approximately 55,000 HIV tests are performed yearly at the demand of GP's in Belgium.
Before extrapolation of these figures, the following criteria were checked for the representativeness of the participating GP's:

- Age and sex distribution of the participating GP's in relation to that of the total Belgian GP's
- Geographical distribution of the SGP's: for this purpose, the 43 Belgian districts are regrouped in 15 homogeneous district clusters. In each cluster SGP's are working and the population covered by this network e.g. in 1987 was about 1.2% of the total population in Belgium (Lobet et al., 1987).

1.2 Reasons for demand

Table 1 shows that 55% of the women who ask for a test do not present any risky behaviour while this proportion is 44% for men. The main reason for demanding a test is anxiety.

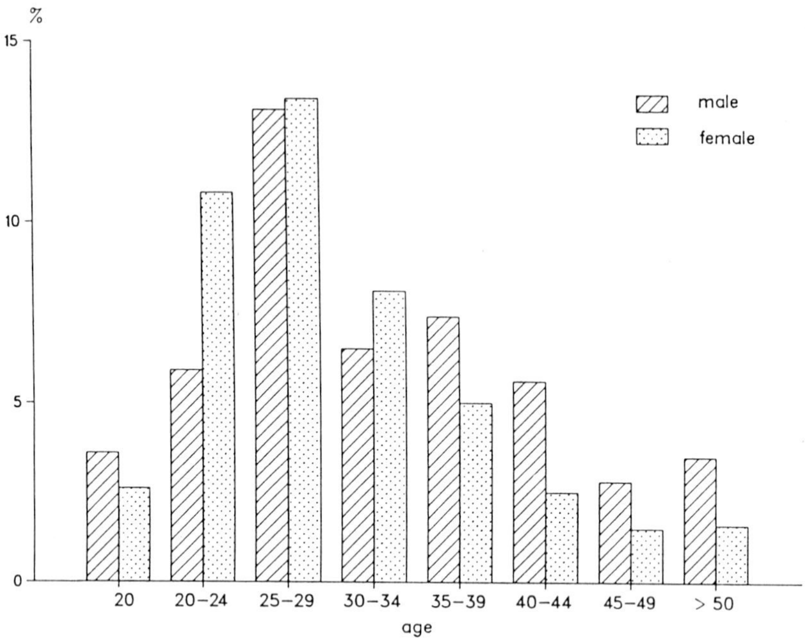

Fig. 1. Age and sex distribution of patients asking HIV tests in Belgian SGP 's

Table 1. Reasons for demanding an HIV test (in %) - Results in Belgium (Period: 02.05.88 - 01.01.89)

Reasons	Male			Female		
	N	%		N	%	
Prostitution	6	1.7		24	7.4	
Contact with prostitutes	43	12.5		...	...	
Multiple heterosexual contacts	66	19.1		67	20.7	
Homosexual contacts	44	12.8	56.5%	...	...	44.9%
STD patient	11	3.2		8	2.5	
IV drug addict	6	1.7		2	0.6	
Other	19	5.5		44	13.6	
Anxiety	86	24.9		80	24.8	
Administrative reason	34	9.9		17	5.3	
Symptoms suggestive of HIV infection	3	0.9	43.5%	...	...	55.1%
Screening before/during pregnancy	...	...		40	12.4	
Screening before marriage	4	1.2		12	3.7	
Other reason	23	6.6		29	9.0	
Total	345	100.0		323	100.0	

The table also shows that 56% of the men who ask for a test present a risky behaviour. These men have either multiple heterosexual partners, homosexual contacts or contacts with prostitutes.
The proportion of women presenting a risky behaviour is 45%. They either have multiple heterosexual partners or they have sexual contacts with persons with a risky behaviour.

1.3 Results of serological tests

Of the 586 HIV tests ordered by the GP's, 581 have actually been performed. For 8 persons the screening test as well as the confirmation test was positive :
- 1 male I.V. drug user
- 3 males with homosexual contacts
- 3 males with multiple heterosexual contacts
- 1 prostitute

1.4 Eurosentinel

The Project Management Group decided to introduce the demand for an HIV test in the first year of registration of the Eurosentinel project. The following countries agreed to participate: Belgium, Denmark, the Federal Republic of Germany, France, Ireland, Italy, Portugal, Switzerland, and The Netherlands. About 15 centres are involved in the project, mainly Institutes of General Practice or Scientific Associations of GP's in these countries. It was proposed to start this registration in October 1989. Agreement to participate is still expected from other interested countries.

The objectives of the registration in each participating country are :
- To get an idea of the frequency and reasons demanding HIV tests in the general practices.
- To identify the population groups consulting for this reason, in terms of age, sex and risk behaviour.
- To follow the evolution of the workload for the GP in view of the expected increase in HIV infection and AIDS patients.

The objective of the international registration is to compare the global patterns in each country for each of the three above-mentioned items.

2. Monitoring HIV seroprevalence in a sentinel population comprising STD patients (Stroobant, 1989)

Recently, it has been decided in Belgium to explore the possibility of developing a sentinel network for monitoring HIV infection trends in specific population groups. As a first step, <u>STD patients</u> have been selected as the <u>sentinel population</u> for the following reasons:

1. STD patients can be easily defined and are accessible.
2. STD patients represent a group at increasing risk situated between the high risk groups and the general population so that the spread of HIV infection into other population groups than the high-risk groups may be apparent first among STD patients. For this reason, sentinel surveillance in STD patients might serve as an early warning system.
3. HIV screening among STD patients raises less ethical questions than in other segments of the population since the physicians taking care of them are usually trained in counseling, tracing contacts and similar activities which are also important for reducing the risk of HIV infection. In addition, in many cases these patients are already routinely tested for HIV or have blood specimens taken for other reasons.

The method for implementing the sentinel HIV monitoring network has been based on the guidelines as proposed by WHO (WHO, 1988). All patients who enter a medical facility for a documented STD are eligible for inclusion in the sentinel population. The sentinel network comprises a sample of all the medical facilities where STD patients seek treatment. In Belgium, the majority of these patients are treated by GP's, gynaecologists and dermatologists, since there are very few specialized STD clinics.

A minimal basic data set has been defined in order to achieve the goals of the surveillance without causing difficulties with ethical issues or excessive workload for the participating physicians.

Data to be collected for each patient include age, sex, nationality, occupation,the diagnosed STD('s), risky behaviour and the result of the HIV 1/HIV 2 test. These basic characteristics are needed to verify whether the study population remains stable over time: this is the most important condition to be considered as a sentinel population, otherwise it would become impossible to interpret the results.

The form used is anonymous and before doing the HIV test, informed consent of the patient is necessary. In case of refusal, the form has to be completed but the serological test is not done. This should allow to assess the bias caused by refusal.

Every participant receives a limited number of forms at the beginning of each month. This number was estimated according to the number of STD patients seen by the different participants in this sentinel network. In this way, before analyzing the data, we can compare the number of forms expected each month with the number really sent.

The sample consists of the first consecutive STD patients, seen by the participants.
The sentinel surveillance network started in December 1988. The months of December and January have been used to test the form and to discuss other organizational points.

In order to illustrate this sentinel network we will give some preliminary results of this first registration period in Belgium (Institute of Hygiene and Epidemiology, 1989a).

2.1 Participation

The participation rate is still irregular. From experience with other networks we know that this situation will improve after a few months of registration, by the time all the non-respondents have acquired a good understanding of the network.

2.2 Medical facilities

Table 2 shows that there is a very important variation in the consistency of reporting between the participating physicians. The return-rate from STD clinics, gynecologists, dermatologists and medical facilities for students is satisfactory. The number of patients reported by GP's and family planning centers is still inadequate.

2.3 Patient characteristics

When we consider the high-risk groups (homosexuals, IV drug users, prostitutes, patients from endemic area, sexual partners of these group(s), syphilis), a significant HIV seroprevalence is found.

Table 2. Participating centers during the first registration period (01/12/88 - 04/04/89)[1)]

Participants	Number of physicians	Number of participating physicians	Estimated number of forms to be sent [2)]	Number of forms really sent	
				N	%
Dermatologists	14	8	96	61	63.5
Family planning centres	12	4	80	21	26.2
Gynecologists	12	6	120	62	51.6
General practitioners	25	10	80	18	22.5
STD clinics	3	3	120	50	41.6
Medical facilities for students	6	5	40	23	57.5
Urologists	6	4	80	31	38.7
Total	78	40	616	266	43.2

1) The figures presented at the workshop covered only the period 1.12.88 - 1.03.89. For the publication they have been completed to cover the period 1.12.88 - 4.04.89.

2) Each participating physician receives a limited number of forms, according to his practice: e.g. dermatologists receive 3 forms, GP's 2 forms and STD Clinics 10 forms, sent at the beginning of each month. The estimated total number of forms to be sent can be estimated by counting the number of physicians for each speciality, multiplied by the duration of the registration period (in months) and the number of forms sent to them each month.

The seroprevalence in non-high-risk groups is 0.5%, 250 times the prevalence found in healthy blood donors. It was stated that HIV seroprevalence in STD patients represents the upper limit of HIV seroprevalence in the general population. The real HIV seroprevalence should then be situated somewhere between these two values.
It is interesting to observe that most seropositives are encountered by dermatologists (see Table 3).

2.4 Diagnostic categories

As shown in Table 4, among men seropositivity is associated with serological evidence of syphilis.

Table 3. Age and sex distribution of patients by category of risk behaviour

Risk factors	Male		Female		Total	
	N	HIV+	N	HIV+	N	HIV+
Homosexual contacts	7	1	0	0	7	1
IV drug use	1	1	0	0	1	1
Prostitution	0	0	1	0	1	0
Originating from endemic area	4	1	6	1	10	2
Sexual contacts with one of these groups	9	0	5	0	14	0
Syphilis	9	1	6	0	15	1
Heterosexual contacts	66	1	126	0	192	1
No risk behaviour identified	6	0	3	0	9	0

Table 4. Distribution of the patients by sex and diagnosis

Diagnosis	Male		Female		Total	
	N	HIV+	N	HIV+	N	HIV+
Urethritis	30	1	4	0	34	1
Vaginitis	0	0	56	0	56	0
Cervitis	0	0	47	0	47	0
Trichomonas vaginalis infection	1	0	27	0	28	0
Syphilis	9	3	6	0	15	3
Chancroid	1	0	1	0	2	0
Condylomata	41	1	28	0	69	1
Herpes genitales	9	0	8	0	17	0
Hepatitis B	2	0	2	0	4	0
Pediculosis pubis	5	0	3	0	8	0
Scabies	0	0	1	0	1	0
Other	5	0	3	1	8	1
Total	103	5	186	1	289	6

Although it is too early for conclusions after the first months of registration, it may be assumed that:

1. The physicians participate without great difficulties, but the regularity of the registration has to be improved.
2. The figures provided by the network give different information than other sources.
3. The monitoring capacity of the network as well as its ability to act as an early warning seems to be already demonstrated.

References

Dondero, T.J. et al. (1988). Monitoring the levels and trends of HIV infection: the public health service's HIV surveillance program. Public Health Reports 103(3), 213-220.

Holland, W.W. (1988). European Community Atlas of avoidable death. CEC, Health Services Research Series no.3, Oxford University Press, Oxford.

Institute of Hygiene and Epidemiology (1989a). Enquête nationale de la seroprevalence HIV chez les patients consultants pour une MST. Rapport trimestriel, avril, Brussels.

Institute of Hygiene and Epidemiology (1989b). Surveillance epidémiologique par les réseaux de médecins généralistes. Rapport trimestriel 1, Brussels.

Lobet, M.P. et al. (1987). Tool for validation of the network of sentinel general practitioners in the Belgian health care system. International Journal of Epidemiology 16(4), 612-618.

National HIV Seroprevalence Surveys Centers for Disease Control (1988). Survey of HIV seroprevalence and assessment of associated risk behaviours in patients attending sexually transmitted disease clinics. February 8.

Stroobant, A. (1989). HIV seroprevalence monitoring based on a sentinel population of STD patients. "European meeting on HIV Seropositivity and AIDS Prevention and Control", Moscow, March 13-17.

WHO (1988). Consultation on information support for the AIDS surveillance system. Tatry-Poprad, 17-19 February (ICP/CDS/032).

Services for the Management of HIV Infection: Problems for Planners

A.M. Johnson

Introduction

Much of the work to date examining the Health Service implications of the HIV epidemic have focused on cost considerations and particularly on cost per case. In conjunction with estimates of the future number of cases, studies have examined the future cost to health care services (Bloom and Carliner, 1988). However, few studies have focused on the overall pattern of care and the cost effectiveness of different care strategies. Furthermore the opportunity costs of investment in management of HIV infection for other sectors of the Health Service have not been examined.

The majority of studies have been carried out in the United States (US) where the provision of health care service is divided between the public and private sectors. In such a health care system estimates of cost per case are essential for the calculation of insurance premiums, and for reimbursement schemes for health care costs. In countries with largely publicly funded health care systems free at the time of need, estimates of cost remain important for central funding, but planning the future organisation of care remains a priority, particularly at a time of contraction in numbers of hospital beds and internal competition for finite resources.

Previous studies (Bloom and Carliner, 1989; Scitovsky et al., 1986; Seage et al., 1986; Johnson et al., 1986) have shown hospital in-patient cost to be a major determinant of cost per case. In cities such as San Francisco the development of community care has been an important strategy for the reduction of in-patient stay (Arno, 1986), although the cost of community care alternatives elsewhere has been poorly documented. In the United Kingdom (UK) over the last two years increasing efforts have been made to reduce hospital stay and to develop services in the community (Kings Fund Centre, 1988), although these services have not been subjected to formal economic evaluation.

The purpose of this paper is to describe the way in which services have developed over time in the UK, and to examine the problems which face health care planners in determining the optimum strategy for service development in the future. Such strategies have been, and will be, determined by estimates of the current and future sizes of the epidemic, the geographical distribution of cases, the existing pattern of health service organisation and the physical and financial constraints upon the health care system.

Epidemiology of HIV and AIDS in the UK: current pattern and future estimates

Any attempt to plan services must take account of the current and estimated future number cases of AIDS and HIV infection.

To the end of December 1988, 1982 cases of AIDS had been reported in the UK, 82% of them occurring in homosexual men. In 1988, a Working Party was convened by the Chief Medical Officer (Chairman, Sir David Cox) to provide current estimates of the number of persons infected with HIV in England and Wales and to make short term estimates of the future number cases of AIDS (Adler, 1987). The report reviewed a number of methods for predicting future cases based on extrapolation techniques and on complex mathematical models. The wide variety of predictions generated by different models underlines the difficulty of making valid estimates even in the short term. Nevertheless, on the basis of mathematical prediction and empirical epidemiological data, the committee concluded that between 20,000 and 50,000 persons were infected in England and Wales at the end of 1987. They provided a "recommended basis for planning" estimate for future cases, calculating 5250 persons alive with AIDS at the end of 1992 in England and Wales.

The geography of the epidemic

Planning for future services also demands an understanding of the geography of the epidemic. As in other countries, the majority of cases of AIDS have been diagnosed in major metropolitan areas. In the UK 73% of cases of AIDS have been reported from the four regional Health Authorities of the Thames Regions surrounding London. Furthermore, the majority of these patients have been looked after in three major hospitals in London. Thus the cost of care of a person infected with HIV has fallen largely on the National Health Service in Central London. Since 1985 the three major centres have received additional central funding for the management of HIV infection. However, over the last year, while the majority of cases have still been diagnosed within the four Thames Regions, there has been some decentralisation of services away from the three major centres. Indeed Regional Health Authorities have encouraged other District General Hospitals to develop services for HIV themselves rather than referring cases to specialist centres.

Service organisation

The development of services for people with HIV infection was in part determined by the history of the service structure. In the UK, there is a network of open access, publicly funded sexually transmitted disease (STD) clinics. These services were popular with homosexual men before the advent of the AIDS epidemic. They were trusted to provide an efficient and confidential service for the treatment of STDs, often without the knowledge of the patient's General Practitioner (GP). Over 80% of cases of AIDS in the UK have been diagnosed amongst homosexual or bisexual men. It is therefore not surprising that the first cases of AIDS were diagnosed in London hospitals with large STD clinics particularly favoured by homosexual men. This service development contrasts with other countries where care of people with AIDS is often primarily undertaken by infectious disease physicians and oncologists. However the emergence of AIDS amongst injecting drug users may in the future place very different demands on the service. This group tend to have poor access to Primary Health Care services and may have less physical and community support than, for example, gay men.

In-patient care

As a result of this situation, in-patient care for AIDS patients fell largely on three London hospitals. Specialist wards were developed in order to centralise medical, nursing and social aspects of care rather than for control of infection reasons. In the early days, the stigma attached to an AIDS diagnosis led to difficulties in nursing patients on open wards. Against the advantages of centralised care were weighted the problems of possible stigmatisation of the ward and concerns about staffing. In practice the ward has been popular with staff and well-accepted by most patients, but there has been no systematic work to evaluate the cost-effectiveness, patient acceptability or clinical outcome for patients managed in specialist rather than generalist facilities. This remains an interesting area for future research.

The shift to community care

One major disadvantage of this "hospital centred" approach to care was the lack of involvement of traditional providers for primary care, i.e. GPs, District Nurses and social services. In addition, hospices were initially reluctant to take on the care of people with AIDS such that those who might be more appropriately cared for in hospice facilities were spending long periods in acute hospital wards (Adler, 1987). Over the last year, hospice facilities have been developed in two specialist units in London, thus relieving the pressure on acute in-patient beds.

There is evidence (Department of Health Working Group, 1988) that HIV positive people may be reluctant to reveal their HIV status to their GP because of fears about confidentiality or a negative reaction from the GP. Inevitably, STD physicians became involved in providing primary care for HIV positive patients, which might be more appropriately provided by GPs. In an attempt to improve links between hospital and community services and to avoid unnecessary hospital admission, Community Care teams have been developed in London. These teams, comprising clinicians, nurses and social workers, have the function of facilitating early discharge from hospital;

organising services and providing assessment at home; and arranging referral for hospice care. They have provided a much needed bridge between hospital services, GPs and voluntary and statutory social services. These evolving patterns of care make future planning for hospital and Community Care facilities a difficult task which is made all the more complicated because of the uncertain magnitude of the future epidemic.

The impact of changing patterns of service on in-patient care

Because of the diversity of service use by people with AIDS, data which accurately measure and cost use of service on an individual basis are laborious to collect and require large sample sizes followed over long periods of time to adequately reflect the variability in use of services from diagnosis to death. The tendency has been to study only hospital care. This is easily measurable, but of course has the disadvantage of ignoring other aspects of care. However, highly detailed costing studies of individuals, which include use of community care, may be of limited usefulness if patterns of care are changing rapidly year by year. Such studies may be out of date by the time they are completed. An alternative approach which provides up-to-date information, at least for hospital planners, is to develop a bed census which estimates the number of hospital beds occupied by patients with HIV infection over time and relates this to the caseload of patients with AIDS at any given point in time.

Such a system is being developed in the three London centres so that comparisons may be made between institutions over time.

The project involves a computerised data base which documents all hospital stays for HIV related disease (both AIDS and Stage IV disease) by date and length of stay. Thus it is possible to generate a census of average number of occupied beds each month. In addition, the data base collects information on each case of AIDS diagnosed in a health district and each case of HIV infection requiring hospital admission. The data base includes demographic data, transmission category information, date of AIDS diagnosis and AIDS indicator diseases. From this a ratio can be calculated of the number of beds occupied to the AIDS caseload (prevalent cases) at a given point in time. The data set in our District (Bloomsbury) now includes data on 349 persons and 886 inpatient episodes. Preliminary analysis of this data set in Bloomsbury Health District shows that, while the AIDS caseload has approximately doubled over the two year period (1987-1989) from the opening of a dedicated ward for HIV infection, the number of beds occupied has remained approximately constant. Thus the ratio of occupied beds to AIDS caseload has fallen from approximately 0.2 in 1987 to 0.1 in 1989. This data set provides constantly updated information for health service planners but illustrates the uncertainties of planning in the rapidly changing field. Even over the short term, estimates of future bed use may be incorrect when patterns of hospital use change rapidly.

The factors which appear to have contributed to reduced hospital in-patient stays include the advent of anti-viral therapy, earlier diagnosis of AIDS indicator diseases, changing treatments for opportunistic infections and the development of hospice care and home care.

Implications of changing patterns of care for economic studies

Studies of individual hospital and medical cost, while useful for hospital bed planning, are restricted in examining the wider economic and planning implications of the HIV epidemic. As care shifts away from hospitals, it may become increasingly important to measure the overall costs of different services and to develop comparative measures of "output" in terms not only of numbers of patients treated, but also in terms of satisfaction of patients, relatives and carers. This may also lead to uncomfortable questions about how much society is prepared to invest in AIDS as compared with other diseases. However, it may also lead to a useful evaluation of care strategies which have implications in service developments in other fields, such as cancer services and care of the elderly.

Conclusions

In a public health care system with finite resources, studies of costs of care and health service use for HIV infection are essential both for the funding and planning of services. Cost per case estimates alone however may be of limited practical use to planners unless they can be linked more closely to patterns of care and the overall development of services. More importantly, much of the service development has occurred without regard to the most cost-effective way of providing services. The time is right for comparing different service "packages" in terms of patient acceptability, costs of care and disease outcome.

Acknowledgement. I wish to thank Carol Shergold for her contribution to data collection and helpful comments on the manuscript, and the Department of Health for project funding.

References

Bloom, D.E. and Carliner, G. (1988). The economic impact of AIDS in the United States. Science 239, 604-610.

Scitovisky, A., Arno, P., Cline, M., and Lee, Ph.R. (1986). Medical care costs of patients with AIDS in San Francisco. Journal of the American Medical Association 256, 3103-3106.

Seage, G.R., Landers, S., Anita, B., Groopman, J., Lamb, G.A., Epstein, A.M., and Barry, M.A. (1986). Medical care costs of AIDS in Massachusetts. Journal of the American Medical Association 256, 3107-3109.

Johnson, A.M., Adler, M.W., and Crown, J.M. (1986). The acquired immune deficiency syndrome and epidemic of infection with human immunodeficiency virus: costs of care and prevention in an inner London district (medical practice; contemporary themes). British Medical Journal 293, 489-492.

Arno, P.S. (1986). The non-profit sector's response to the AIDS epidemic: community-based services in San Francisco. American Journal of Public Health 76, 1325-1330.

Kings Fund Centre (1988). AIDS: Models of care. London.

Adler, M.W. (1987). Care for the patients with HIV-infection and AIDS. British Medical Journal 295, 27-30.

Department of Health Working Group (1988). Short-term prediction of HIV infection and AIDS in England and Wales. HMSO, London.

Costs of AIDS and HIV Infection

Economic Evaluation of Programmes for AIDS and HIV Infection: Methodological Issues

M. Drummond, L. Davies

1. Introduction

AIDS is not only a disease of great social concern; it also has major resource implications. In most of the developed countries governments have been concerned about the costs of treating an increasing number of cases and the costs of mounting major public information campaigns to prevent the spread of the disease. The increased expenditure on treatment has raised questions about the relative priority that should be assigned to interventions for AIDS and HIV infection, when there are many other potential uses of scarce health care resources. The relative value for money of alternative treatment packages has also been a source of debate.

In principle economic evaluation can assist those making choices in the allocation of health care resources at national, regional and local levels. A number of studies of the costs of treating AIDS and the related consequences of HIV infection have been published in recent years. Given the increasing concern about the economic impact of AIDS and the growing economics literature, this paper:

- Briefly outlines the methods of economic evaluation of health care programmes
- Reviews and interprets existing studies of the costs of treating AIDS
- Specifies how one would undertake an economic evaluation of a programme for the treatment of AIDS, using the example of drug therapy.

2. Methods for the economic evaluation of health care programmes

The methods for the economic evaluation of health care programmes have been extensively documented elsewhere (Weinstein and Stason, 1977; Warner and Luce, 1982; Drummond et al., 1987), so only a few methodological issues pertinent to the evaluation of AIDS programmes will be highlighted here.

First, economic evaluation should embody a comparison of alternatives. These may be alternatives in prevention, diagnosis, treatment or the organization of services. Therefore, cost of illness studies (Scitovsky and Rice, 1987) are not of themselves full economic evaluations, although they may provide useful background data for discussions of priorities in research or treatment (Black and Pole, 1975).

Secondly, economic evaluations require an assessment of the effectiveness of the health treatments or programmes concerned. Ideally, this should be established through controlled studies, such as randomised controlled trials. However, the difficulties in mounting trials in a disease like AIDS/HIV should not be under-estimated. Being a life-threatening condition it has inevitable emotional overtones which militate against random allocation of subjects to receive, or not receive, a new treatment technology. Also, treatment practices have changed rapidly, making the strict adherence to trial protocols difficult. However, the danger is that new treatments may not be properly evaluated and economists will have to use guesswork in assessing the cost-effectiveness of treatments or programmes.

Thirdly, an appropriate range of costs and consequences needs to be considered. Fig. 1 gives the relevant range for the evaluation of options from the viewpoint of society. Other viewpoints include those of the hospital, health care system, government or patient. Different viewpoints imply consideration of different costs and consequences so it is important that the viewpoint of the evaluation be stated explicitly. Economists argue that the societal viewpoint, being the broadest, should always be considered by health policy makers.

In particular, significant amounts of voluntary and informal care resources are being consumed in AIDS/HIV programmes in many developed countries. Therefore it is important that health policy is not determined solely by economic studies that focus on a more narrow hospital or health care sector perspective. Indeed one of the most interesting issues for economic evaluation is the comparison, in terms of value for money, of comprehensive community-based care, using voluntary support, with traditional hospital-based regimens.

Finally, more effort needs to be placed on the interpretation of study results for decision making purposes. Given the comments made earlier about uncertainties in assessment of the effectiveness of interventions and the additional difficulties of interpretation of results from one setting to another, it is important that economic evaluations incorporate a sensitivity analysis, where the estimates are produced using a range of values for the key parameters.

Also, given the need to assign priorities between programmes for AIDS/HIV and other diseases, it is important that the results of economic evaluation be comparable across different health care interventions. One promising approach is the calculation of the cost per quality adjusted life-year gained (QALY) from different interventions (see Table 1). If the results for AIDS/HIV programmes are to be included in such tables in the future, data will be required not only of the extension of life from treatment or prevention, but also of the quality of that life (see Fig. 2). Economists and others have developed a number of approaches for measuring the quality of life (Katz, 1987; Teeling Smith, 1988; Walker and Rosser, 1988).

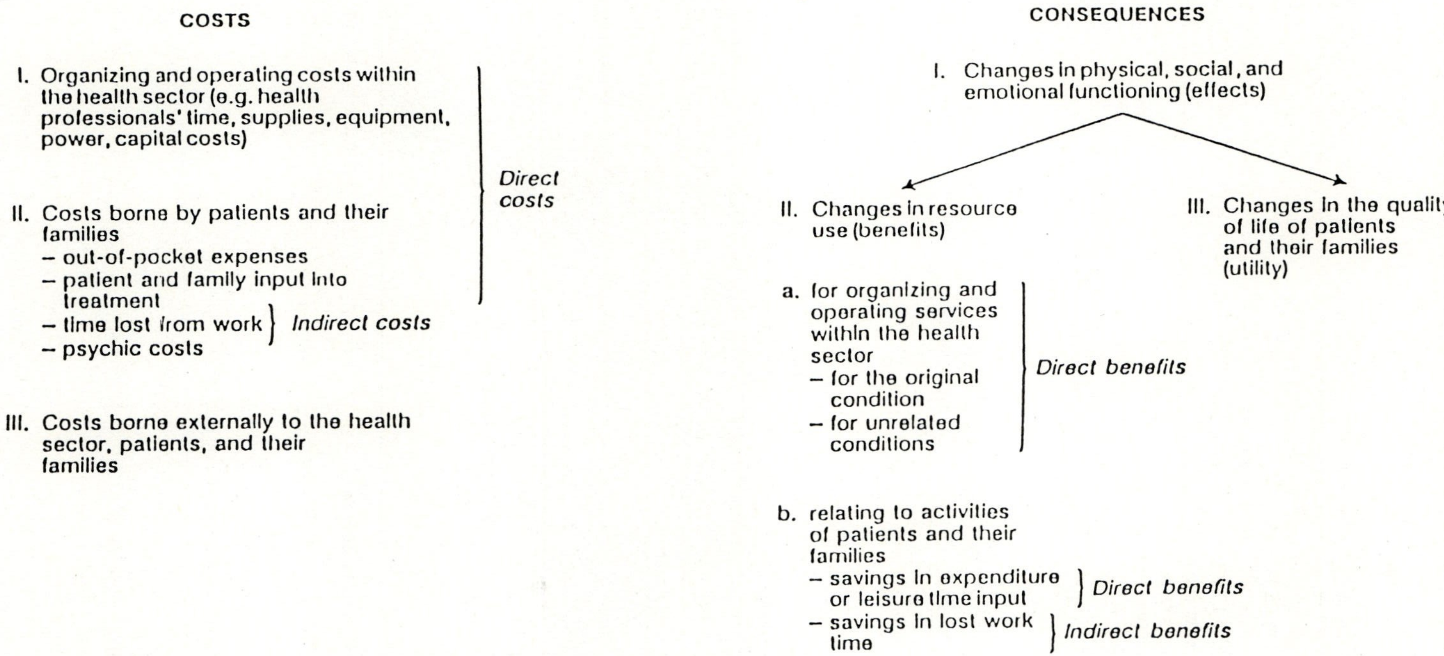

Fig. 1. Types of costs and consequences of health services and programmes (from Drummond et al. 1987)

Table 1. 'League table' of costs and QUALYs for selected health care interventions (1983-84 prices)

Intervention	Present value of extra cost per QUALY gained (£)
GP advice to stop smoking	170
Pacemaker implantation for heart block	700
Hip replacement	750
CABG for severe angina LMD	1,040
GP control of total serum cholesterol	1,700
CABG for severe angina with 2VD	2,280
Kidney transplantation (cadaver)	3,000
Breast cancer screening	3,500
Heart transplantation	5,000
CABG for mild angina 2VD	12,600
Hospital haemodialysis	14,000

Adapted from Williams, 1985, 1986

CABG: Coronary Artery Bypass Graft; LMD: Left Main Disease; 2VD: Two Vessel Disease

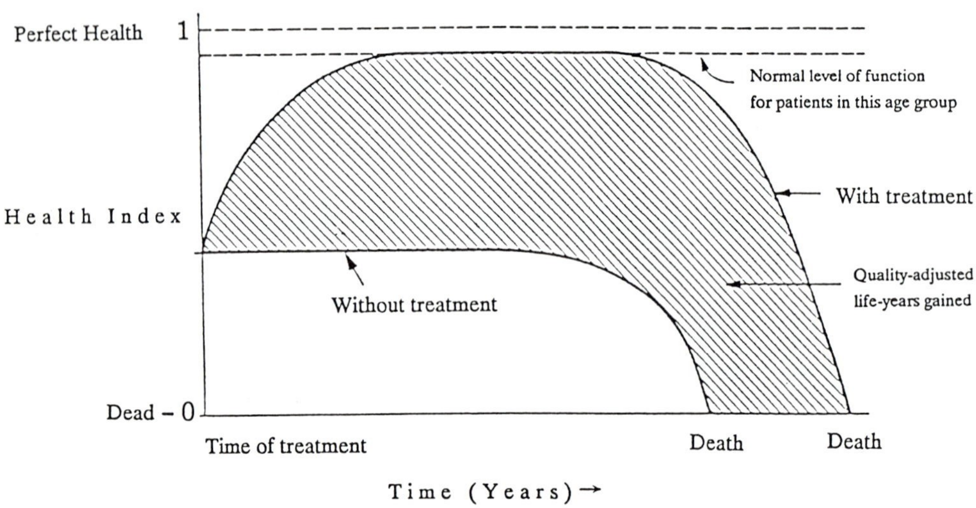

Fig. 2. Quality-adjusted life-years added by treatment

3. Interpreting existing studies of the costs of AIDS/HIV programmes

A number of studies of the costs of AIDS/HIV programmes in developed countries have been published (Scitovsky and Over, 1988; Drummond and Davies, 1988) (see Table 2). These relate almost exclusively to hospital-based treatment or care and confine their consideration to health sector costs. It is important to bear a number of points in mind when interpreting these studies.

Table 2. Costs of treating AIDS (1986 prices) [1)]

Source	Year of estimate	Lifetime cost per person ($)	Length of survival (months)	Cost/person per year ($)
USA				
Hardy et al., 1986	1984	155,400	13.0	143,400
Scitovsky et al., 1986	1984	29,200	7.4	46,700
Seage et al., 1986	1984	NA	NA	49,200
Andrulis et al., 1987	1984	NA	NA	38,300
Kizer et al., 1986	1985	92,800	18.0	61,900
Kizer et al., 1987	1986	70,000	18.0	46,700
Lafferty et al., 1988	1985	19,600	7.2	32,700
Scitovsky and Rice, 1987	1986	NA	NA	33,700
Pascal, 1987	1986	94,000	15.0	75,200
Hay et al., 1987	1987	32,900	12.0	32,900
Hellinger, 1988	1985	58,100	24.0	29,100
Hiatt et al., 1988	1987	33,900	15.1	24,200
France				
Debeaupuis and Tcheriatchoukine, 1987	1986	NA	NA	21,800
Germany				
AUK (Berlin), 1987 [2)]	1986	36,600	18.0	24,400
Universitäts Poliklinik (Munich) 1987 [2)]	1986	11,400	6.6	20,900
United Kingdom				
Johnson et al., 1986	1984	13,400	5.2	31,000
Cunningham and Griffiths, 1988	1986	47,200	12.0	47,200
Rees et al., 1988	1987	NA	NA	24,600
Australia				
Whyte et al., 1987	1986	17,300	7.2	28,800
Canada				
Fanning et al., 1987	1983	NA	NA	33,900-47,500

1) These costs have been adapted from the papers by Drummond and Davies (1988) and Scitovsky and Over (1988). Discrepancies in the costs reported in these papers and the costs presented here are due mainly to our use of a more recent version of OECD purchasing power parity exchange rates (OECD, 1987).

2) Personal communication

First, most studies report merely the current costs of care for people with AIDS or related conditions. Few discuss the question of alternative methods of care, or the effectiveness of the treatments being given.

Secondly, in order to make informative comparisons, the raw cost data reported in individual studies needs to be adjusted. It has been suggested that the best method of adjustment is to calculate the cost per person per year and to use purchasing power parities in making exchange rate conversions (Scitovsky and Over, 1988; Drummond and Davies, 1988).

Thirdly, there are important differences in study methodology that are likely to affect the estimates obtained. These include the categories of patients included in the study, the range of costs considered (hospital costs only, or including ambulatory care) and the methods of cost calculation (average daily hospital cost, or more detailed study).

Finally, the studies differ both in their date and setting. Therefore, it is likely that they reflect different treatment technologies, which have changed through time and varied by location. For example, there have been significant changes in drug therapy and a shift towards community-based care. The studies also reflect key features of the health care systems in which they were undertaken. For example, longer hospital stays are likely in a country like the Federal Republic of Germany, where secondary and primary care services are not closely linked. Also, the availability of drugs may differ from country to country.

Nevertheless, a fairly constant pattern appears to emerge from the existing studies. Namely, the cost of caring for a person with AIDS is similar to that of caring for people with other end-stage diseases, such as cancer or chronic renal failure. As yet there are no data on the cost per QALY gained from treatment for AIDS to compare with that of other health care interventions.

4. Economic evaluation of programmes for AIDS/HIV: the case of drug therapy

Given the need for data on the value for money of programmes for AIDS/ARC and the difficulties in interpreting existing cost estimates, how should economic evaluations be carried out? This issue is addressed below, using the example of drug therapy. Drug therapy has been chosen because of the concerns about the cost of medicines for AIDS, most notably zidovudine (Retrovir^{R}).

The first methodological issue concerns the alternatives for comparison. Zidovudine is now widely prescribed for patients with AIDS and AIDS related complex (ARC), following the extension in the length of life of patients shown in earlier clinical trials (Fischl et al, 1987). It would therefore now be considered unethical to compare zidovudine to no treatment in these patients, although such a comparison could and should be made in persons with earlier stages of the disease. The main alternatives for patients with more advanced stages of the disease are between zidovudine as monotherapy and combination therapy with other medicines. Even so, it may be difficult to undertake controlled trials at the present time, for the reasons stated earlier.

Ideally economic evaluation should be based on sound evidence of the effectiveness of the medicines concerned. Therefore, where possible the evaluation should be conducted alongside a clinical trial, or based on evidence gained in earlier clinical studies. The main measure of effectiveness in clinical trials for AIDS/ARC patients is length of survival. This would enable a cost-effectiveness analysis to be performed, giving an estimate of incremental cost per life-year gained.

However,it may be better to adjust the years of life gained by a measure of the quality of the extra years, thereby conducting a cost-utility analysis. The advantage of this approach would be that drug therapy for AIDS/ARC could be compared with other health care interventions in terms of its incremental cost per QALY gained. This approach should clearly be considered since the quality of the added years may be less than perfect. Patients may suffer infections, be considerably distressed, or experience side effects of therapy. Therefore trials of drug therapy for AIDS/ARC should either include a measure of health-related quality of life, or collect clinical symptomology data in a way that would enable the health status of patients to be categorised on a generic scale, such as that developed by Kind, Rosser and Williams (1982) (see Table 3).

Table 3. Valuation matrix for 70 respondents

Disability rating		Distress rating			
		A No distress	B Mild	C Moderate	D Severe
I	No disability	1.000	0.995	0.990	0.967
II	Slight social disability	0.990	0.986	0.973	0.932
III	Severe social disability and/or slight physical impairment	0.980	0.972	0.956	0.912
IV	Physical ability severely limited (e.g. light housework only)	0.964	0.956	0.942	0.870
V	Unable to take paid employment or education, largely housebound	0.946	0.935	0.900	0.700
VI	Confined to chair or wheelchair	0.875	0.845	0.680	0.000
VII	Confined to bed	0.677	0.564	0.000	-1.486
VIII	Unconscious	-1.028	*	*	*

Source: Kind et al. (1982)

Notes: healthy = 1.0; dead = 0.0; * = not applicable

Trials of drugs in the earlier stages of the disease, such as in people who are merely HIV positive, may use progression to AIDS/ARC as their primary end-point. This is acceptable providing there is no reason to suppose that earlier administration of drugs affects the survival of patients in the later stages of disease. Otherwise the length and quality of survival should also be assessed in these studies.

The relevant range of costs to be considered in an evaluation of drug therapy would include not only the cost of the drugs themselves but also:

- The number of inpatient hospitalizations and the length of stay by category of ward.
- The number of hospital outpatient visits.
- The number and type of laboratory tests, either to assess suitability for drug therapy, or to monitor the effects of therapy.
- The costs of diagnosing and treating opportunistic infections and the side effects of drug therapy.
- The number of blood transfusions, and whether these are performed on an inpatient or outpatient basis.
- The costs of care given outside the hospital by other governmental, private or voluntary agencies.

A key issue in the analysis of these data would be to assess whether drug therapy adds further to costs, through the need for close patient monitoring and blood transfusions, or, alternatively, whether there are savings in the use of health care resources which partly offset the cost of the drug. For example, patients whose health status is being better maintained may require fewer hospitalizations.

Other items that are relevant include the patients' work status and the social security payments received. The latter items are particularly relevant to the government's viewpoint, although therapy in the advanced stages of disease may not affect them very much.

Finally, the study design should pay attention to the need to interpret the results in different settings. This is important since the opportunities to undertake controlled evaluations of drug therapy for AIDS/HIV are likely to be few and many trials are themselves undertaken in a number of centres, often spanning a number of countries. The potential for interpretation and synthesis of economic evidence from a number of locations or settings is the subject of one of the sub-projects of another European Community Concerted Action in the field of health technology assessment (Drummond, 1987). A particularly important point is that resource consumption should be recorded in terms of the physical quantities (e.g. hours of nursing time) as well as the financial amounts. In addition, in health care systems with extensive financial transactions between providers and third party payers, it is important to distinguish between costs and charges (Finkler, 1982).

5. Conclusions

Because interventions for AIDS/HIV consume scarce health service resources, they should be subjected to economic evaluation. Such evaluation will be helpful in searching for more cost-effective strategies and in assigning the appropriate priority to this disease compared to others.

If evaluations are to be carried out it is important that they are methodologically sound. Several features of a good economic evaluation have been specified, including the comparison of alternatives, the assessment of effectiveness through a controlled study, the enumeration of a wide range of costs and consequences, and the appropriate interpretation of study results.

Several studies of the costs of treating AIDS and the related consequences of HIV infection have already been published. Care needs to be exercised in interpreting study results and the key issues in undertaking this task have been identified. A fairly constant pattern appears to emerge from the existing studies. Namely, the cost of caring for a person with AIDS is similar to that of caring for people with other end-stage diseases, such as cancer or chronic renal failure.

Finally the example of drug therapy has been used to illustrate how the key methodological features of economic evaluation can be incorporated into study design. It is recommended that this be done more often in the future.

Acknowledgement. We are grateful to The Wellcome Foundation Ltd for a research grant to study the economic aspects of AIDS. However, we alone are responsible for the views expressed.

References

Andrulis, D.P., Beers, V.S., Bentley, J.D., and Gage, L.S. (1987). The provision and financing of medical care for AIDS patients in US public and private teaching hospitals. The Journal of the American Medical Association 258, 1343-1346.

Black, D.A.K. and Pole, J.D. (1975). Priorities for biomedical research: indices of burden. British Journal of Preventive and Social Medicine 29(4), 222-227.

Cunningham, D. and Griffiths, S.F. (1987). AIDS: counting the cost. British Medical Journal 296, 921-922 (letter to the editor).

Debeaupuis, J. and Tcheriatchoukine, J. (1987). Report on the cost of hospital treatment for AIDS. Inspectorate General of Social Affairs, Paris.

Drummond, M.F. (1987). EC project on the methodology of economic appraisal of health technology. Proposals for concerted action. Health Services Management Centre, Birmingham.

Drummond, M.F. and Davies, L. (1988). Treating AIDS: the economic issues. Health Policy 10, 1-19.

Drummond, M.F., Stoddart, G.L., and Torrance, G.W. (1987). Methods for the economic evaluation of health care programmes. Oxford University Press, Oxford.

Fanning, M.M., Harmon, T., Shepherd, F.A., Vellend, H., and Minnick, S. (1987). Influence of disease and casemix severity on the hospital costs of caring for AIDS patients. III International Conference on AIDS, Washington DC (abstract MP 209).

Finkler, S.A. (1982). The distinction between costs and charges. Annals of Internal Medicine 96, 102-109.

Fischl, M.A., Richman, D.D., Grieco, M.H. et al (1987). The efficacy of azidothymidine (zidovudine) in the treatment of patients with AIDS and AIDS-related complex: a double-blind, placebo-controlled trial. New England Journal of Medicine 317(4), 192-197.

Hardy, A.M., Rauch, K., Echenberg, D., Morgan, W.M., and Curran, J. (1986). The economic impact of the first 10,000 cases of acquired immunodeficiency syndrome in the United States. The Journal of the American Medical Association 255, 209-211.

Hay, J.W., Osmond, D.H., and Jacobson, M.A. (1988). Projecting the future medical costs of AIDS in the United States. IV International Conference on AIDS, Stockholm, June (abstract 9578).

Hellinger, F.J. (1988). Forecasting the personal medical care costs of AIDS from 1988 through 1991. Public Health Reports 103, 309-319.

Hiatt, R.A., Fireman, B., Quesenberry, C.P., and Selby, J.V. (1988). The impact of AIDS on the Kaiser Permanente Medical Care Program (Northern California Region). Paper 4, OTA Series on AIDS-related issues, Office of Technology Assessment, Washington DC.

Johnson, A.M., Adler, M.W., and Crown, J.M. (1986). The acquired immune deficiency syndrome and epidemic of infection with human immunodeficiency virus: costs of care and prevention in an inner London district. British Medical Journal 293, 489-492.

Katz, S. (ed.) (1987). Special issue on measuring the quality of life. Journal of Chronic Diseases 40(6).

Kind, P., Rosser, R.M., and Williams, A. (1982). Valuation of quality of life: some psychometric evidence. In: The value of life and safety (ed. M.W. Jones-Lee). Elsevier/North Holland, Amsterdam.

Kizer, K.W., Rodriguez, J., McHolland, G.F., and Weller, W. (1986). A quantitative analysis of AIDS in California. Department of Health Services, State of California, Sacramento.

Kizer, K.W., Rodriguez, J., and McHolland, G.F. (1987). An updated quantitative analysis of AIDS in California. Department of Health Services, State of California, Sacramento.

Lafferty, W.F., Hopkins, S.G., Honey, J., Harwell, J.D., Shoemaker, P.C., and Kobayashi, J.M. (1988). Hospital charges for people with AIDS in Washington State: utilization of a statewide hospital discharge data base. American Journal of Public Health 78, 949-952.

Pascal, A. (1987). The costs of treating AIDS under Medicaid: 1986-1991. A rand note prepared for the Health Care Financing Administration. US Department of Health and Human Services, Santa Monica.

Rees, M., Hawkins, D.A., Gazzard, B.G., and Roberts, B. (1988). The impact of AIDS/HIV on the activities and costs of St Stephen's Hospital, London. IV International Conference on AIDS, Stockholm, June (abstract 9601).

Scitovsky, A.A., Cline, M., and Lee, P.R. (1986). Medical care costs of patients with AIDS in San Francisco. The Journal of the American Medical Association 256, 3103-3106.

Scitovsky, A.A. and Over, M. (1988). AIDS: costs of care in the developed and developing world. AIDS 2, Suppl. 1, 571-581.

Scitovsky, A.A. and Rice, D.P. (1987). Estimates of the direct and indirect costs of acquired immunodeficiency syndrome in the United States, 1985, 1986 and 1991. Public Health Reports 102(1), 5-17.

Teeling Smith, G. (ed.) (1988). Measuring health; a practical approach. John Wiley and Sons, Chichester.

Walker, S.R. and Rosser, R.M. (eds.) (1988). Quality of life: assessment and application. MTP Press, Lancaster.

Warner, K.E. and Luce, B.R. (1982). Cost-effectiveness and cost-benefit analysis in health care: principles, practice and potential. Health Administration Press, Ann Arbor (Mich.).

Weinstein, M.C. and Stason, W.B. (1977). Foundations of cost-effectiveness analysis in health care. New England Journal of Medicine.

Williams, A.H. (1985). Economics of coronary artery bypass grafting. British Medical Journal 291, 326-329.

Williams, A.H. (1986). Screening for risk of coronary heart disease: is it a wise use of resources? In: Screening for risk of coronary heart disease (eds. M. Oliver, M. Ashley-Miller, and D. Wood). Wiley, London.

Whyte, B.M., Evans, D.B., Shreurs, E.J., and Cooper, D.A. (1987). The costs of hospital-based medical care for patients with the acquired immunodeficiency syndrome. Medical Journal of Australia 147, 269-272.

The Economic Analysis of Prevention of HIV Infection: Evaluation of Programmes and Decision Support for Priority Setting in Health Policy. Case Study. Sweden

M. Lagergren

In the absence of an effective cure or vaccine for AIDS, prevention still stands out as the only way to combat the spread of the epidemic. WHO has developed a Global Programme on AIDS for this purpose, and all countries in Europe are by now engaged in fighting the disease through a range of prophylactic methods.

Possible preventive measures against AIDS include among others:

- Screening of blood and blood products from blood donors
- Organization of information campaigns aimed at behaviour modification in the general public or specifically targeted at persons with risk behaviour
- Provision of testing for HIV antibodies, either voluntary or mandatory and either for special groups or for the general public
- Contact tracing
- Organization of campaigns to encourage the use of condoms, for instance including free supplies
- Supply of clean needles to intravenous drug users

A programme of prevention will have to include several or all of these measures in order to be efficient. In designing the programme it is essential to try to estimate costs as well as effects on the spread of the disease for the different preventive measures. These estimates can then be used as a basis for evaluation of alternative programmes. The concept "costs" should be interpreted in this context in the broadest sense including direct and indirect economic costs as well as political and ethical considerations.

Direct economic costs for preventive measures include e.g. costs for blood screening, advertising campaigns, HIV antibody testing, supply of free condoms etc. These costs are normally easy to estimate. Table 1 shows governmental expenditure on different items for 1987 in Sweden.

As can be seen from Table 1 the 1987 governmental expenditures on prevention in Sweden were far from insignificant. The total amount, 256 million Swedish kronen (MSKr), can be compared to the cost for treatment of HIV/AIDS patients, which in the same year amounted to 57 MSKr. Such a relationship between costs for prevention

Table 1. Costs for HIV prevention. The case of Sweden, 1987

	Total cost (MSKr)	Cost per inh. (SEK)
Testing blood donors	46	6
Other HIV testing	78	9
Information campaigns	40	5
Other costs for prevention (counselling, research, etc.)	92	11
Total	256	31

Source: Brorsson and Herlitz, 1988

and costs for care are almost unique for HIV/AIDS. The general rule in the health services is that expenditures for prevention - albeit difficult to obtain a true estimate - amount to a few percent of the total health care expenditures. The only rational explanation for this discrepancy must be the general belief that successful prevention will save much larger costs in the future.

Even if the economic costs of prevention, as can be seen from Table 1, are quite high they are by no means unsurmountable in a developed country. The situation is very different in developing countries. Even such obvious and relatively cheap preventive measures as the testing of blood donors may in some cases be too expensive to implement.

In developed countries other obstacles rather than pure economic costs obstruct the path for the introduction of preventive measures (Lee and Moss, 1987). These stumbling blocks may be ethical in nature, as e.g. promotion of condom use in countries where moral and religious beliefs run contrary to such practice. HIV prevention policies might come in conflict with other aims of society, e.g. supplying free needles to IV-drug abusers, which carries the risk of promoting drug abuse. Preventive measures could also be opposed on the grounds that they circumscribe individual freedom or infringe on individual rights. Hard-hitting information campaigns carry the risk of raising unnecessary anxiety and fear among the general population with low or non-existent risk of ever catching the disease. On the other hand those who run a real risk may tend to ignore a too soft message. The formulation of efficient, behaviour changing messages is thus a very delicate task.

The benefits of HIV prevention are as a rule much more difficult to assess than the costs. To acquire some kind of quantitave estimation one has to rely upon a mathematical model, that will calculate the effect of different preventive measures in terms of e.g. reduced number of deaths in a specific period of time given certain specified assumptions. The problem is that precise calculations of this kind require data concerning infectivity, rate of contacts and partner change, patterns of relationships between different groups etc, that we do not have and in all probability will never get - at least not in the required detail. Precise cost benefit evaluations of different preventive measures will therefore not be possible to make.

This does not mean, however, that mathematical modelling is useless as a tool for programme evaluation. It only means that we must use the mathematical models in a different way - rather to obtain qualitative insight into the epidemiological process and the ways a preventive measure will interfere in the spread of the disease than to get a precise estimate of the outcome. With this general philosophy in mind we have developed a family of HIV epidemiological computer models at the Karolinska Institute, starting from the simplest situation of one group of subjects and moving gradually into the description of more complex patterns. Using these fairly simple models the effects of different preventive measures can be illustrated and some general conclusions can be drawn. The basic principle behind the epidemic spread of all contagious diseases is that propagation of an epidemic requires that each afflicted person will infect at least one other person. When this holds there will be an epidemic and the epidemic will continue as long as the condition is fulfilled. When it does not, the epidemic will not arise or, if it has already started, will gradually taper down.

This basic concept, the estimated number of persons infected by each infected person, is in the case of HIV transmission in a homogeneous group given by the expression (Andersson and May, 1987)

$$R = C*B*D$$

where C is the number of partners
B the probability of transmission per partner
D the duration time of infectiousness and
R the Basic Reproduction Rate

If R is greater than 1 we will get an epidemic, if it is less than 1 we will not. The magnitude of R will determine the speed of the epidemic spread. If R is near one the spread in a group may take many decades but if it is above, say 5, it will be a matter of years.

In theory, to prevent an epidemic breaking out simply means controlling R so that it stays less than one.

In practice there are many problems to be considered. The population can not be regarded as homogeneous. It consists of a great number of different approximately homogeneous sub-groups which are distinguished with respect to sexual behaviour, partner selection and change rate, presence of cofactors with relevance for infectivity and susceptibility etc. These subgroups are more or less connected to each others by way of partner exchange and in this way the epidemic may spread from group to group.

One way of describing the HIV epidemic is then to describe the incidence and prevalence of HIV infection in the different groups involved and the rate of infection that is carried between the groups. Some general conclusions from modelling the epidemic spread within and between such groups can then be stated. These conclusions all stem from the concept of the basic reproduction rate.

1. In a group where the conditions for an epidemic exist, i.e. $R > 1$, once the epidemic has started it will not end until everyone in the group is infected, or the basic conditions have changed.
2. If the conditions for an epidemic do not exist in a group, i.e. if $R < 1$, the number of infected will only continue to increase as long as infections are brought in from outside the group. When these cease to come, the epidemic in the group will gradually taper off.

This means that if the incidence rate is falling to nearly zero in a group before the saturation level is reached either some behaviour change has occurred in the group, or the group was not properly defined in the first place, i.e. it was not a homogeneous group with regard to partner selection. In the latter case the "real" homogeneous subgroup has become saturated and the infection of the rest of the group will depend on what relations they have with the saturated subgroup. If the conditions for epidemic spread are fulfilled in the remaining subgroup, a small number of contacts with the infected group will be sufficient for the epidemic to continue and gain speed after a time lag of perhaps several years.

When it comes to prevention it is obviously very important to know which one of these alternatives is true. If behaviour has changed in the whole group prevention must be geared at maintaining that good situation. In the other case it becomes paramount to identify the subgroups and direct the preventive efforts towards the non-infected group.

Preventive efforts could have as a goal to

1. Reduce the number of contacts with (potentially) infected partners
2. Reduce the probability of transmission of HIV virus

One of the purposes of HIV testing is to identify the infected individuals so that their behaviour can be modified - voluntarily or by coercion - in order to stop or reduce their contribution to the further spread of the infection.

The question then is: What effect will testing a certain proportion of the population (or groups at risk) have on the development of the epidemic, given that a certain proportion of those tested and found HIV positive will stop spreading the virus?

A computer simulation on a homogeneous group with high-risk behaviour (10 partners/year; risk of infection per partner 0.2) yielded the results shown in Fig. 1. (Lagergren, forthcoming). The chosen effect measure is percentage reduction in the number of persons in the group dead because of AIDS within 20 resp 40 years. As can be seen the death number in 20 years will be reduced by more than 50% if 30% in the group are tested each year and 50% of those found HIV positive stop spreading the disease.

It is important to note that the result will not be as favourable if the period of time is stretched to 40 years. The reason for this is that this preventive measure will not be sufficient to bring the basic reproductive rate below one. The effect will then only be to slow down the spread. The epidemic will be postponed but not inhibited.

One way of reducing the risk of transmission per sexual contact is the use of condoms. The efficacy of condoms has been debated. A very conservative measure derived from studies of unwanted pregnancies is that condoms will reduce the risk for transmission of the HIV virus by a factor of 10 (Hearst and Hultey, 1988). What effect will it then

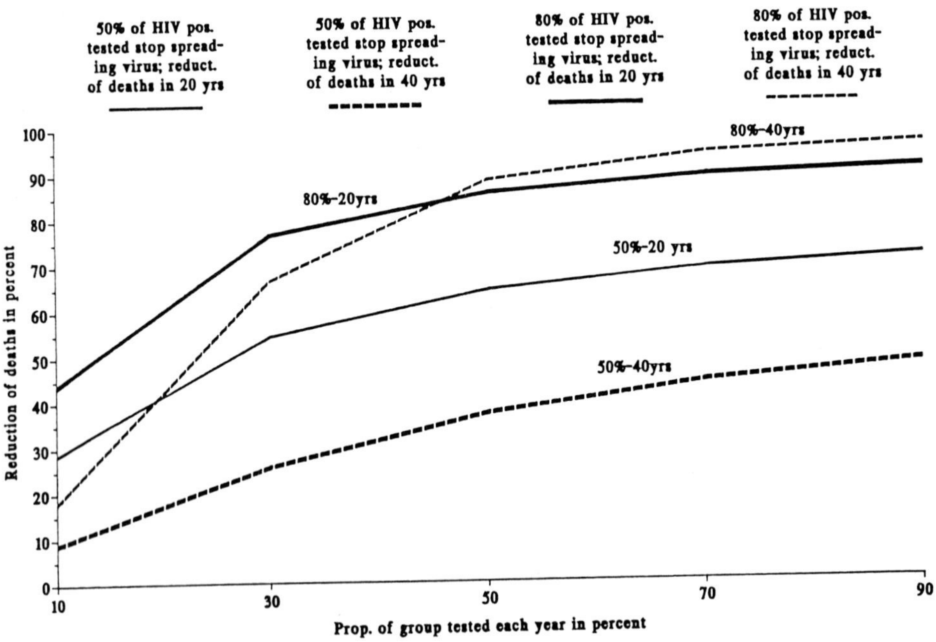

Fig. 1. Reduction of the number of deaths in AIDS by testing and behaviour modifications

have on the spread of the epidemic if a certain percentage of all members of a group use condoms? The result is shown in Table 2 for two different groups: one high risk group with 10 partners per year and one low risk group with 3 partners. Both groups are initially above the critical reproduction rate but the spread of the infection will take a considerable time in the second group. The outcome measure is again the percentage reduction of the number of deaths because of AIDS in 20 resp 40 years.

Another way of describing the effects of condom use is by showing the prevalence of HIV infection as a function of time in the different cases. It will be noted here that even with 75% condom use in the high risk group the epidemic is not brought to a standstill but only postponed. In the low risk group, however, 75% of condom use is sufficient and the prevalence of HIV infection will actually be decreasing over time (see Fig. 2a and Fig. 2b).

Given the basic mechanisms of the epidemic it is important to be able to evaluate the relative effects of barring entrance to a group compared to changing conditions in that same group through different behaviour modifications. In the last figure the HIV prevalence is shown in a certain group as a function of time under four different assumptions.

Alt. A The members of the group have 3 partners per year. Of these 0.1 partners are from a high risk group with a total of 10 partners per year and initial HIV prevalence of 0.001.

Table 2. Reduction of the number of deaths because of AIDS by condom use

Rate of condom use per contact	High risk group (10 partner/year) Perc. reduction of no. of AIDS deaths		Low risk group (3 partner/year) Perc. reduction of no. of AIDS deaths	
	20 yrs	40 yrs	20 yrs	40 yrs
0	0	0	0	0
0.25	61%	23%	25%	57%
0.5	85%	72%	44%	81%
0.75	94%	97%	58%	90%
1	97%	99.7%	68%	95%

Assumed rate of infection/partner

	High risk group	Low risk group
Without condom	0.08	0.16
With condom	0.01	0.03

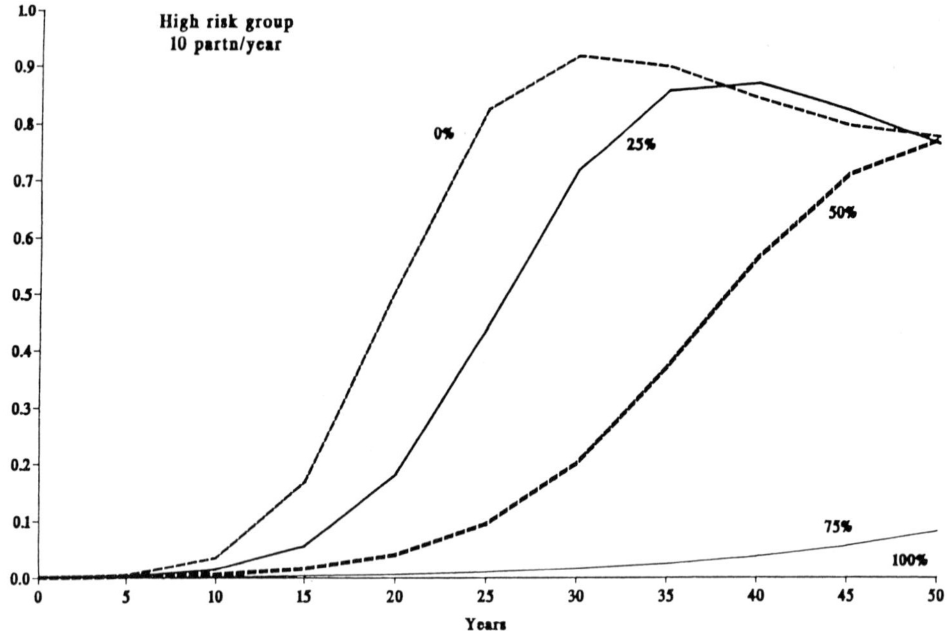

Fig. 2a. HIV prevalence as a function of time depending on rate of condom use

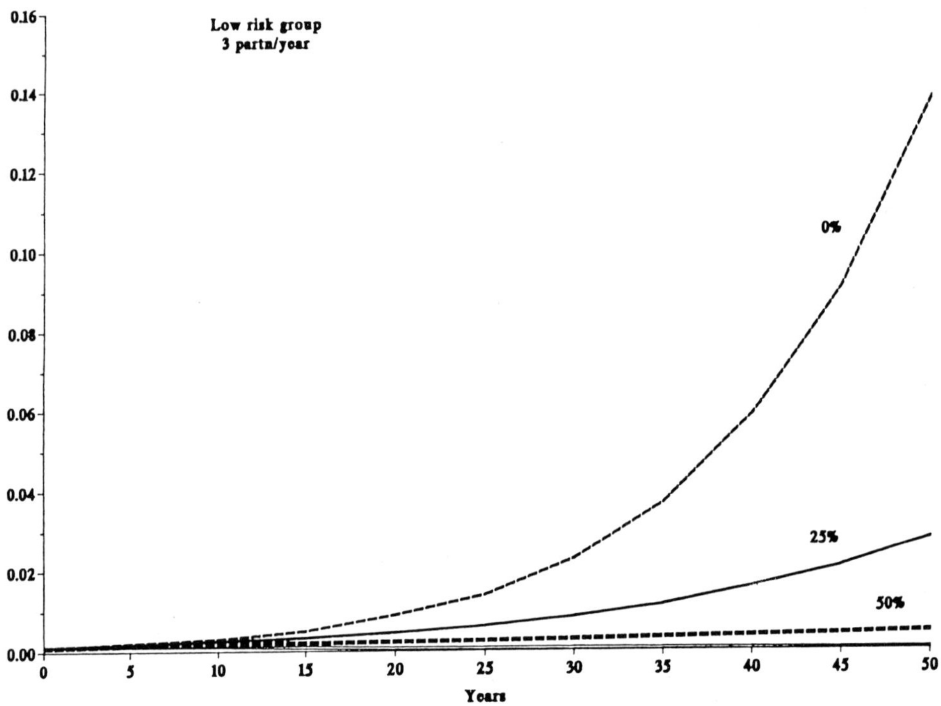

Fig. 2b. HIV prevalence as a function of time depending on rate of condom use

Alt. B As alt. A, but the number of partners from the high risk group is reduced by a factor of 10 to 0.01. The number of partners from the low risk group remains the same.

Alt. C As alt. A, but the number of partners from the low risk group is reduced to 0.9. The number of partners from the high risk group remains the same (meaning that their proportion has increased).

Alt. D As alt. C, but the total number of partners is reduced to 1 per year with the proportion of partners from the high risk group remaining the same.

The difference in outcome between the strategies can clearly be seen as a question of time-perspective. Barring contacts with the high risk group has positive short term effects but if basic conditions for the epidemic spread are unchanged, the epidemic will gather speed in the long run despite narrowing the "channel" between the groups. On the contrary reducing the number of partners within the low risk group shows small advantages in the short run - especially if no corresponding cuts are made in the contacts with the high risk group - but in the long run this strategy still comes out more efficient. Most efficient of course is the fourth alternative with reduction in partner frequency both within and outside the group.

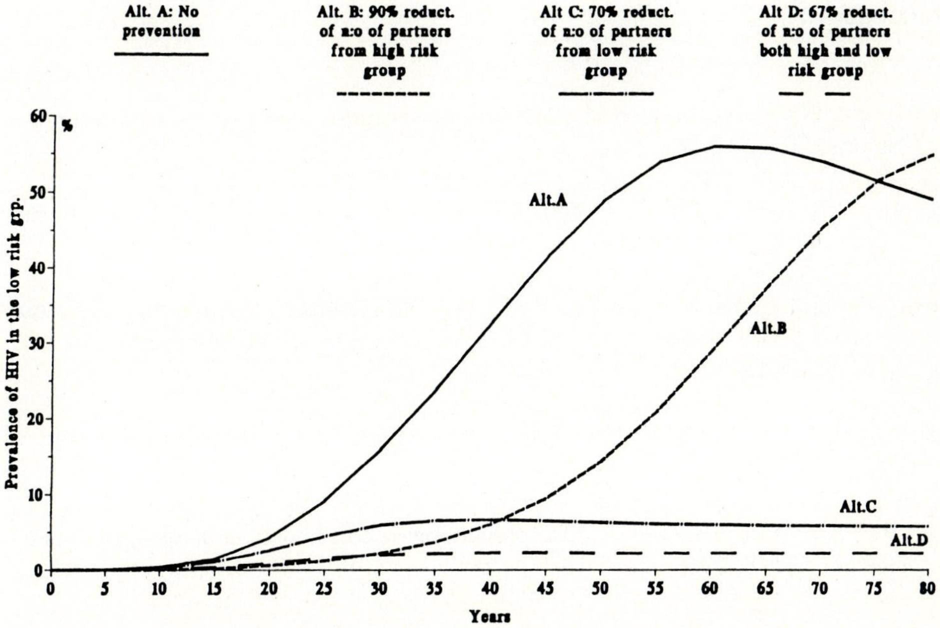

Fig. 3. HIV prevalence of a group as function of time depending on prevention strategy

Some lessons can be learned when it comes to designing preventive strategies from these rather simple computational exercises. Due to the long incubation period the time-constant involved in the development of the epidemic is very long. All measures must be considered in a time perspective which lies outside most of the affairs we handle. Sometimes there might be a conflict depending on which perspective we apply. What seems good in the short run might be devastating in the long run. Since the spread in the population goes through a number of subgroups or strata it becomes important to try to define these groups and direct the prevention efforts towards them. General surveys of sexual behaviour seem less to the point in this case than selective investigations directed toward different groups that are especially at risk.

The risk for a general spread of the epidemic in the total heterosexual population seems at present low since the conditions for epidemic spread do not seem to be met. The preventive effort must then be directed towards halting the spread within groups at high risk and reducing as much as possible the accidental infections that these groups might spread out to other groups. These efforts justify quite substantial expenditures. The problem is to maintain these efforts in the long run when the public arousal triggered by the first appearance of the epidemic has subsided.

References

Andersson, R.M. and May, R.M. (1987). Transmission dynamics of HIV infection. Nature 326, 137-142.

Brorsson, B. and Herlitz, C. (1988). The AIDS-epidemic and costs for the health services (in Swedish). DFR report 1988:1, Dalarnas Forksningsråd, Borlänge.

Hearst, N. and Hultey, S.B. (1988). Preventing the heterosexual spread of AIDS. Are we giving our patients the best advice? Journal of the American Medical Association 259, 2428-2432.

Lagergren, M. (to be published). A systems dynamic model for analyzing the spread of HIV.

Lee, P.R. and Moss A.R. (1987). AIDS prevention: Is cost-benefit analysis appropriate? Health Policy 8, 196-198.

The Cost of AIDS and HIV Infection: Public Expenditures for AIDS Prevention in the Federal Republic of Germany

A. Jenke, A.-M. Reinkemeier

1. Introduction

Since 1985 the analysis of the economic impact of the AIDS epidemic has been increasing in importance. One aim of this research is to provide an estimate of the financial effects of AIDS as early as possible. Existing studies assess mainly the costs for treatment of AIDS patients in different health care settings (Drummond and Davies, 1989).

Currently, we have neither an effective vaccine against the HIV infection nor an effective treatment for AIDS in its different stages. To delay the advance of the HIV epidemic, preventive measures are of central importance. The costs of preventive measures must therefore be included in the analysis of the socioeconomic aspects of AIDS. To meet this objective, the Institute for Health Systems Research conducted a study to evaluate the various measures for AIDS prevention in the Federal Republic of Germany and estimate the costs incurred by various institutions during 1987. The research was sponsored by the Federal Ministry of Health.

2. AIDS prevention measures

To carry out this research, the current AIDS prevention measures were divided into three categories. The first category comprises common information about the infection. Special counselling and educational work is offered to specific risk groups, HIV positive persons and their relatives. A HIV antibody test is also provided free of charge. Most information and counselling are offered by state and local health offices, voluntary non-profit organisations, health care associations and self-help groups. The work of these institutions is largely financed by federal and state governments.

The second category consists of additional hygienic measures taken within health care institutions to protect staff and patients. Hygienic measures for the police, penal institutions and certain parts of the services sector have also to be taken into account. The third category comprises research aimed at developing a vaccine, improving treatment or prevention and establishing meaningful figures on the AIDS epidemic.

Some of the government measures against AIDS induce private expenditures. One example of private expenditure to prevent AIDS is the requirement that all motor vehicles be equipped with safety gloves. Since there are no data on the yearly consumption of safety gloves, no estimate of costs was made. Another example is the increase in expenditure associated with the use of condoms. These are not easily apparent and cannot be attributed solely to AIDS prevention.

3. Methods

First, we identified the institutions engaged in AIDS prevention in the Federal Republic of Germany. Secondly, a survey was conducted among persons responsible for AIDS prevention measures to inquire into their relevant expenditures in 1987.

The survey results provide an estimate of the cost of AIDS prevention from an institutional viewpoint (Leidl, 1988). The measures were estimated according to the expenditure data submitted by the various institutions. The survey was carried out between March 1st and October 30th 1988.

A complete enquiry of all federal and state administrations involved, health insurance funds, welfare organisations, professional groups and other health care associations was carried through. 42 out of 48 institutions adressed replied. To assess the expenditures of local governments, a short questionnaire was sent to 46 municipalities and 50 county administrations. Answers that could be evaluated were returned by 37 county administrations and 34 municipalities. To gain insight into the costs of AIDS prevention in the hospital sector, 11 hospital administrators and physicians who have experience in treating of AIDS patients were interviewed. In addition, 24 universities with medical faculties were questioned. To assess the expenditure on AIDS research, the universities were also asked to include AIDS related research in non-medical faculties. 23 universities answered.

Most AIDS prevention measures are financed in part by federal or state subsidies. The amount of these subsidies was established to prevent double counting when federal and state funds were added. This means that those expenditures mentioned in the following are always from the institutions' own funds. The quality of the data is varied. The information given by the regional administrative bodies can be expressed in figures and is comparable to a large extent. Health insurance funds, welfare organisations and some of the universities sent a mainly verbal description of their activities. The federal expenditures for some sectors could not be extrapolated. If not otherwise mentioned, the following details refer to 1987. The results presented are a conservative estimate of the public costs of AIDS prevention in the Federal Republic of Germany.

4. Results

The first section includes expenditure for the production and dissemination of information, counselling and financial support of AIDS education centres. Fig. 1 shows the financing institutions and their expenditure. A total of 118.4 million DM was spent on AIDS information, education and assistance. About 63% of these funds came from the Ministry of Health. 43 million DM were spent on the information campaign by the Federal Centre of Health Education. In the same year, the states spent 30.5 million DM, or 25.5% of all AIDS related expenditure for information and counselling on AIDS.
Approximately 9 million DM, or 7.6% of the expenditure for information and personal counselling, was spent by the municipal governments. Half of the expenditure arises in towns with more than 500,000 inhabitants. Most of the towns' resources for AIDS

Institution	Issue	Expenditure in Mio. DM	Percentages
Ministry of Health	Financial support of counselling centres	30.9	
	Information campaign by the Federal Centre of Health Education	43.5	
States	Financial support of counselling centres, Information	30.2	
Municipalities	Personal counselling	9.0	
Voluntary non-profit organisations	Personal counselling, Information	4.6	
Ministry of Defence	Information	0.2	
Total		118.4	100 %

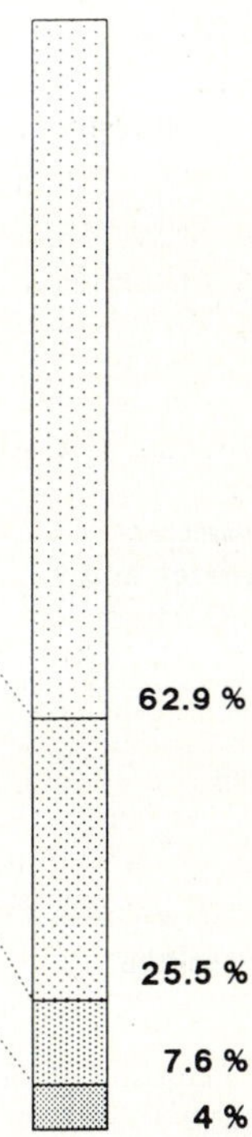

Fig. 1. AIDS prevention 1987, expenditure on information, counselling, financial support of counselling centres

prevention measures were raised by local public health agencies and by social welfare agencies. Expenditures for the municipalities resulted from:

- HIV tests, precautionary measures, information
- Subsidies for local AIDS education centres
- Equipment for local AIDS education centres.

The second sector includes expenditure for AIDS research. Fig. 2 shows the financing institutions and the money spent in 1987. A total of 33 million DM was calculated for research work. The largest amount was support given for research in medical science and epidemiological studies. The Ministry of Health and the Ministry of Research and Technology funded most of this research. No evaluation could be made of the expenditure in private industry and private research. Thus total expenditure on research in AIDS exceeds the amount calculated here.

Institution	Issue	Expenditure in Mio. DM
Ministry of Health	Federal Health Office research programs	15.0
	Evaluation of counselling programs and the national information campaign	6.5
Ministry of Research and Technology	Research funding (life sciences)	8.0
Berlin	Local research funding	2.2
Universities	Research projects not funded by other authorities	1.3
Total		33.0

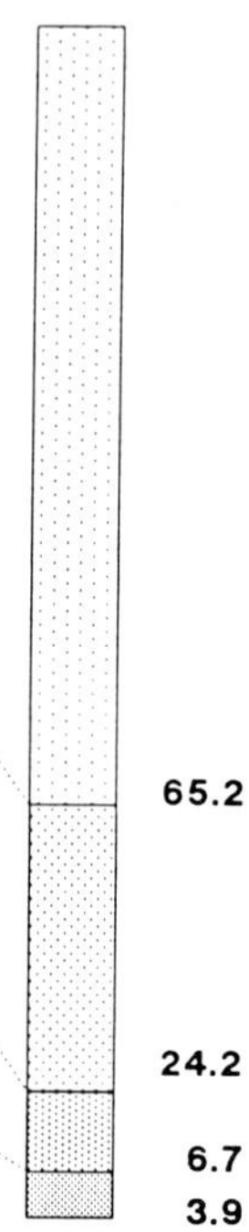

Fig. 2. AIDS prevention 1987, public expenditure on research and development

Hygienic safety measures are the third sector which showed high expenditure. Figures are available for safety measures in emergency services and precautions with donated blood. To protect staff, emergency services need safety gloves and additional artificial respiration devices. Expenditure of approximately 1.1 million DM for the Federal Republic of Germany was extrapolated from the figures given by Schleswig-Holstein. Expenditure that results from screening measures for blood products can be determined without great difficulty. A screening method capable of excluding all contaminated blood has been in use in all blood donation centres since 1985. The blood donation service of the German Red Cross in Hamburg and Schleswig-Holstein indicates additional costs of 3.89 DM for each blood sample. Assuming for 1987 a demand of 3.5 million units for blood samples or other blood products (Beske and Hanpft, 1986), a total expenditure of 13.6 million DM was estimated.

We also evaluated reports of other expenditure from two federal ministries which do not fit in any of our categories. The Federal Ministry for Labour and Social Affairs distributed 4 million DM in support to institutions providing care to AIDS patients. The same amount was spent by the Ministry for Economic Cooperation in supporting long-term prevention programmes in developing countries.

If all expenditure mentioned above is counted as for preventive measures, it amounts to 174.1 million DM. The expenditure is shown in Table 1 for the main areas of AIDS prevention and the financing institutions.

In a further step, we tried to evaluate the expenditure on hygienic safety measures in physicians' and dentists' offices and in hospitals. Three kinds of safety measures were included:

- Additional mechanical barriers to prevent contacts with blood and other bodily fluids
- Disinfection measures
- Longer set-up time for endoscopes.

Here only a slight expenditure increase was attributable to AIDS. This is due to the already high standard of hygienic safety measures in all sectors of health care. Hygienic safety measures as a precaution against various infectious diseases do not differ greatly (Flatten and Allhoff, 1988; Greenspan et al., 1986).

A marked difference in expenditure was reported from hospitals. Here expenditure depends on the estimated number of AIDS patients. No influence was reported by hospitals that have less than 10 AIDS patients per year. If a hospital has 10 to 250 AIDS patients per year, an increase of 0.10 to 2.00 DM per day of care for material expenditure can be assumed. This was calculated with the help of a model.

Table 1. AIDS prevention 1987, estimated total public expenditure in million DM

Issue	Institution	Expenditure	Remarks
I Research and development	Ministry of Health	15.0	Research projects funded by the Federal Health Office
		2.7*	Evaluation of new prevention programmes
		3.8*	Evaluation of the information campaign of the Federal Centre for Health Education
	Senate of Berlin	2.2	Local research funding
	Universities	1.3	Research not funded by other authorities
	Ministry of Research and Technology	8.0	Research funding
	I	33.0	
II Information, counselling work HIV testing, financial support of counselling centres and self help groups	Ministry of Health	30.9	New prevention and counselling programmes
		43.5	Information campaign by the Federal Centre for Health Education
	Federal States	30.2	
	Municipalities	9.0	
	Ministry of Defence	0.2	Counselling and HIV testing within the army
	Associations in the health care sector	4.6	
	II	118.4	
III Hygienic safety measures in the emergency services and blood donor centres	III	14.7	Safety gloves, special precautionary measures, screening of blood donors
IV Other expenditures	Ministry for Labour and Social Affairs	4.0	Financial support to institutions providing care to AIDS patients
	Ministry for Economic Cooperation and Development	4.0	Prevention programmes in developing countries
	IV	8.0	
Total sum		174.0	

* 8% of the total amount, examination based on information given by the Federal Ministry of Health

The expenditures for AIDS prevention evaluated in this study were mainly those of federal, state or municipal administrations. With the exception of the municipalities, the expenditures planned for 1988 were also reported. These are compared in Fig. 3.

The total federal and state expenditure for AIDS prevention measures in 1987 amounted to approximately 153.5 million DM. The expenditure increased to 272 million DM in 1988, towns excluded. As in 1987, the largest portion, or 132 million DM, was financed by the Federal Ministry of Health.

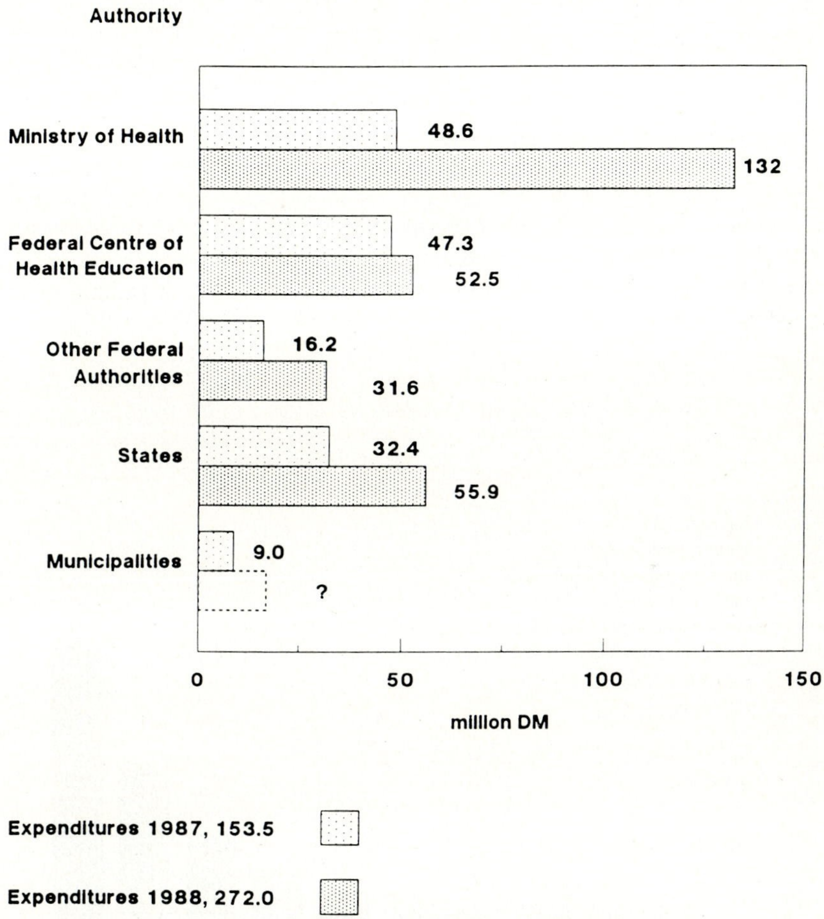

Fig. 3. AIDS prevention 1987-1988: expenditures of public authorities in the Federal Republic of Germany in million DM

5. Discussion

In contrast to studies on the costs of the treatment of AIDS patients, a comparison of the expenditures for AIDS prevention measures lacks a defined reference figure. It is only possible to compare the expenditure per capita for certain regions. Differences in the regional expenditure per capita may be seen as differences in the regional counselling and information work.

A regional categorisation was possible for the expenditure of the state governments. The comparison included expenditure for information and counselling only. There were great differences in 1987 as to the regional per capita expenditure between the various states. In Hesse, the expenditure on information and counselling about AIDS was 920 DM per 10,000 inhabitants; Hamburg spent 15,000 DM and Berlin 26,000 DM per 10,000 inhabitants. The differences can be partly explained by the different prevalence of AIDS in these cities.

For further research on the effects of AIDS prevention measures it would be interesting to compare regional differences in expenditures with the changing incidence of the HIV. At present, no figures are available for such comparisons in the Federal Republic of Germany.

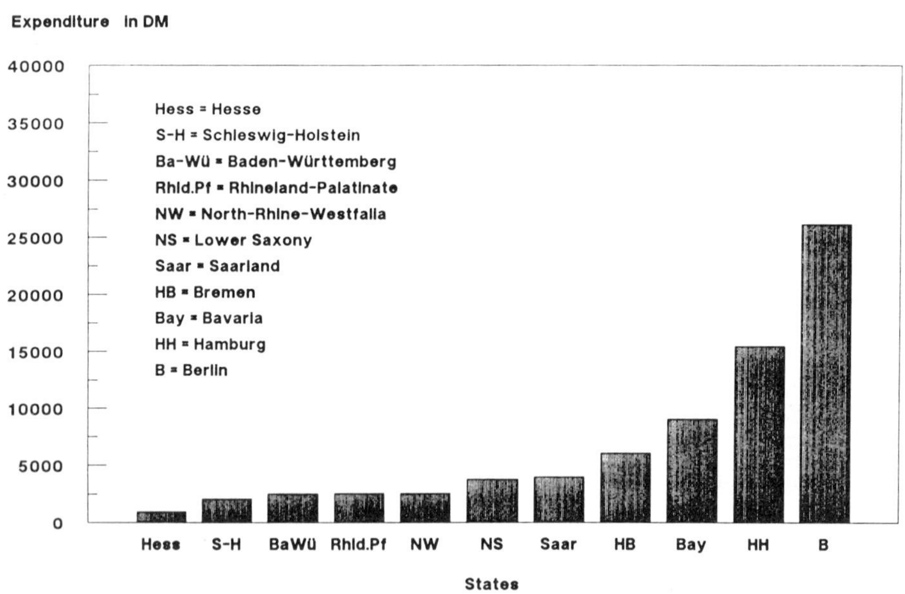

Fig. 4. States' expenditure for AIDS prevention in 1987 per 10,000 inhabitants

References

Drummond, M. F. and Davies, L. (1989). Treating AIDS: the economic issues. Health Policy 10, 1-19.

Leidl, R. (1988). Ökonomische Aspekte (XI-3). In: AIDS und HIV-Infektionen; Diagnostik, Klinik und Praxis (ed. H.Jäger). Ecomed, Landsberg a.L.

Beske, F. and Hanpft, R. (1986). Gesundheitsökonomische Aspekte zum erworbenen Immundefektsyndrom (AIDS). I. Blutspendewesen. Schmidt & Klaunig, Kiel.

Flatten, G. and Allhof, P.G. (1988). AIDS als Problem in der kassenärztlichen Versorgung. Deutscher Ärzte Verlag, Köln.

Greenspan, D., Greenspan, J. S., Pindborg J. J., and Schiodt. M. (1986). AIDS and the dental team. Munksgard, Kopenhagen.

The Costs of Hospital Care of AIDS Patients at the Teaching Hospital of the University of Amsterdam

P.R.E. Bijlsma

1. Introduction

The acquired immune deficiency syndrome (AIDS) is a relatively new infectious disease, transmitted mainly through blood and sexual contact, which first appeared in the US in 1980 and in Western Europe a few years later.

In the Netherlands there were 450 AIDS cases known by spring 1988. Approximately 60% of these were treated at the teaching hospital of the university of Amsterdam (AZUA/AMC), while the rest were treated in different hospitals in the country. The AZUA/AMC hospital was designated as the national "super-centre" hospital for AIDS. This means that, in addition to the care and treatment of patients, the hospital also has the responsibility for researching into new methods of treatment and for giving information about the implications for hospital management of caring for AIDS patients.

Of the 450 known AIDS patients 95% are homosexual men, while the remaining 5% are IV-drug users, haemophiliacs and people who had received a blood transfusion with infected blood.

Research on the costs of care of AIDS patients has been mainly carried out in the US. There are large differences in the results of individual research projects. In the Netherlands it was totally unknown until now what the costs of care of AIDS patients amounted to.

In this article are presented the first results of a research project which aims to give an insight into the costs of hospital care of AIDS patients and to determine the factors which influence these costs. This article gives an orientation into the size and components of the costs of hospital care of AIDS patients in the AZUA/AMC hospital between 1982 and spring 1988.

2. Data and methodology

2.1 The data

In order to gain an insight into the illness and treatment process, a database was developed based on individual patient information. This database consists of all the individual data of all 230 patients who were treated between 1982 and spring 1988 for AIDS, ARC and HIV^+ with opportunistic infections at the AZUA/AMC hospital. The data were taken out of different parts of the hospital information system (ZIS) and from medical and nursing records. In order to take into account the privacy aspects, the data were made completely anonymous. An extensive analysis by the AIDS unit under the supervision of Dr. S. Danner showed that the database contained approximately 95% of all treatment data.

The following patient information was collected:

- Personal data: sex, date of birth, place of domicile.
- Characteristics of illness: date and description of main and secondary diagnoses (ICD9 and CDC).
- Characteristics of treatment: date and description of hospitalization, nursing days, interventions, blood transfusions, use of Retrovir and other medication.

Because the data about consultations, Retrovir and other medication, and external laboratory tests were not available per patient in computerized form, an estimate was made from a sample of the records of twenty patients.

For the calculation of hospital costs, national sickness fund tariffs were used. For the calculation of the costs of Retrovir, other medication and external laboratory tests, the actual cost prices were used.

2.2 Methodology

In a survey article Drummond and Davies (1988) give some possible reasons for the large differences between the results of research done up to now on the costs of hospital care of AIDS patients. Especially differences in methodology and in the composition of the patient population appear to have had a large influence on the results found. Because of this we divided the total population of patients into four groups:

<u>Subgroup I:</u> Patients who have already died and who had already received treatment at the AZUA/AMC hospital before AIDS was diagnosed (n=105);
<u>Subgroup II:</u> Patients who have already died and who received no treatment at the AZUA/AMC hospital before AIDS was diagnosed (n=44);
<u>Subgroup III:</u> Living patients who had treatment at the AZUA/AMC hospital before AIDS was diagnosed (n=58);

Subgroup IV: Living patients, who had had no treatment at the AZUA/AMC hospital before AIDS was diagnosed (n=23).

The costs are directly dependent on the medical treatment which patients receive. The way patients are treated is closely linked to the progression of the disease. The progression of the disease and corresponding treatment are in turn influenced by the characteristics of the patient, the treatment protocol and a large number of other factors. These inderdependent relationships are shown in Fig. 1.

A preliminary exploration was done with the help of the Kruskall-Wallis test in order to test the possible relationship between the kind of treatment of patients received on the one hand and the age at which patients first made contact with the AZVA/AMC hospital, the possible use of Retrovir, the main diagnosis at first contact with the hospital, the year in which treatment started and finally a subdivision of the AIDS diagnosis into CDC categories on the other.

3. Results

3.1 Some characteristics of hospital care

In Table 1 are shown some characteristics of the treatment of all 230 patients treated at the AZUA/AMC in the period from 1982 till spring 1988. From Table 1 it appears that

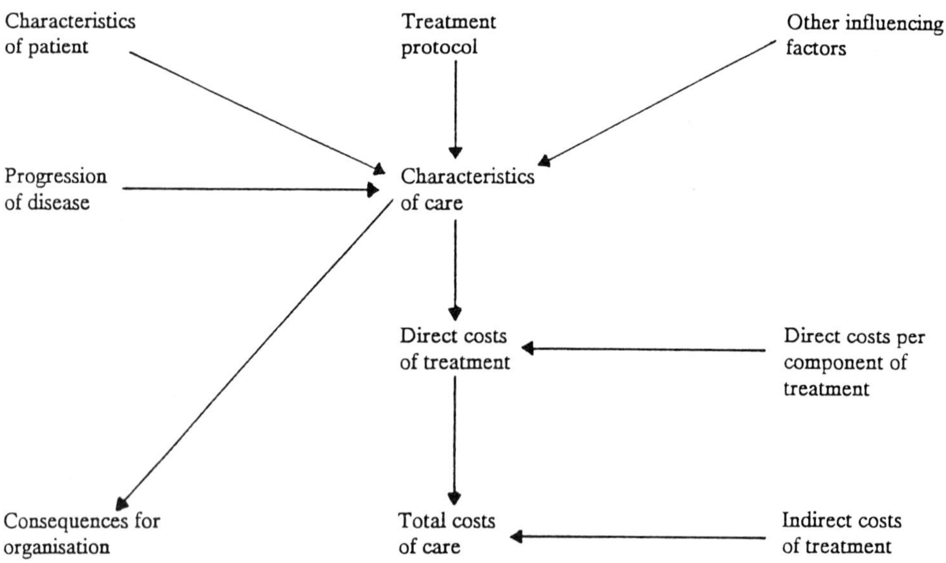

Fig. 1. Characteristics of care and the relationship with treatment costs and consequences for hospital organization

all the characteristics of treatment show a large variation. Minimum and maximum lie far apart. This is not due to outliers, as can be seen from the fact that the standard deviation is relatively large in proportion to the mean. The median (the value above and below which 50% of observations lie) lies below the mean for all characteristics. This means that the frequency distribution of the characteristics is positively skew. Most patients score lower than average on the various characteristics of treatment, while a small proportion score much higher than average.

Table 1. Some characteristics of hospital care (total population: n = 230)

	Average	Median	Minimum	Maximum	Standard deviation
Total length of care at AZUA/AMC hospital (in days)	526.0	374.0	1	2162	491.0
Number of hospitalizations	3.1	2.0	1	22	2.9
Number of nursing days	60.0	41.0	1	507	66.0
- Of which number of days in intensive care, resuscitation and isolation	9.0	0.0	1	375	39.8
Number of nursing days per hospitalization	23.6	14.6	1	375	36.1
Number of doses of blood (total)	9.0	3.0	1	134	17.4
Total number of tests/interventions	209.0	123.0	2	1601	267.0
- Of which:					
Laboratory test	182.0	102.0	2	1480	247.0
X-ray	8.5	6.0	1	96	10.2
In-patient interventions	164.0	75.0	2	1579	268.0
Out-patient interventions	45.0	34.0	1	477	48.0

Fig. 2 gives the frequency distribution of the number of nursing days. Another source of variation is due to the fact that some characteristics, such as the number of hospitalizations and nursing days, laboratory tests and X-ray examinations, are to be found for almost all patients, while other characteristics, such as blood transfusions and nursing days in special units (intensive care, resuscitation and isolation), are only to be found for a minority.

Table 2 shows some characteristics of treatment given for the four subgroups of the total population. There appear to be some large differences between the separate subgroups. The living patients (subgroups III and IV) appear to be under treatment for a much longer period on average than the patients who have already died. The patients who were already undergoing treatment at the AZUA/AMC hospital before AIDS was diagnosed (subgroups I and II) also show on average, as one might expect, a longer period of treatment than the others. Differences between the subgroups with respect to the average number of hospitalizations are not markedly large.

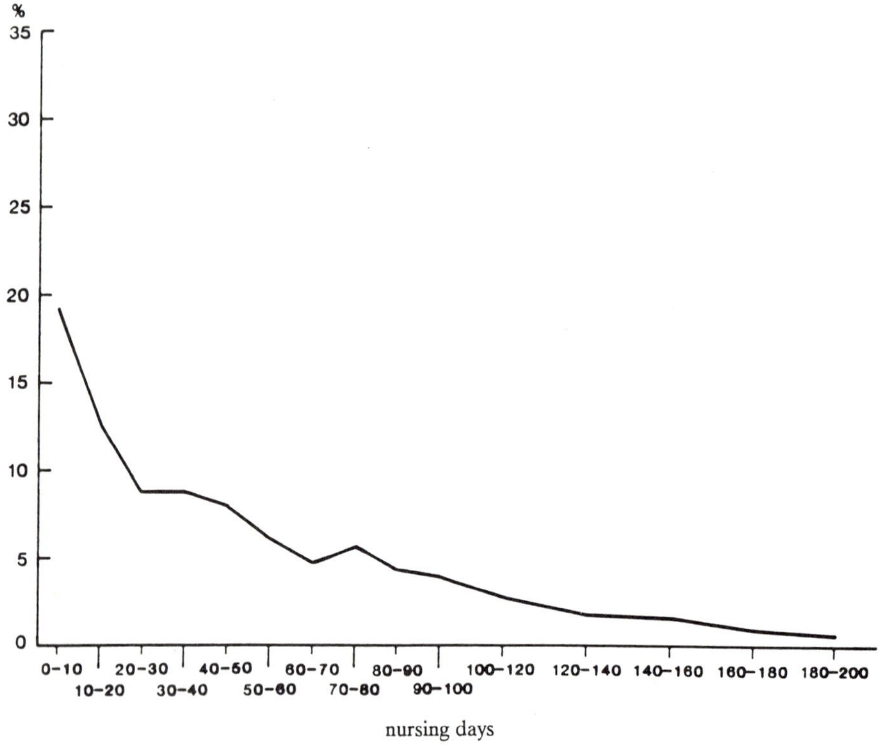

Fig. 2. Frequency distribution of the number of nursing days. Total population (n = 230)

Table 2. Some characteristics of hospital care per subgroup (AZUA/AMC hospital)

	Mean	Median	Minimum	Maximum	Standard deviation
Number of days in care from first contact with hospital					
Subgroup I	533.0	344.0	6	2162	486.0
Subgroup II	196.0	152.0	1	1048	205.0
Subgroup III	826.0	635.0	1	2121	549.0
Subgroup IV	363.0	419.0	1	715	218.0
Number of hospitalizations					
Subgroup I	3.4	3.0	1	22	3.2
Subgroup II	2.5	2.0	1	15	2.6
Subgroup III	2.9	2.0	1	10	2.7
Subgroup IV	3.1	3.0	1	10	2.9
Number of nursing days					
Subgroup I	84.0	64.0	1	507	80.0
Subgroup II	42.0	34.0	4	155	37.0
Subgroup III	36.0	25.0	2	132	36.0
Subgroup IV	43.0	13.0	1	203	57.0
Number of nursing days per hospitalization					
Subgroup I	34.7	19.0	1	375	48.6
Subgroup II	18.3	15.5	4	59	14.8
Subgroup III	12.0	9.9	2	64	12.8
Subgroup IV	12.5	6.3	1	102	21.2
Number of doses of blood					
Subgroup I	11.3	3.0	1	134	21.8
Subgroup II	8.9	3.0	2	82	15.8
Subgroup III	6.2	0.0	1	42	9.9
Subgroup IV	6.4	2.0	2	36	10.3
Number of test/interventions					
Subgroup I	295.0	173.0	23	1601	322.0
Subgroup II	214.0	138.0	3	1308	274.0
Subgroup III	93.0	74.0	2	276	63.0
Subgroup IV	101.0	88.0	6	328	91.0

The situation is different for the number of nursing days: the average for patients who came to the AZUA/AMC hospital after the diagnosis AIDS (subgroups II and III) lies slightly below that of other patients. There is furthermore a visible difference between the two groups who were treated at the AZUA/AMC hospital before AIDS was diagnosed: the patients who have already died (subgroup I) had on average twice as many nursing days as the patients who are still alive (subgroup III). The number of interventions is two to three times higher for the patients who have died (subgroups I and II) than for the others.

Fig. 3 shows the frequency distribution of the number of nursing days for the four separate subgroups. It can be observed on Fig. 3 that the frequency distribution is less positively skew for the patients who have already died (subgroups I and II) than for the others.

For the patients with the most extensive treatment at the AZUA/AMC hospital (subgroup I) a further investigation was done in order to discover whether there were possible relevant factors which might be linked to the number of nursing days and a number of interventions. These factors are:

- The age of the patient at first contact with the hospital.
- The possible use of Retrovir.
- The main diagnosis according to ICD9.
- The subdivision of the AIDS diagnosis into CDC categories.
- The year in which treatment started.

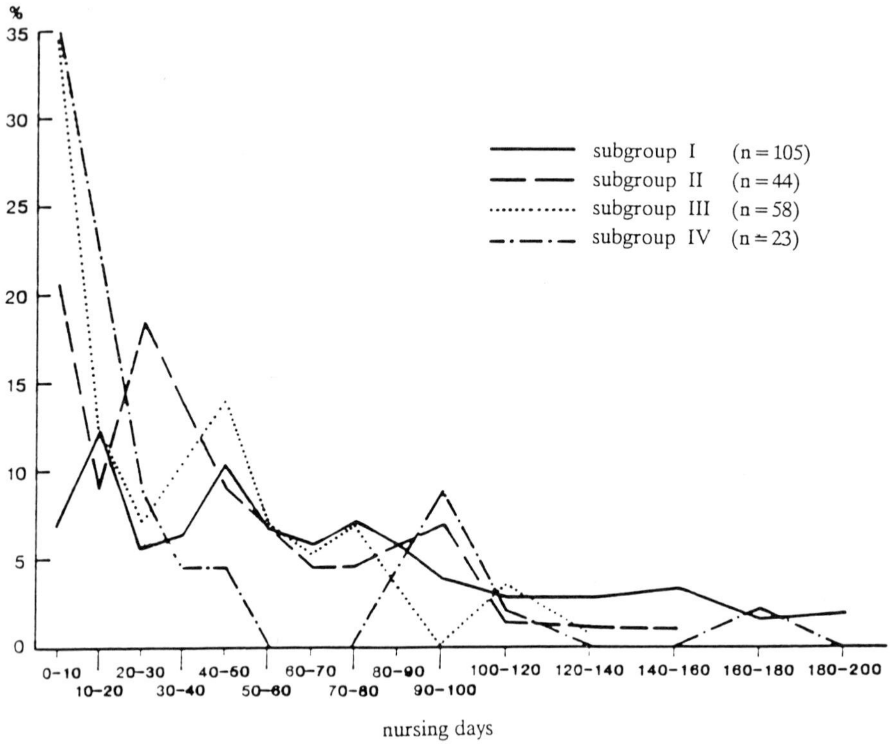

Fig. 3. Frequency distribution of the number of nursing days per subgroup

This investigations led to the following results:

- With respect to the age at which first contact with the hospital was made:
  - patients up to the age of thirty had the greatest number of hospitalizations per patient, followed by those of the age group 31-40 years; patients in the 41-50 years age group had the least number of hospitalizations per patient, while patients in the age group 50^+ fell somewhere in between;
  - patients in the 50^+ age group had the greatest number of nursing days per patient while the patients below the age of thirty had the smallest;
  - the same pattern was observed for the number of interventions: the patients from the age group 50^+ had the highest number of interventions per patient, the patients below the age of thirty had the smallest.

- With respect to the use of Retrovir:
  - the number of hospitalizations of patients who were given Retrovir is clearly greater per patient than for the other patients;
  - this also holds for the number of nursing days per patient;
  - the number of interventions per patient was clearly lower, however, for patients who had received Retrovir than for the others.

- With respect to the main diagnosis at the first hospitalization: (the main diagnoses have been subdivided into the following five categories: AIDS (pneumocystosis), AIDS (kaposi), AIDS (other), ARC, and "other diagnoses")
  - the number of hospitalizations per patient was the lowest for AIDS (kaposi) and "other diagnoses". The diagnoses AIDS (other) and ARC give the highest number of hospitalizations per patient;
  - AIDS (other) and ARC have the longest treatment period per patient, while AIDS (kaposi) the shortest;
  - the number of interventions per patient is the greatest for ARC patients, but the lowest for AIDS (pneumocystosis).

- With respect to the CDC classification: (this classification is only known for patients receiving Retrovir)
  - the number of hospitalizations per patient was the highest for the category IV-CI, D (opportunistic infections and secondary malignancies), followed by the category IV-CI (opportunistic infections); the number of hospitalizations per patient was the lowest for the patients who received no Retrovir and hence were not included in a CDC category;
  - the category IV-CI, D had the greatest number of nursing days per patient, while the patients who received no Retrovir had the lowest;
  - the number of interventions per patient was highest for the category IV-CI, D and lowest for the category IV-CI and for the other patients receiving Retrovir.

- With respect to the year in which hospital treatment was started (because this is a relatively new disease for which no effective treatment has yet been found, the treatment protocol is constantly being adjusted on the grounds of new experience):
  - the number of hospitalizations per patient appears to be clearly lower in 1987 and 1988 than in the previous years.
  - the number of nursing days per patient shows a falling trend since 1984.
  - the number of interventions per patient shows no clear pattern, except that they tend to be lower in 1987 and 1988 than in previous years.

3.2 The hospital costs

Table 3 shows the results of the calculations made for different categories of hospital costs. These costs have been calculated for the whole patient population and for subgroup I, in the group of patients who had the most complete life-time treatment at the AZUA/AMC hospital.

Table 3 shows that the average hospital costs per AIDS patient amount to Fl. 68,000 (in 1988 prices), while the life-time costs of subgroup I are Fl. 90,000 per patient, a difference of more than Fl. 20,000.

4. Discussion

The care of AIDS patients at the AZUA/AMC hospital shows large individual variation. The frequency distribution of the various characteristics of treatment shows that it is

Table 3. The average medical costs (in Fl.) of hospital care per patient at the AZUA/AMC hospital (1988 prices)

Categories of costs	Total population (n = 230)		Subgroup I (n=105)	
	Subtotal	Total	Subtotal	Total
Nursing days		44,400		64,300
Laboratory tests	2,200		3,000	
X-ray	1,000		1,400	
Other tests/interventions	3,000		3,900	
Total tests/interventions		6,200		8,200
Blood transfusions		700		800
Retrovir (in-patient)		8,000		6,200
In-patient consultations	500		600	
Out-patient consultations	800		800	
Total consultations		1,300		1,400
External laboratory tests		2,800		2,800
In-patient medication		4,600		6,300
Total costs		68,000		90,000

not advisable to work with total averages as such as representative of the treatment procedure. The subdivision into more homogeneous groups helps to overcome some of these problems.

Furthermore another remark should be made at this point. Approximately 80% of the patients whose hospital treatment started before and up to 1986 have now died. For the patients who first received treatment in 1987, the figure is almost 50%, while it is 30% for those who first received treatment in 1988. This means that for the patients who are still alive, only part of the treatment has been included in the calculations. The patients whose treatment started in more recent years and who have died are those patients with a relatively short survival time.

The costs per patient which have been calculated for those patients whose treatment started recently are therefore an underestimate of the costs which will arise in the future until the whole cohort has died. This problem is even more significant because the proportion of patients whose treatment has recently started is relatively higher because of the recent fast growth in the patient population.

We have been able to establish that the five factors which we examined were all linked to the characteristics of treatment. Not in all cases, however, is there a clear proportional relationship to be established. A further analysis which takes into account the possible interrelationships between these five and other factors is therefore desirable.

In this study an indication of the hospital costs has been given by means of sickness fund tariffs. It would have been better to have used real costs. However, the data required for these calculations do not exist. This would also have entailed a detailed time check of the number of working hours spent on each activity and an insight into the special prevention measures taken against the risk of infection of AIDS inside the hospital.

For this reason tariffs had to be used in this study. These are based on the "average" care of the "average" patient in the hospital. The care of AIDS patients, however, is much more intensive than that of the "average" patient. The number of nursing staff per bed, for example, is twice as high in the AIDS wards as the number found in an "average" ward.

That the care of AIDS patients is more intensive than the care of average patients is not only to be seen in the special AIDS units, but also in the supporting units. Because the activities carried out on AIDS patients are also more intensive there, one can speak of a loss of production capacity. This means that the costs calculated by means of tariffs will be an underestimate of the true costs. How large this underestimate is will have to be established in further research.

The results presented here give an indication of the size and components of the costs of hospital care at the AZUA/AMC hospital between 1982 and spring 1988. Because treatment has only just begun for the majority of patients who have recently been admitted to the hospital for the first time, the results found cannot be interpreted as a correct estimate of the costs of hospital care for an average AIDS patient without due caution. The database which was developed for this study is based on the treatment and care of the majority of AIDS patients known in the Netherlands. The database was set up in such a way as to enable the total progression of the disease and its treatment to be followed through time. This database therefore offers a good starting point for further economic analysis.

When the research results are compared internationally with other economic analyses on the care of AIDS patients, attention can be drawn to the following points:

- With respect to the size and methodology of the study:
  This study has the largest complete population (230 patients) and the longest research period (6.5 years). The study of Andrulis et al. (1988) had data on 5393 patients, but was based on questionnaires. Other studies were less up to date (1984/1985) and were based on a much shorter research period. In this study we have been able to establish that an underestimate of life-time treatment costs can arise from these kinds of studies.
- With respect to the components of costs and variables included in the study:
  This study includes by far the most extensive range of cost components and variables. This is directly related to the possibilities offered by this database.
- With respect to the composition of the patient population:
  In international studies little analysis has been done of such patient characteristics as age and sex. Where this has taken place, the results are comparable with the results of this study. Approximately 90% of patients are male and the majority are between 31 and 40 years old.
- With respect to the characteristics of treatment:
  - number of hospitalizations:
    The average number of hospitalizations per patient found in our study corresponds best with the results of the studies of Scitovsky et al. (1986) and Seage et al. (1986). The study of Lafferty (Lafferty et al., 1988) gives a much lower number, while that of Kizer et al. (1986) gives a much higher number.
  - length of hospitalizations:
    The average length of hospitalizations in the various studies shows a large variation. The average number of nursing days per hospitalization that we have calculated is rather high.
  - number of nursing days:
    There are similarities with respect to the average number of nursing days between this research and that of Kizer et al. (1986), Drummond et al. (1988) for Germany and Seage et al. (1986). Extremely high outcomes are to be found in the study of Hardy et al. (1986) and extremely low in the study of Scitovsky et al. (1986).

Table 4. International comparisons (in Dutch guildus)*

	San Frans. Scitovsky	Mass. Seage III	Teach.hosp. Andrulis	Washingt. Laferty	FRG Drummond	France Drummond	UK Drummond	CDC Hardy	Californ. Kizer	AZUA Wiggers /	AZUA Bijlsma
										Total	No longer alive
Number of population N =	201	45	5,393	165	19	-	33	-	-	230	105
total number of admission	-	-	-	-	-	100	-	-	-	700	360
Period (years)	1 ('84)	1 ('84)	1 ('85)	1.5	-	-	-	-	-	6.5 Y	6.5 Y
- average costs per hospitalization	18,000	-	25,000	18,000	-	-	-	-	-	22,000	26,500
- average costs of total treatment	14-47,000	100,000	-	-	-	-	6,800	295,000	118,000	68,000	90,000
- average life-time costs	55,000	-	-	-	24,000	-	-	-	-	-	90,000
- average costs per nursing day	1,500	-	1,300	-	800	600	-	-	1,200	1,100	1,100
- average costs per person per year	88,000	85,000	40,000	64,000	28,000	26,300	124,000	270,000	80,000	45,500	60,000
- average number of hospitalizations	3.2	3.3	1.6 pY	2.1	-	-	-	-	6	3.1	3.4
- average length of hospitalization (in days)	11.7	21	19	13.3	20	-	10	31	14	19	35
- average number of treatments (in days)	224	390	-	-	540	-	157	392	540	1.5 Y	1.5 Y
- average number of nursing days	35	62	32 pY	-	78	-	50	168	89.6	60	84
- average number of consultations	-	18.4	-	-	-	-	10.2	-	-	20	20
- average number of IC days	-	4	-	-	-	-	-	-	-	9	-
- average number of doses blood	-	-	-	-	-	-	-	-	-	9	-

* exchange rate: $1 = Fl. 2

pY = per year

- length of treatment:
  An average length of treatment of eighteen months corresponds with that found in with that the studies of Kizer et al. (1986) and Drummond et al. (1988) for Germany. In those two studies, the length of treatment was not based on a direct calculation, as with our study, but it was indirectly estimated. Scitovsky et al. (1986) and Drummond et al. (1988) for Great Britain estimate the length of treatment to be less than one year.
- With respect to the costs:
  Mention was already made of the fact that the results of various international studies showed great variation in the characteristics of treatment. The variation is even greater when it comes to cost calculations. One exception to this is the calculated average cost per hospitalization.

The results of the studies compared here show large differences. This variation is largely due to differences in
- The methodology.
- The (length of) period observed.
- The composition of the patient population.
- The basis on which costs have been calculated (tariffs or real costs).

It is interesting to note that the results of the Dutch situation fall within the range of the international results, with respect to the characteristics of treatment, as well as with respect to the costs.

5. Conclusions

Hospital care of AIDS patients is characterized by large individual variation. These variations in hospital care appear to be linked to the following factors: age at first contact with the hospital, the use of Retrovir, the main diagnosis at the first hospitalization, the year in which the treatment started and the subdivision of the AIDS diagnosis into further CDC categories.

The lifetime costs of hospital care were calculated for the patients treated in the AZUA/AMC hospital in the period between 1982 and spring 1988 and amounted Fl. 90,000 per patient.

The costs of hospital care consist of 70% hospitalization costs, while the remaining 30% are made up of costs related to in- and out-patient interventions and tests, medication, external laboratory tests and blood transfusions.

The costs have been calculated using sickness fund insurance tariffs. This implies an underestimation of the real costs of treatment of Aidspatients. The treatment of AIDS patients is far more intensive than that of the average patients and the tariffs are based on the treatment of average patients.

AIDS is a relatively new and fast-growing disease. The majority of patients who recently started being treated are therefore not yet at the end of the treatment. This is another reason why the calculated costs probably will be an underestimation of the true costs of hospital treatment of the average AIDS patient. The results that have been found for the Dutch situation are within the ranges given by a number of international studies.

A dynamic database was set up for the purpose of this study, in which the complete progression of the disease and the treatment per patient were registered from the moment of first contact with the AZUA/AMC hospital. The way in which this database is organized gives a good starting point for further and more in-depth analysis.

Acknowledgement. The authors wish to thank Dr. S.A. Danner, Prof. Dr. R.M. Lapré, the computer department of the AZUA/AMC hospital, Drs. F.J.M. Werner and colleagues at the AZUA/AMC hospital and the NIPG/TNO for their helpful comments on this article.

References

Andrulis, D.P., Beers, V., Bentley, J.P., and Gage, L.S. (1987). The provision in US public and private teaching hospitals. Journal of the American Medical Association 258, 1343-1344.

Drummond, M. and Davies, L. (1988). Treating AIDS: the economic issues. Health Policy 10, 1-19.

Hardy, A.M., Rauch, K., Echenberg, D., Morgan, W.M., and Curran, J. (1986). The economic impact of the first 10,000 cases of acquired immune deficiency syndrome in the United States. Journal of the American Medical Association 255, 209-211.

Kizer, K., Rodrigues, J., McHolland, G.F., and Weller, W. (1986). A quantitative analysis of AIDS in California. California Department of Health Services.

Lafferty, W.E., Hopkins, S.G., Honey, J., Harwell, J.D., Shoemaker, P.C., and Kobayashi, J.M. (1988). Hospital charges for people with AIDS in Washington State: utilization of a statewide hospital discharge data base. American Journal of Public Health 78, 949-952.

Scitovsky, A., Cline, M., and Lee, P.H. (1986). Medical care costs of patients with AIDS in San Francisco. Journal of the American Medical Association 256, 3107-3109.

Seage III, G.R., Landers, S., and Barry, A. (1986). Medical care costs of AIDS in Massachussets. Journal of the American Medical Association 256, 3107-3109.

Direct and Indirect Costs of AIDS in Belgium: A Preliminary Analysis

J. Lambert, G. Carrin

1. Introduction

In this note, we present an analysis of direct and indirect costs of AIDS in Belgium. Direct costs comprise the costs of medical treatment and the non-personal costs of public information campaigns and other governmental assistance serving the general public. Indirect costs contain the costs of morbidity only. Incomplete information precluded us from also considering the indirect costs due to premature mortality.

The costs of medical treatment are based on detailed data related to 24 patients that were treated at the hospital unit of Antwerp's Institute of Tropical Medicine (ITM). The latter unit is located on the premises of the University Hospital of Antwerp. The data sources are patient records and bills concerning inpatient and outpatient care provided at the hospital unit. All 24 patients had AIDS as defined by the Centers for Disease Control (CDC) and the World Health Organization (WHO).

The purpose of this paper is to inform decision-makers in Belgium about the cost implications of AIDS treatment. This information will hopefully be an incentive to use resources as effectively as possible, aiming at preventing AIDS and at improving existing patients' lives. In the following section, we restrict ourselves to the analysis of the sample of patients treated at the ITM: we discuss patient characteristics and present the medical cost per patient and the medical cost per patient per year. In the third section, these cost figures are used to estimate the global cost of AIDS for the country as a whole. The final estimates and their implications are examined in the final section.

2. Patient characteristics and medical costs

2.1 Patient characteristics

Initially we selected 20 patients who received treatment during the period between April 1, 1987 and March 31, 1988. The prime reason for considering this time frame was that nearly all hospital bills related to costs incurred during that particular period could be made available. These 20 patients are further divided into three subgroups: group A contains five patients who died during the above mentioned period; group B consists of six patients who were already being treated before April 1, 1987; group C is composed of nine patients whose treatment started during the selected period. It is important to note that all patients of groups B and C were still alive on March 31, 1988.

We emphasize that 15 patients were still alive at the end of the considered period. This means then that our data set may contain insufficient information about terminal costs. There is also the fact that three patients of group A died in a hospital other than the ITM's hospital unit. We therefore decided to partially remedy this bias by adding group D, comprising four deceased patients that were treated in 1984-1986, to the initial sample of 20 patients. The costs related to this particular group were adjusted to 1987-1988 price levels.

2.2 Cost analysis of medical treatment

2.2.1 Medical cost per patient (MCP)

We present, in Table 1, the MCP based on the hospital bills concerning the period April 1, 1987- March 31, 1988 (for groups A to C) and the period 1984-1986 (for group D). The costs comprise those of hospital services (viz. nursing care and hotel services), medication and blood transfusions, physicians' care and clinical biology. Note that the costs are related to both inpatient and outpatient care at the ITM. We will also make a distinction between the costs borne by the Belgian Health Insurance Scheme (HIS) and those paid by patients themselves. Because of lack of accurate information, we were not able to take into account the cost of medical treatment outside the ITM, such as health care provided by general practitioners or care given at another hospital unit. For the same reason, the cost of outpatient care for patients of group D was not incorporated in the cost analysis. Table 1 also gives the total number of months of treatment per patient group.

Table 1. Medical cost per patient (MCP), in BEF

Patient group	Cost			Total number of treatment months
	Financed by HIS	Total by patient	treated	
A	120,564	12,911	133,475	20
B	218,911	14,662	233,573	72
C	669,869	24,240	694,109	59
D	592,605	189,914	782,519	36
All patients	429,813	47,098	476,911	187

The MCP in group A is the lowest. However, it is also underestimated due to the lack in the data on the terminal cost of three patients. The relatively low level of the MCP in group B has several causes: first, five patients were ARC patients for several months; secondly, none of the six patients were terminal; and thirdly, the initial treatment costs, which are generally high as a result of exhaustive observation and diagnostic procedures, are not included in the considered period. Group C entails a significant amount of costs, the initial treatment costs now being part of the total cost picture. In addition, group C's high cost level can be explained by the substantial cost of medicines (in particular zidovudine and interferon A) and the completeness of the data. The cost of group D is the highest. Yet it is still underestimated due to missing bills for outpatient care. The part of the costs paid by these patients is higher than that for other groups because they were mostly accommodated in single hospital rooms that involve higher payments.

2.2.2 Medical cost per patient per year (MCPY)

Seage et al. (1986) have proposed calculating the MCPY. This method consists of dividing the medical cost by the number of months of treatment and multiplying subsequently by twelve. The use of this method over the one above is frequently recommended. It avoids the disadvantage of the MCP method whereby one disregards all costs incurred before and after the study period. It also does not take account of the difference between a patient treated over a 12 month period and another treated, say, over only one month. However, one unfavourable characteristic of the present method is that the MCPY in certain groups of patients may be subject to an upward or downward bias. On the one hand, this is the case for the groups that contain terminal patients and patients that start their treatment: the significant cost of treatment may be translated into an overestimated MCPY. This method also overestimates the yearly costs of terminal patients, as soon as their treatment is stopped, due to death, before the end of the sample period. On the other hand, there can be an underestimation in the case of patients who are still in the non-terminal stages of AIDS.

In order to apply the MCPY method, we used all available data in the hospital bills related to the period between 1984 and 1988; all costs were adjusted, if necessary, for inflation. The results obtained by means of the method of Seage et al. (1986) are presented in Table 2.

We observe indeed that the MCPY for group C is the highest amongst four groups, due in part to some overestimation. The MCPY for the whole sample amounts to 917,374 BEF. We judge that the latter figure is quite plausible. First, in the calculation of this average cost, a possible overshooting due to the costs of terminal patients is compensated by the lower costs induced by patients in the non-terminal stages of AIDS. Secondly, it is also acceptable in view of the relatively high cost of the most recent drug therapies.

Table 2. Medical cost per patient per year (MCPY), in BEF

Patient group	Cost		
	Financed by HIS	Total by patient	
A	821,505	94,856	916,361
B	260,932	22,605	283,537
C	1,279,001	46,520	1,325,521
D	753,836	197,225	951,061
All patients	841,645	75,729	917,374

We also draw the attention of the reader to the amount paid by patients themselves, viz. an average of 75,729 BEF per year. We can compare the latter with earnings in Belgian industry, for instance; the mean yearly wage in 1987 varies between 583,680 BEF and 893,328 BEF for blue and white collar workers, respectively (Ministerie van Economische Zaken, 1988). Hence, we find that the proportion of average annual wages payed by patients themselves varies between 8.5% (for white collar workers) and 13% (for blue collar workers). It thus appears that AIDS treatment is fairly costly for patients themselves.

We now present additional information on the cost shares of the medical inputs. Using the hospital bills, we were able to divide total cost into the following categories: 46.3% of the total cost is spent on the cost of hospital services, 28.1% on medication and blood products, 5.1% on physician fees and 17% on lab tests. Notice that the share of drug costs turns out to be very significant. A further increase in drug costs can be expected in the near future because of the growing use of expensive treatments such as zidovudine and interferon A treatment. Zidovudine is generally prescribed on a continuous basis, at an average cost of 1300 BEF per day. Interferon A is normally used in a once-and-for-all episode of treatment, at an average total cost of 750,000 BEF per treatment.

The shares of inpatient and outpatient care in total costs are 83.1% and 16.9%, respectively. Note further that 88.2% of the total cost is paid by the HIS, the remainder by the patient. Given that the inpatient cost occupies a large share of total cost, it is certainly informative to calculate the mean cost per hospital bed-day. Remark that the latter cost incorporates all costs of inpatient care, including the use of drugs, blood transfusions, physician activities etc.

First, we observe that the mean cost per hospital bed-day of groups A and D (which contain terminal patients) is below that of groups B and C. This indicates that it is the required length of hospitalization that finally determines total cost, of course. Secondly, the main reason for the higher cost of group C is the use of new and expensive drug therapies.

Table 3. Mean cost per hospital bed-day, in BEF

Patient group	Cost		
	Financed by HIS	Financed by patients	Total
A	5,698	1,672	7,370
B	6,677	699	7,376
C	14,380	499	14,878
D	4,826	1,451	6,277
All patients	7,529	1,155	8,684

2.2.3 Pathology-specific costs per patient per year

We next present the MCPY according to the different dominant pathologies: Kaposi's sarcoma (5 patients), Pneumocystis carinii infection (5 patients) and other pathologies (other opportunistic infections or HIV encephalopathy) (14 patients). Both MCPY and the cost per hospital bed-day are computed; see Tables 4 and 5. When using these cost figures, however, the small sizes of the subgroups from which they were generated have to be taken into account, especially when thinking of representativity.

Table 4. Medical cost per patient per year (MCPY), in BEF

Patient group	Cost		
	Financed by HIS	Financed by patients	Total
Kaposi's sarcoma	1,273,531	85,423	1,358,954
P. carinii infection	639,237	38,691	677,928
Other pathologies	759,688	85,494	845,182
P. carinii infection and other pathologies	727,990	73,178	801,168

Table 5. Cost per hospital bed-day, in BEF

Patient group	Cost		
	Financed by HIS	Financed by patients	Total
Kaposi's sarcoma	16,192	2,129	18,321
P. carinii infection	6,575	450	7,025
Other pathologies	5,957	1,130	7,087
P. carinii infection and other pathologies	6,082	993	7,075

Notice that the treatment of Kaposi patients entails considerably higher costs. This result is opposite to the findings of Seage et al. (1986) and Scitovsky et al. (1986). A very likely explanation is that the newer therapeutic methods such as interferon A were not yet incorporated in the treatment cost recorded in the mid eighties. However, like Seage et al. (1986), we only observe a slight difference between the groups with Pneumocystis carinii and other opportunistic infections. The costs per hospital bed-day of both groups are also quite similar. The latter confirms the results obtained by Scitovsky et al. (1986).

The data also allowed us to identify the treatment period and related costs of patients with Aids Related Complex (ARC). We counted 8 patients and 38 months of treatment in the ARC stage of the HIV infection. The medical cost per patient per month of treatment amounts to 12,666 BEF. The latter cost is far less than that of treatment of a full blown AIDS patient. It again indicates how large differences can be between the various stages in the treatment of AIDS.

3. Estimation of the total yearly cost of AIDS in Belgium

The total yearly cost will be composed of direct costs (viz. medical costs and non-personal costs) and indirect costs (viz. morbidity costs). Only the costs of resident patients are considered. Note that a resident is a person who has been living in Belgium for at least five years.

First, we estimated medical costs by combining the pathology-specific MCPY with epidemiological data from the Institute of Hygiene and Epidemiology (IHE) of the Ministry of Public Health. Note that on the 31st of December 1986, 68 resident cases were registered in Belgium, 31 of whom had died already. On December 31, 1987, 126 resident cases had been registered, 64 of whom had died. Thus in 1987, 95 (=126-31) patients were treated and 33 (=64-31) had died. Of those 95 patients, 25 had Kaposi's sarcoma while 70 had Pneumocystis carinii infection or other pathologies. The appropriate MCPY figures were then used to estimate the total yearly medical cost for Belgium, presented in Table 6.

Table 6. Estimates of the total yearly medical cost of AIDS in Belgium, in BEF

Patient group	Cost		
	Financed by HIS	Total by patients	
25 patients with Kaposi's sarcoma	31,838,275	2,135,575	33,973,850
70 patients with P. carinii infection or other pathologies	50,959,300	5,122,460	56,081,760
All patients	82,797,575	7,258,035	90,055,610

Secondly, we calculated the morbidity cost, viz. the loss of income due to illness and disability during the treatment episode. Given the information on the occupation of the 16 resident patients in our sample, yearly earnings could be estimated. Use was made of earnings data published by the Ministerie van Economische Zaken (1988a, 1988b). We next identified the degree of disability of each patient from patient records. We also supposed that the patient was disabled during 20% of the time he resided at home and only received outpatient care. Combining then the earnings data with the morbidity pattern, the morbidity cost per patient per year was estimated to be 269,908 BEF. The latter figure has to be understood as a minimum: almost half of the patients' records showed treatment over only a few months. Considering now that there were 95 resident patients in 1987, the morbidity cost is estimated to be 25,641,260 BEF.

Thirdly, we identify the non-personal costs. These include government expenditures for research (20 million BEF) and blood screening and testing (232 million BEF, including 48 million BEF in support of specialized control laboratories), for special aid to international organizations and developing countries (87 million BEF), and for information campaigns (46 million BEF). We thus obtain a total amount of 385 million BEF.

Adding the three components of the yearly cost of AIDS, we arrive at a total figure of 500,696,870 BEF. The latter represents 0.02% of national income in 1987.

4. Discussion

Several lessons can be learnt from the present exercise. First, from the cost estimates it can be derived that the burden of the medical treatment of AIDS on the HIS amounted to 0.034% of its overall budget in 1987. Considering that this share of the budget may increase as a result of a growing number of AIDS patients, it is understandable that the future demand for cost-effective treatments will be high on the HIS's agenda. The need for cost-effective treatment is also likely to be spurred by the relatively high burden of copayments on patients' incomes. Earlier we have seen that inpatient care accounted for the largest part, viz. 83.1%, of the medical cost of AIDS. The latter indeed illustrates the need to search for appropriate and cost-effective substitutes for lengthy hospital treatment. In fact, recent data already reveal a reduction in hospital-based treatment. The latter trend can only sustained by the establishment of new ambulatory treatment methods or the development of innovative drugs that entail a downward effect on the need for hospitalization.

Secondly, the urge to find new ways of treatment not only originates in the desire for cost-containment, of course. They are also wanted for their potentially beneficial impact on the quality of life of AIDS patients and on the lengthening of their life expectancy.

Thirdly, how do we have to assess the government budget for information campaigns and research in 1987, viz. 66 million BEF ? Let us remind ourselves that the medical and morbidity cost of the 95 resident AIDS patients amounted to 115,696,870 BEF (=90,055,610 BEF + 25,641,260 BEF), or 1,217,862 BEF per patient per year. A substantial amount of costs will therefore be avoided as soon as information campaigns result in a lower incidence of AIDS. At present, however, there is hardly any information on the impact of Belgian information campaigns on the behaviour of risk groups. It is thus premature to say that this budget should be increased in order to bring costs further down.

Fourthly, in the present analysis, we were not able to take account of the indirect costs, or foregone earnings, due to premature mortality. Scitovsky and Rice (1987) have pointed out that this particular category of indirect costs is even greater than the cost of medical treatment. The latter is not surprising since the main group of patients consists of normally active men aged between 25 and 45 years. Therefore, the fact that these particular indirect costs will also be averted in the event of efficient information campaigns adds to the economic rationale of efforts in the area of prevention. Apart from ethical reasons, research activities also find an additional justification in the potential for lengthening life expectancy and, therefore, for reducing the indirect cost due to premature mortality.

To summarize, countries are well advised to inquire into the desired level of budgets for research and preventive campaigns, in view of their potential for reducing future costs and for enhancing patients' quality of life. Research in particular needs to concentrate on improvement of the knowledge of the pathology itself, the therapeutics and on the possibility of vaccination.

In spite of the limited sample of patients and the simplifying assumptions that were made, we believe that these preliminary estimates of the direct and indirect costs of AIDS in Belgium are informative and can contribute to the discussion and elaboration of future health policies.

Acknowledgement. Our sincere thanks go to Professor H.Taelman of the Institute of Tropical Medicine who was so kind to help us with setting up the databank needed for this study. We also thank Mrs. Van Hemeldonck of the IHE for updating us on the epidemiological data. Thanks also to D.De Graeve for her pertinent comments on earlier drafts of this article. The present note is based on the first author's B.A. thesis, which was awarded a special prize by the Dr.Paul Janssen Institute. All remaining errors are our responsibility, of course.

References

Ministerie van Economische Zaken (1988). Statistisch Overzicht van België 1988. Nationaal Instituut voor de Statistiek, Brussels.

Ministerie van Economische Zaken (1988a). Sociale Statistieken, nr.1, 79.

Ministerie van Economische Zaken (1988b). Statistisch Tijdschrift 74(3), 171.

Scitovsky, A.A., Crine, M., and Lee, P.R. (1986). Medical care costs of patients with AIDS in San Fransisco. Journal of the American Medical Association 256(22), 3103-3106.

Seage, G.R., Landers, S., Barry, M.A., Groopman, J., Lamb, G.A., and Epstein, A.M. (1986). Medical care costs of AIDS in Massachusetts. Journal of the American Medical Association 256(22).

Hospital Costs for AIDS Patients

B. Olesen, P. Gøtzsche, I. Bygbjerg, L. Møller, V. Faber

Introduction

AIDS was first diagnosed in Denmark in 1981. By 1 March 1989, 380 AIDS patients had been diagnosed, of whom 202 have already died. The management of patients with AIDS is very costly, but it is largely unknown how the expenses are divided between the basic cost of in-hospital care and the variable costs of diagnostic procedures and treatment. When planning the health care system, knowledge about these relations is essential. The aim of this study was to clarify the distribution of expenses involved in diagnostic procedures and treatment of AIDS patients.

Material and methods

Hospital expenses from the first admission to the Department of Infectious Diseases until death were determined for the first 33 AIDS patients in a retrospective study of patient records. The patients, 32 males and 1 female, were admitted to the department in the period from May 1980 to January 1986. The average age at the time of death was 38 years (range 28-54, median 37). One female and one male were without known risk factors, another male had many sexual relationships with women in Central Africa, and the rest were homo- or bisexual males.

The patients were hospitalised for an average time of 95 days (7-352, 82), distributed over 4 admissions per patient (1-32, 3). From the first admission the patients spent an average of 53% of their remaining lifetime as in-patients. The expenses were all calculated in 1986 prices.

Results

The total expenses of hospital care from the first admission to death were on the average $ 50,000 or $ 526 per day. The basic hospital fee made up more than 2/3 of the total. It consisted mainly of personnel, inventory, laundry, administration, etc. and amounted to $ 34,037 per patient. Laboratory costs, made up of microbiology, serology / immunology and clinical chemical tests, amounted to $ 4,784 or 9.6% of the total.

Microbiology

The average costs per patient amounted to $ 1,979. Virus culturing, which mainly consisted of cytomegalovirus, from respiratory passages, urine and stool was estimated at 23% and was, together with bacterial culturing from the respiratory passages with another 23%, the most expensive item. Bacterial culturing from the blood was estimated at 19%. Bacterial culturing and protozoan examinations from stool and rectum came to 16%. The rest of the costs was made up by bacterial culturing from various places such as spinal fluid and bone marrow, catheters and ulcers, tissue biopsies and urine. All of them each made up 5% or less.

Serology and immunology

This amounted to $ 1,675 per patient. Approximately half of this was made up by qualitative and quantitative lymphocyte investigations.

Clinical chemical tests

These amounted to $ 1,130 per patient. Because of the frequency with which the tests were made (every 3-4 days) hemoglobin and leucocytes were the most expensive parts.

Out-patient treatment

This amounted to 3.9% or $ 1,975 per patient. Most patients received regular out-patient treatment, on average 8 visits per patient.

Private duty nurse

This amounted to 2.8% or $ 1,420 per patient. 19 patients had a private duty nurse for 9 days on average.

Medicine and blood products

This amounted to 8.1% of the total and $ 4,077 per patient. 88% of this was made up by drugs. Range of the cost of drugs was $ 10 - 23,941, median $ 16,075. None of these patients had been treated with Retrovir. 26 patients received transfusion with a blood product, on average 8 (0-48, 4).

Other diagnostic procedures

This amounted to 2.6%. Gastric, bronchial and rectoscopic examinations incl. biopsies were $ 291 per patient. Taking and histologically examining the biopsies made up approximately 2/3 of the cost. On the average 7 biopsies were taken per patient. The

most frequent examination was bronchoscopy performed on average 0.8 times per patient.
X-ray and CT scan costs amounted to $ 1,033 per patient. 61% of this was made up by CT scan (most frequently of thorax and brain), the rest mainly by X-ray of thorax. Apart from CT scan 15 X-rays were made per patient (2-45, 13).

Autopsy

These costs amounted to 2.3% of the total or $ 1,135 per patient. 23 autopsies were carried out; in the remaining 10 patients autopsy was prohibited. The price of one autopsy was $ 1,627, of which microbiological examinations of material from the autopsy made up 59%.

Consultants

This expense amounted to 1.8% of the total or $ 910 per patient. Each patient was on average examined by 21 consultants, most frequently a surgeon (6), an eye specialist (4), a dentist (3) and a dermatologist (1). Most patients received physiotherapy, but it was not possible to estimate the exact number of treatments.

Surgery

This amounted to 0.5% of the total or $ 238 per patient. On the average 0.9 operations were performed per patient. 4 patients had an open lung biopsy taken, 3 patients a brain biopsy, and 2 patients underwent laparatomia.

Other expenses

These amounted to 0.1% of the total or $ 70 per patient.

Discussion and conclusions

In conclusion, the greatest expense in the hospital treatment of AIDS patients was the basic hospital fee, which was 2/3 of the total, while the expenses of treatment and diagnostic procedures comprised only about 1/3 of the total costs. The expenses calculated cannot be used for future economic assessments without adjustment. Both the number of diagnostic examinations, particularly within virology and immunology, as well as expenses for medical treatment are increasing. Treatment with the drug Retrovir, which most AIDS patients now receive, will cost up to $ 12,500 per patient per year. Moreover, this calculation does not take into consideration the large nursing requirement of these patients, and in particular the basic hospital fees are uncertain, and the assessment is probably too low.

To reduce the hospital costs in the future, it is essential to reduce the length of the in-hospital stay. This could be achieved by an increased access to diagnosis and treatment for out-patients, better homecare like the one in San Francisco led by the well-organized gay community (Schietinger, 1986), and by better psycho-social support, since some admissions of AIDS patients are mainly due to psycho-social problems. Cost-benefit analyses of diagnostic procedures and treatment (Gøtzsche et al., 1988) would also be useful. Apart from the economic aspect, the AIDS patients themselves would highly benefit from all proposals mentioned above.

In Rigshospitalet Copenhagen the average number of days spent in hospital per AIDS patient has already been reduced in step with the growing experience with AIDS. For patients who died in 1980-85 the admission time was 95 days, in 1986 it had been reduced to 72 days, in 1987 to 54 days, and for patients who died up until March 1989, the average time as in-patients was 32 days. The department has now employed a psychologist exclusively for AIDS patients, and an extra social worker has been engaged.

References

Gøtzsche, P.C., Bygbjerg, I.B., Olesen, B., Møller, L.H., Salim, Y., and Faber, V. (1988). Yield of diagnostic investigations of opportunistic infections in AIDS: a survey of 33 patients. Scandinavian Journal of Infectious Diseases 20, 395-402.

Schietinger, H. (1986). AIDS beyond the hospital. 1. A home care plan for AIDS. American Journal of Nursing 86, 1021-28.

Comparing Inpatient and Outpatient Costs for HIV, LAS and AIDS: Methodology, Results and Consequences from a Study in Germany

R. Hanpft, F. Reinecke, F. Beske

Introduction

For some years now, the Institute for Health Systems Research in Kiel has been studying some economic aspects of the HIV infection in the Federal Republic of Germany. An investigation into expenditures for testing blood donations was finished in early 1986 (Beske and Hanpft, 1986; Beske and Hanpft, 1987). A study concerning the public expenditures for preventive measures is published in this volume (cf. Jenke and Reinkemeier). Results are also available from a study that compared the expenditures for the treatment of LAS/AIDS patients by inpatient as opposed to outpatient medical services in a West German hospital (Kook-Walewski et al., 1988). Another study, which is presented here, has provided data on the costs and expenditures for diagnosis and therapy of HIV infected patients in the Federal Republic of Germany (Reinecke et al., 1988).

1. The groups of patients under study

In order to calculate the costs of, and expenditures for, medical care for a selected group of patients, hospital and general practitioners' services were recorded in retrospect. The patients were assigned to the three stages of infection as defined by the original CDC classification: HIV positive incubation, LAS stage and AIDS stage.

Fig. 1 shows the distribution of the 57 patients whose medical care records were evaluated. The distribution proved to be fairly equal, both with regard to the stages of infection and to the place of treatment. For each patient, the treatment records of 12 months were covered. As the data are from 1985 and 1986, they do not reflect most recent forms of AIDS therapy. For example, none of the patients was treated with azidothymidine (AZT). Furthermore, it must be pointed out that the records evaluated are not necessarily representative of all HIV infected patients.

Stage according to CDC classification	Treatment by General Practitioner	Hospital Treatment	Total
HIV positive incubation	10	9	19
LAS	10	10	20
AIDS	8	10	18
Total	28	29	57

Fig. 1. Groups of patients under study

2. Evaluation of the treatment by general practitioner

To calculate the expenditures that resulted from the general practitioner's treatment, the services rendered were assessed and then added. In addition, the prices of the drugs prescribed were added as they are recorded in the Red List, a drug index of the German pharmaceutical industry (Bundesverband der Pharmazeutischen Industrie e. V., 1987). For the medical care provided by the general practitioner, only the crude expenditures, i. e. the prices of services charged to the health insurance funds, were considered (Welzel and Liebold, 1986). These figures give an appropriate estimate of ambulatory services.

3. Evaluation of the hospital treatment

Hospital treatment was evaluated under two different aspects. It had to be considered that the expenditures of the health insurance funds and the hospital's operating costs may differ greatly. So, on the one hand, the expenditures of the health insurance funds for the required days of medical care were calculated, and, on the other, the costs of the hospital were assessed as far as possible. Expenditures for inpatient care follow from multiplying the patient's length of stay with the daily rate for care to be covered by health insurance.

To assess the costs of the hospital, its services were itemized as shown in Fig. 2. The total costs consist of those for the physician, nursing accommodation and food ('hotel' costs), special diagnostic tests (medical costs) and drugs and physical therapy (cost of

Cost Sector	Data Source
physician costs	cost accounting centre
nursing costs (rated according to intensity)	cost accounting centre (corrected by own rating)
'hotel' costs	cost accounting centre
medical costs	own evaluation
cost of materials	own evaluation

Fig. 2. Evaluation of hospital treatment costs

materials) (Tauch, 1986). The annual costs of physician, nursing and 'hotel' of the ward in which the patients lay were taken from the cost accounting centre of the hospital. Dividing those costs by the number of patient days results in the average cost for a single day. It has to be taken into account that the ward also consisted of patients not infected with HIV.
While average costs of the ward were used to evaluate physician and the 'hotel' costs, the average daily nursing costs were rated according to the assumed nursing intensity of patients in the different stages. For HIV positive patients, the average nursing costs were multiplied by the factor 0.6, for LAS patients by 1 and for AIDS patients by 1.6.

This rating resulted from the following considerations:

- According to studies, an intensity of 0.6 of the average time for nursing can be assumed when a patient is still able to stand up by himself, at least most of the time, and to eat, etc. by himself (Deutsches Krankenhausinstitut, 1987).
- It was assumed that a LAS patient requires the average time for care.
- According to a study by Zöllner in Munich, the time of care for an AIDS patient is 1.6 times as high as that of an average patient.

The costs for special diagnostic tests (medical costs) and for drugs and physical therapy (costs of material) were evaluated in detail and separately for each patient. The medical services were assessed using the DKG-NT. This is a schedule of charges issued by the German hospital society for the determination of fees-for-services (Deutsche Krankenhausgesellschaft, 1987). The costs of drugs were calculated from the purchase price of middle-sized packages for hospital pharmacies. Certain medical costs also comprise services rendered on the ward such as entrance examinations and taking the costs of the medical and care personnel had to be excluded, as those costs were already included in the costs for physicians' services and nursing costs. These medical costs were assessed by subtracting the costs for personnel, which responds to the difference between full costs and costs for material in the scale of charges from the German hospital society.

4. Expenditures and costs

The average treatment expenditures and treatment costs of the patients during the evaluation period are shown in Fig. 3.

The results are classified according to the three infection stages. The expenditures for treatment by general practitioner are DM 1,567 for patients in the LAS stage; this is about one and a half times more than for patients in the HIV positive incubation stage, which amounts to DM 977. The ambulatory treatment of patients with AIDS resulted in lower expenditures than for those in the LAS stage - a reflection of the fact that patients with AIDS are mostly treated in hospital.

To calculate the expenditures for hospital treatment, an average care rate of DM 348.85 from seven German hospitals accommodating an above-average number of HIV infected patients was used. A comparison between the average expenditures for hospital treatment and the approximate average costs shows that HIV positive and LAS patients led to costs of DM 6,712 and DM 8,286 respectively; this is slightly less

		CDC stage		
	Place of treatment	HIV positive	LAS	AIDS
Expenditures	general practitioner	977	1,567	1,201
	hospital	7,012 1) 2)	8,442 1) 3)	23,164 1) 4)
Costs	hospital			
	- per year	6,712 2)	8,286 3)	28,344 4)
	- per day	334	343	427

1) daily care rate DM 348.85
2) length of stay 20.1 days
3) length of stay 24.2 days
4) length of stay 66.4 days

Fig. 3. Average treatment expenditures and treatment costs per year and patient in DM

than the expenditures of DM 7,012 and DM 8,442. The average costs for AIDS patients, however, exceed the average expenditures by about 20%.

These ratios are also reflected in the amounts per patient day. The average costs for treatment per day of care for HIV positive and LAS patients, DM 334 and DM 342, are slightly less than the expenditures, which are based on a daily care rate of DM 348.85. The daily costs for the AIDS patients are DM 427, thus exceeding the daily care rate by about 20%.

5. Costs in various categories

It is interesting to observe those five cost categories in which, depending on the stage of the infection, differences are so considerable that they obviously affect the total costs for hospital treatment. The share these categories have in the total costs of each stage of the illness is shown in Fig. 4.

As mentioned before, average figures for physician's as well as 'hotel' costs were assumed in all stages. The costs for nursing increase, according to the rating, from the HIV positive stage through the LAS stage to the AIDS stage. For the development of those two cost categories where each single individual service was accounted and summed up, it is typical that the costs for drugs and physical therapy, very small in the first two stages, are about 30 times higher in the AIDS stage, whereas the costs for

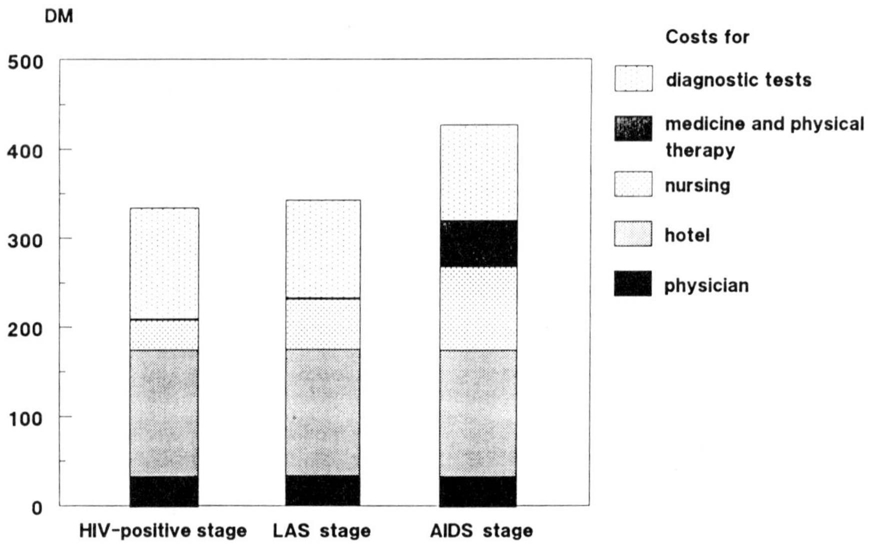

Fig. 4. Cost categories of hospital treatment

diagnostic examinations decrease absolutely and relatively from the HIV positive stage through to the AIDS stage but, on the whole, remain at a high level.

6. Expenditures for a HIV infected person during the total time of infection

To be able to sum up the expenditures for one HIV infected patient during the whole length of infection, hypothetical careers of illness and treatment were regarded. The calculation was made under the following assumptions:

1. Although the sums for the average yearly expenditure in an infection stage were calculated by recording the treatment of several patients, they were added to one sum for a "model patient".
2. The maximum amount of hospital treatment during the HIV positive incubation stage was restricted to 1 year, even though it was assumed that this stage lasts several years.
3. For the LAS stage and the AIDS stage yearly expenditures for hospital treatment and for treatment by the general practitioner were estimated.
4. While the HIV positive stage and LAS stage were assumed to have a length of 1 year to several years, the AIDS stage was assumed to be 1 year only.

Due to this premise and depending on the course of the illness and the varying demand for treatment, different results may occur in the expenditures for a HIV positive person during the whole period of infection. This is shown by two examples in Fig. 5. An infection period of 10 years is assumed in both cases.

Example 1 shows a patient with a 3-year HIV positive stage, a 6-year LAS stage and a 1-year AIDS stage. The patient is hospitalized once during the HIV incubation. This results in expenditures of DM 94,000.

Example 2 shows a patient in which the LAS stage follows an 8-year HIV positive stage, lasts 1 year and is, in turn, followed by an AIDS stage of 1 year. The expenditures amount to DM 42,000.

When calculating the treatment of different extreme cases which all have an infection period of 10 years, this model results in expenditures of DM 33,000 to 114,000 during the whole period of infection.

7. Conclusions

1. It has to be taken into account that the calculations rely on data from one hospital and one general practitioner as well as from a relatively small number of patients, also that since the survey period 3 years have passed.

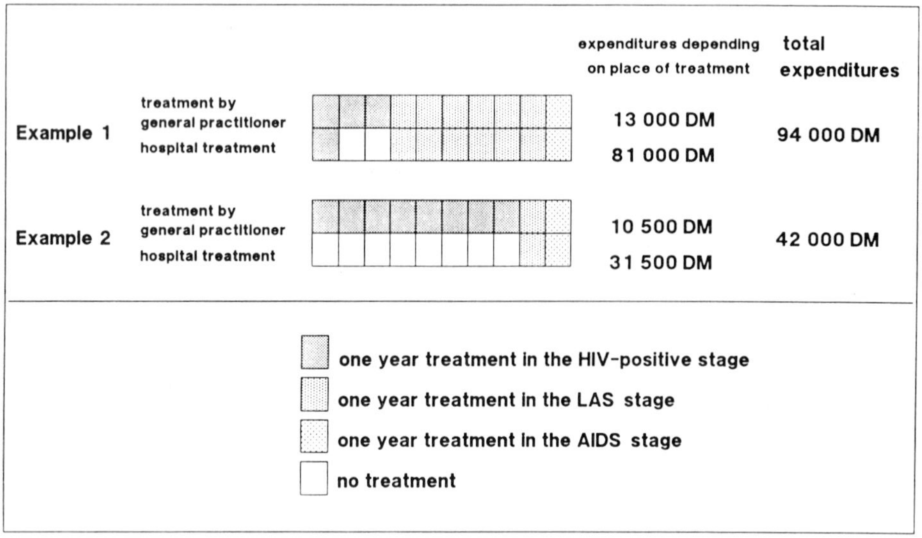

Fig. 5. Model calculation of the treatment expenditures during the whole period of infection

2. As 20% higher hospital treatment costs than expenditures for AIDS patients were determined, it can be assumed that if the number of AIDS patients increases, the daily rates of hospital care will not cover the costs. The greatest cost increase during the progression of the disease can be expected in the cost categories therapy and nursing.
3. It was shown that the expenditures for diagnosis and therapy of HIV infected patients vary greatly, depending on the course of the illness and the demand for care. When using these calculations for further forecasts, different results may be expected, depending on the frequency distribution of the infection stages and on the degree of demand for care.

References

Beske, F. and Hanpft, R. (1986). Gesundheitsökonomische Aspekte zum erworbenen Immundefektsyndrom (AIDS). I. Blutspendewesen. Schmidt & Klaunig, Kiel.

Beske, F. and Hanpft, R. (1987). Gesundheitsökonomische Auswirkungen des erworbenen Immundefektsyndroms (AIDS) im Bereich des Blutspendewesens. Das Öffentliche Gesundheitswesen 49, 99-101.

Bundesverband der Pharmazeutischen Industrie e.V. (ed.) (1987). Rote Liste 1987. Editio Cantor, Aulendorf.

Deutsche Krankenhausgesellschaft (ed.) (1987). DKG-NT, Tarif der Deutschen Krankenhausgesellschaft, zugleich BG-T, vereinbarter Tarif für die Abrechnung mit den gesetzlichen Unfallversicherungsträgern. 17. Auflage. Kohlhammer, Köln.

Deutsches Krankenhausinstitut (ed.) (1987). Patientenbezogene Leistungs- und Kostenbudgetierung. Bertelsmann Stiftung, Gütersloh.

Kook-Walewski, A., Wilke, K., Wegner, R., and Stille, W., (1988). Kostenanalyse von LAS- und AIDS-Patienten in der Universitätsklinik Frankfurt. Deutscher AIDS-Kongreß, München (abstract).

Reinecke, F., Hanpft, R., and Beske, F., (1988). Gesundheitsökonomische Aspekte zum erworbenen Immundefektsyndrom (AIDS) II. Diagnose und Therapie. Schmidt & Klaunig, Kiel.

Tauch, J.G. (1986). Budgetierung im Krankenhaus. Bertelsmann Stiftung, Gütersloh.

Welzel, H. and Liebold, R. (1986). Handkommentar. BMÄ '78 EGO, GOÄ. 5. Auflage, 16. Lieferung, Stand: 1. Januar 1987. Asgard Verlag, St. Augustin.

Medical Services and Costs of AIDS Patients in an Outpatient Clinic for Infectious Diseases, Frankfurt University Hospital

I. Gschrey-Düver, H. Exner-Freisfeld, A. Koock-Walewski,
C. zur Lippe, R. Müller, S. Staszewski, W. Stille

Introduction

Since 1986, medical services and the resulting costs for AIDS patients at our outpatient clinic have been analysed (the term "medical services" includes consultations, physical as well as technical examinations, laboratory tests, counselling). For this particular question, there are hardly any data available in the Federal Republic of Germany. Except for the cost analysis regarding ARC and AIDS patients, performed by Koock-Walewski (Koock-Walewski and Stille, 1989), only a few comparable studies (e.g. Hanpft et al., 1988) are known to us. However, these studies mainly researched expenditure for inpatient care and, only to a lesser extent, services performed for outpatients.

There are a number of US studies analysing costs per patients, some of them based on high caseloads (e.g. Andrulis et al., 1987), but again, these studies mainly deal with costs arising during inpatient treatment. As the results of these studies vary significantly between different US regions, they are hardly, if at all, comparable with the situation in other countries. This is also true for cost analyses performed by other countries, e.g. Great Britain (Johnson et al., 1986). The differences of national health and social security systems as well as differing prices for pharmaceutical products, etc., make a comparison and a useful interpretation even more difficult. Furthermore, the professional know-how of medical staff will play a most important role regarding the extent of medical expenditures arising.

The diagnostical and therapeutical standards which have been found to be useful and necessary for the treatment of the different stages of HIV infection will have a determinative influence on length as well as frequency of hospitalisations. Another important determinant on cost development is the improvement of life quality, i.e. patients' ability to work and support themselves. Thus, in order to fight possibly occurring financial bottlenecks, it is necessary to carry out retrospective as well as prospective studies on service-expenditure development. Such a study is being done in a specialised health care institution, the AIDS Outpatient Clinic (AOC). This outpatient clinic, to which a 15-bed ward is attached, has existed since 1987. Starting in 1982, regular office hours for HIV-infected persons were offered.

The aim of the study mentioned is to investigate the expenditure necessary for the outpatient treatment of HIV infected persons with manifest illness. To this end, we shall present a study of costs of medical expenditure for an AIDS patient who was solely treated on an outpatient basis. We shall further discuss data presented in two service-cost analyses performed by the Department of Infectious Diseases Frankfurt (Koock-Walewski and Stille, 1989; Exner-Freisfeld and Helm, 1987) which evaluate medical interventions performed on patients with full-blown AIDS. After a short survey of these studies, we shall compare the respective data dealing with the expenditure for outpatients with AIDS. This means that only medical interventions performed by the AOC will be taken into account.

Cost analysis I

This study assesses medical services performed by the AOC for an outpatient under azidothymidine (AZT, zidovudine, Retrovir). The evaluation of services was based on the patient's medical record, which was analysed retrospectively until August 1988, and from then on prospectively. The registration of data was based on the charges according to the fee-for-service schedule for office-based physicians (GOÄ) as of July 1, 1988. Pharmacotherapy was calculated on the grounds of "Lauer tax", the German standard price list valid from February 1989.

Medical performances were registered separately for the following areas:
- Services carried out by an outpatient doctor
- Laboratory tests
- Diagnostic services by means of technical equipment
- General pharmacotherapy
- Anti-retroviral therapy (AZT)

Services performed by consultants from other specialities were not taken into account.

Patient's history
At first examination (17 September 1986), the 35-year-old, homosexual patient already showed slight focal symptoms (paresthesia left thigh) of toxoplasmosis of the brain which soon became clinically significant. CD4 and CD8 cell counts were significantly pathological with 126/µl and 399/µl, respectively. Thus, the patient already met the CDC criteria for full-blown AIDS at first presentation at the AOC.

The patient was treated with AZT (average dosage per day: 1 g) for 444 days. He was not hospitalised during the entire time of monitoring. The acute treatment of not very severe toxoplasm encephalitis (early 1987) was also done on an outpatient basis. The study was conducted over a period of 900 treatment days (equalling 10 treatment quarters) until the end of 1988.

Results

For services performed by doctors, laboratory tests and diagnostical services by means of technical equipment, expenditures totalled DM 17,745. In this sum, the highest amount by far was caused by laboratory tests (DM 15,233 = 86%). The total of pharmacotherapy amounts to DM 31,500, 70% of which (DM 22,200) is due to the AZT therapy over 444 days. The entire expenditure for medical services over 900 outpatient treatment days (10 quarters) had amounted to DM 49,244 - including AZT therapy - by the end of 1988. Expenditure development for the investigated treatment quarters is shown in Table 1.

The medical services carried out by consultants from other specialities, which were not included in the registration of services performed by the AOC, were: 10 neurological interventions (follow-up after cerebral toxoplasmosis), 8 dermatological interventions (diagnosis and therapy of a disseminated Kaposi's sarcoma, having occurred under AZT), 1 ophthalmological intervention due to suspected CMV retinitis, performed by the end of the last treatment quarter investigated.

Discussion I

Not unexpectedly, anti-retroviral therapy (AZT), with 70% of pharmacotherapy and 45% of total outpatient treatment costs, has a significant influence on expenditures. Also, the proportionally rather high costs for laboratory tests may be seen in connection with the monitoring of a newly introduced pharmacotherapy which causes a significant number of side effects needing treatment. In this case, however, no costs for interventions due to therapy arose. Considering that survival time after diagnosis of AIDS was more than 900 days and that the patient was treated entirely on an outpatient basis over the whole monitoring period - which is quite extraordinary - expenditures up to now do not seem unreasonably high.

An assessment of 74 medical records of patients with full-blown AIDS who had died before June 30, 1987 (Helm et al., 1987) showed a mean survival time of 25 weeks after AIDS diagnosis (the manifestation being CNS toxoplasmosis; n=9), with a minimum of 3.1 and a maximum of 77.1 weeks (=540 days). At present, it is not certain if the achieved prolongation of survival times with a rather high quality of life is partly due to improved diagnosis and therapy of opportunistic infection as well as to more adequate psycho-social care.

In this context, we should like to mention the 55 consultations in the 10 quarters and the connected medical services performed by doctors of the AOC, which, with regard to costs, hardly show in the books at all (2.2%). In spite of this, regarding substance and time consumption, they represent the most expensive medical service.

Table 1. Case example: outpatient with AZT therapy

	Laboratory test	Services by doctors	Services performed by means of technical equipment	Subtotal in DM	Pharmaco-therapy	AZT therapy	Pharma-ceutical products in DM	Total
III 86	1,137.20	28.16	-	1,165.36	-	-	-	1,165.36
IV 86	505.48	116.71	83.49	705.69	-	-	-	705.68
I 87	1,024.39	252.89	917.62	2,194.90	4,309.92	-	4,309.92	6,504.82
II 87	1,702.22	81.29	26.62	1,810.13	934.26	1,450.00	2,384.26	4,194.39
III 87	2,666.68	148.72	53.24	2,868.64	493.72	4,600.00	5,093.72	7,962.36
IV 87	2,360.37	104.50	-	2,464.87	784.20	4,550.00	5,334.20	7,799.07
I 88	1,577.51	63.91	-	1,641.42	592.72	4,550.00	5,142.72	6,784.14
II 88	1,124.40	59.40	-	1,183.80	566.20	4,200.00	4,766.20	5,950.00
III 88	1,244.15	71.39	83.44	1,398.98	771.46	-	771.46	2,170.44
IV 88	1,890.87	187.33	232.54	2,310.74	847.50	2,850.00	3,697.50	6,008.24
Total	15,233.27	1,114.30	1,396.95	17,744.52	9,299.72	22,200.00	31,499.72	49,244.24

Analysis of consultations conducted by doctors of the AOC

An unpublished study investigating "Consultations performed by doctors at the outpatient clinic - duration and substantial emphasis" (Frankfurt University Clinic, Department of Infectious Diseases) shows that doctor-patient conversations are highly time-consuming. The investigation was based on consultations of three outpatient clinic doctors who were all experienced in the treatment of HIV infected persons and was carried out during main office hours on various days.

The investigation was based on 135 consultations, 35 female and 100 male patients. 30% of the patients had AIDS, 45% PGL/ARC, and 14% were asymptomatic HIV-positive persons. In the remaining 11%, the stage of disease was unclear at the time of investigation, or patients were seronegative for HIV but lived under circumstances which put them at risk of an HIV infection. Infection risk was homosexuality in 69 patients, and anamnestic i.v. drug abuse in 52 patients. Of the remaining 14 patients, 6 were heterosexual, 6 were bisexual, 1 patient was a hemophiliac, and another patient had received an infective blood transfusion after polytrauma. Table 2 shows duration of consultation listed according to different groups of patients.

In four cases, hospitalisation right after consultation at the outpatient clinic became necessary due to acute symptoms. The reasons were:
- Necrotic scrotal lesions due to herpes
- Somnolent patient; neurological symptoms
- Icterus in stage PGL/ARC
- CMV relapse (retinitis).

In one case, an acute blood transfusion was necessary, which was carried out at the AOC.

A total of 28 so-called crisis-management consultations was registered, the average duration being 40 minutes (minimum 15, maximum 90 minutes). The most common reasons for crises were:
- Danger of suicide,
- Acute relapse into drug abuse,
- Impending psycho-social decompensation,
- Problems in connection with pregnancy,
- Progression to AIDS.

In 27 cases, patients were accompanied by a life companion, spouse, sibling, or another person helping them because they suffered from amaurosis, walking disability due to paresis, etc.

Table 2. Duration of consultation according to different groups of patients. Analysis of 135 individual consultations at AIDS Outpatient Clinic (AOC), Frankfurt University[1)]

	Time in minutes																	
	5	10	15	20	25	30	35	40	45	50	55	60	65	70	75	80	85	90	(~Ø)
Total (n = 135)	5	21	23	20	20	17	6	5	5	4	1	4	-	1	-	-	1	2	(26)
Homosexual (n = 69)	3	7	12	15	10	7	2	2	5	-	1	2	-	1	-	-	1	1	(26)
IVDA (n = 52)	2	12	9	4	9	8	1	3	-	2	-	1	-	-	-	-	-	1	(23)
Other risks (n = 14)	-	2	2	1	1	2	3	-	-	2	-	1	-	-	-	-	-	-	(30)
AZT patients (n = 57)	1	4	12	13	12	6	3	-	1	3	1	1	-	-	-	-	-	-	(24)
Follow-ups (n = 122)	4	20	23	20	20	15	6	4	3	3	1	1	-	1	-	-	-	-	(24)
Patient in crisis (n = 28)	-	-	2	2	7	4	1	2	1	2	1	3	-	1	-	-	1	1	(40)
New patients (n = 12)	(1)	(1)[2)]	-	-	-	2	-	1	2	-	-	3	-	-	-	-	1	1	(55)
Female IVDA (pos.) (n = 31)	-	8	8	3	5	4	1	1	-	1	-	-	-	-	-	-	-	-	(21)
AIDS (n = 44)	1	2	9	8	7	8	2	2	1	-	1	2	-	1	-	-	-	-	(26)
PGL/ARC (n = 44)	2	11	9	10	12	5	4	1	4	3	-	-	-	-	-		-	-	(24)
Asympt. HIV-pos. persons (n = 19)	1	4	4	2	1	3	-	1	-	-	-	1	-	-	-	-	1	1	(28)

1) Overlaps were not taken into account
2) Intensive examination later

99 patients mentioned somatic complaints, 49 patients gave psycho-social problems as reasons for their visit at AOC. This means that in more than 50% of cases, somatic as well as psycho-social reasons were given.

Patients' histories were investigated in detail in 14 cases. In 14 cases, a complete physical examination was carried out, and in 74 patients, examinations related to symptoms were performed. The latter mainly concerned examination of skin and mucosa, palpation of lymph node sites and abdomen, and percussion and auscultation of lungs.

From 67 patients, blood samples were taken, in a number of cases for extensive laboratory tests (57 of these patients were reveiving AZT). Swabs were done in 4 patients, faeces examinations for pathogens in 1 patient. In 18 patients, urinary tests were done.

12 patients were referred to a consultant specialist: 2 to a neurologist, 7 to a dermatologist, 1 to a hematologist/oncologist, and 2 to a surgeon.

In 27 cases, telephone calls by doctors had to be made. For 21 patients, short medical statements or certificates were written, 64 patients received prescriptions, and 5 patients were given a certificate of disability to work.

Medical services planned and/or carried out by means of technical equipment were: 2 rest spirographies (during consultation), 5 abdominal sonographies, 4 chest X-rays. The following table lists the medical services which are reimbursed according to the fee-for-service schedule [Gebührenordnung für Ärzte (GOÄ), 1988].

Discussion II

The average time of consultation was 26 minutes (from the time the patient entered the doctor's office to the time he left). In 5 cases, the consultations lasted only 5 minutes each; mainly these had the function of making an appointment for a later date. In 2 cases, the outpatient doctor had conversations lasting longer than 1 1/2 hours. The average duration of consultation or examination (26 minutes; minimum 5, maximum 90 min.) did not differ significantly between the members of the main risk groups:

Homosexuals: 26 min (minimum 5, maximum 90)
IVDA: 23 min (minimum 5, maximum 90).

14 patients with a risk background other than homosexuality or i.v. drugs had an average of 30 minutes' (minimum 10, maximum 60) consultation time.

Table 3. According to fee-for-service schedule for doctors (GOÄ) of July 1, 1988, the following reimbursable services were performed by doctors in 135 consultations

# GOÄ	Service	# Services	Price	Total (DM)
1a	Short information prescription	5	3.96	19.80
1	Counselling/examination < 20 min.	21	7.92	166.32
806	Crisis management > 20 min.	28	27.50	770.00
14	Short certificates, i.e. work disability	5	3.41	17.05
1b	Detailed counselling > 25 min.	66	16.50	1,089.00
65	Detailed examination	66	11.66	769.56
1b	Detailed counselling/ examination > 15 min.	43	16.50	709.50
605	Rest spirographies	2	26.62	53.24
Intermediate total: services performed by doctors during consultation				3,594.47
15	Medical statements with assessment med. letter	19	5.50	104.50
20	Written certificates	3	12.50	36.30
250	Blood tests without BSR	22	4.40	96.80
286	Blood transfusion incl. biological pre-testing	1	39.93	39.93
407	Abdominal sonographies	5	66.00	330.00
5135	Chest radiographies	4	33.00	
	Survey plus			227.48
5137	Additional radiograph		23.87	
Intermediate total: service performed by doctors in addition to consultation				835.01
Total for all services performed by doctors for 135 individual consultations				4,429.48

Time of consultation for newly admitted patients (n=12) differs significantly from the above mentioned findings: average consultation time was 55 minutes (minimum 30, maximum 90) not regarding two initial organisational conversations lasting 5 and 10 minutes.

Patients who are treated at the AOC on a regular basis (so-called follow-ups; n=122), need an average consultation time of 24 minutes (minimum 5, maximum 90). Female IVDA (n=31) have the shortest consultation times: ca. 21 minutes (minimum 10, maximum 50).

Only counselling is remarkably rare in consultations; in most cases, physical examinations and laboratory tests became necessary.

The remarkably long duration of consultations for all risk groups shows that the group of patients treated at the AOC is not comparable with the usual patients of a GP. This is also confirmed by the subjects the consultations and examinations focus on. The particular problems connected with HIV infection need a substantial infectiological know-how. Doctors must be able to diagnose opportunistic infections at an early stage and treat them adequately; they must be able to render psychological counselling; and they must have knowledge about socio-medical aspects. As we found out in our study, for a high number of patients, the outpatient doctor is one of the first places they turn to if they have questions concerning life support, impending loss of work, problems with administration (social security, application for acknowledgement of disability). Furthermore, there are groups of patients who need particular treatment, e.g. IVDA, whose addiction demands detailed knowledge. This boils down to the fact that the outpatient treatment and care of HIV-positive persons or persons at risk for HIV infection demands specialist knowledge to a high degree.

Cost study III

In 1987, still before the actual onset of anti-retroviral therapy with AZT, a service-cost analysis on ARC/AIDS patients of Frankfurt University Clinic was performed (Koock-Walewski and Stille, 1989). This study calculated care expenditure for AIDS in- and outpatients at DM 39,000.00, based on the average total costs and the mean survival time of 243 days.

According to this study, the average medical costs (inpatients and outpatients) amounted to the following sums per patient per year:

Patients with PGL/ARC:	DM 11,070.00
Patients with AIDS:	DM 26,977.00

Average hospitalisation costs:

Patients with PGL/ARC:	DM 7,917.00
Patients with AIDS:	DM 18,191.00

Average outpatient treatment costs were retrospectively calculated on the grounds of services performed for a group of 16 PGL/ARC patients and 10 AIDS patients. Consultative services from other specialities were included.

Services performed by doctors on an outpatient basis (diagnostics and therapy) were again calculated on the basis of the fee-for-service schedule (GOÄ). Pharmacotherapeutical costs were calculated according to Lauer tax.

Care expenditures amounted to the following totals per patient per year:

Patients with PGL/ARC:	DM 3,153.00
Patients with AIDS:	DM 8,786.00

This investigation does not separately list special therapies (e.g. anti-retroviral) or length and frequency of hospitalisations for outpatients.

For 10 AIDS outpatients, services performed by the AOC could be calculated separately per patient per year:

DM	391.00	medical services performed by doctors
DM	4,105.00	laboratory tests
DM	405.00	services performed by means of technical equipment
DM	2,618.00	pharmacotherapy
DM	7,519.00	per patient per year

Cost study IV

Also in 1987, the expenditures for in- and outpatient treatment (diagnostics, therapy) arising for one AIDS patient of Frankfurt University Clinic were investigated (Exner-Freisfeld and Helm, 1987). This study also considers the increasing complex of social problems and investigates social security expenditures from time of diagnosis to patient's death.

At first examination on 28 February 1986, the 26-year-old patient fell ill with pneumocystis carinii pneumonia (PCP), this disease also being the AIDS manifestation. He soon suffered a relapse, and later developed CNS toxoplasmosis. The monitoring period from AIDS diagnosis to death was 580 days.

Sickness benefits and a number of social security benefits received by the patient (he was not entitled to claims on statutory pension insurance fund) amounted to DM 23,300.00. In addition, costs for hospitalisation were also calculated. The entire medical expenditure for 269 hospital treatment days amounted to DM 46,420.68. According to survival time and number of complications in the course of disease, this individual case is in the average range of patients with manifest disease. This sum is

Table 4. Comparison of service-cost analyses of Frankfurt University Clinic: AIDS outpatients (sums in DM). AIDS Outpatient Clinic (AOC), Dept. of Internal Medicine (Prof. Stille)

	III 10 Patients (1987) outpatient treatment costs, no AZT		IV 1 Patient (1987) outpatient treatment costs, no AZT		I 1 Patient (1986-1988) only outpatient treatment + AZT	
	per pat./quart.	per pat./year	311 days	per year	900 days	per year
Services performed by doctors	102.68	391.21			1,114.30	452.60
Laboratory tests	1,077.42	4,104.97	7,782.00	9,132.00	15,233.30	6,179.45
Services performed by means of technical equipment	106.24	404.77			1,396.35	565.75
	1,286.34	4,900.96	7,782.00	9,132.00	17,744.52	7,197.80
+ 4% 1)		196.04		365.28		
		5,097.00		9,497.28		
Pharmacotherapy	687.12	2,617.93	5,262.00	6,176.00	9,299.72	3,770.45
Total		7,714.93		15,673.28	27,044.00	10,968.00
+ Azidothymidine					22,200.00 2)	18,250.00 3)
					49,244.00	29,218.00

1) Rate increase in fee-for-service schedule for doctors (GOÄ) of July 1, 1988
2) 444 days of AZT therapy (0.1g/day)
3) 365 days of AZT therapy (0.1g/day)

III Koock-Walewski (1987)
IV Exner-Freisfeld and Helm (1987)
I Gschrey-Düver (submitted)

based on the fee-for-service schedule for doctors (GOÄ). It does not include the costs for housing, catering, medical care and services performed by doctors.

Considering a calculation based on daily care expenditure rates (169 days x DM 352.65, and 100 days x DM 382.08), the entire hospitalisation costs amounted to DM 97,806.00. After subtraction of costs calculated according to GOÄ, there is a total of DM 51,385.00 for 269 days' care, housing, catering and the additional personnel expenditures. This results in DM 191.00 per day.

The outpatient treatment costs for 311 days (interrupted by 14 hospitalisations with a total of 269 days of care) amounted to DM 7,782.00 for medical care and diagnostics. The expenditures for pharmaceutics prescribed on an outpatient basis amounted to DM 5,262.00. Thus, for this individual patient there was a total outpatient cost of DM 13,044.00. The patient spent a considerable part of his survival time (46.4%) after diagnosis of AIDS in a hospital. No special anti-retroviral therapy was performed.

Finally, the different studies on cost-service relations performed at Frankfurt University Clinic were be compared with regard to AIDS outpatients (costs per patient per year).

Study III is based on data of 10 patients but does not mention any interruptions of outpatient treatment by hospitalisations. Compared with studies IV and I we estimate the lower total expenditures to be due to less service-intense treatment intervals between hospitalisations. In the calculation of total average cost, the average duration of AIDS stage is assumed to be one year. In the meantime, this assumption is outdated. A special anti-retroviral therapy is not listed, as this therapy was just about developing at the time of cost analysis.

In study IV, the monitoring period of 580 days is interrupted by hospitalisations 14 times, the total days of care being 269. Medical services performed by doctors and diagnostic services were listed together; a subtraction of consultative services for improving comparability could not be carried out. A special anti-retroviral therapy was not performed.

In study I, the monitoring period of 900 days is not interrupted by any hospitalisation. This represents quite an uncommon course of disease. The patient had been randomly chosen out of a group of AIDS patients treated with AZT; usually patients with full-blown AIDS need a number of hospitalisations per year. The anti-retroviral therapy (444 days; average dosage: 1 g/d) is listed separately.

Résumé and outlook

Looking at the three different cost studies with regard to total expenditures per patient per year, we get a rather homogeneous picture of a health care institution treating AIDS outpatients and making use of accumulated medical knowledge.

The opportunistic infections and tumors, which are very likely to occur during the course of disease in HIV-positive persons, cause extensively high medical expenditures concerning diagnosis as well as therapy.

However, the duration and frequency of expensive hospitalisations can be lowered by means of regular, professional medical monitoring of the patients. This includes laboratory tests as well as services by means of technical equipment. By these measures, complications in the course of this rather variable disease can be diagnosed early, and adequate therapies can be applied.

Early diagnosis and exact monitoring of patients which helped to improve therapeutical schemes in consequence led to an improvement of patients' life quality.

A special therapy aiming at the cause of disease by means of the anti-retroviral agent azidothymidine (AZT) was started at AOC in early 1987 (at that time as phase II study).

By this therapy, which represents a substantial cost factor in the outpatient treatment, the patients' state of health and course of disease could be significantly improved, especially during the first 200 days of treatment (Staszewski et al., 1989). On the other hand, the considerable side effects of AZT cause additional expenditures with regard to monitoring and possibly therapy (e.g. blood transfusion). AZT therapy, which in the future will be partly applied in a modified way (therapeutical intervals), will need - for reasons of medical carefulness - quite an amount of medical monitoring. This of course is also true for other, newly introduced anti-retroviral agents.

The progress in diagnostics and therapy of AIDS and associated diseases which has been achieved during the last two years, together with positive effects of AZT therapy, relieves the hospital sector. It also promotes treatment on an outpatient basis, which is preferred by most of the patients.

Due to these facts, for specialised health care institutions like the AOC, there will be the substantial problems as to financing the necessary health care services in future. Expenditures for services performed by doctors, laboratory tests and services performed by means of technical equipment were calculated by the different studies as follows:

Study III:	DM 5,100.00 per patient per year	(n=10)
Study IV:	DM 9,500.00 per patient per year	(311 days, individual care)
Study I:	DM 7,200.00 per patient per year	(900 days, individual care)

The services mentioned above are refunded according to the institutional contract between AOK Frankfurt (statutory health insurance scheme) and the University Clinic Administration (via association of statutory health insurance physicians; Kassenärztliche Vereinigung). The presently valid lump sum per treatment quarter per

HIV-positive or AIDS patient of AOC amounts to DM 330.00. This total of DM 1,320.00 per patient per year does by no means cover the actual costs.

With increasing caseload, the deficient cover will lead either to a financial gap or to a reduction of health care quality for other patients (Leidl 1988). A deficient cover seems extremely likely because an increasing number of diseases associated with HIV infection are treated on an outpatient basis. This means that severeness of disease as well as degree of complication within the individual patient's course of disease will rise significantly within the respective main health care institutions. Tendencies in accordance with this assumption have already been noted in the outpatient as well as the inpatient sector.

For these reasons, we believe that a service structure similar to one already existing and well-functioning for other chronically ill people (leukemia, renal deficiency, etc.) should also be established for HIV-infected persons. The main structures in these schemes are day-care centres, teams of experts, high-level consultative services and adequate refund for medical services for AIDS patients performed by specialists.

References

Andrulis, D.P., Beers, V.S., Bentley, J.D., and Gage, L.S. (1987). The provision and financing of medical care for AIDS patients in US public and private teaching hospitals. Journal of the American Medical Association 258(10), 1343-1346.

Exner-Freisfeld, H. and Helm, E.B. (1987). HIV-Infektion (AIDS) unter dem Aspekt des SchwbG. Deutsches Ärzteblatt 84(15), 989-993.

Exner-Freisfeld, H. and Helm, E.B. (1989). Ambulante und stationäre Kosten für Diagnostik und Therapie eines AIDS-Patienten der Frankfurter Universitätsklinik, unter Berücksichtigung der zunehmenden Sozialproblematik, einschließlich der Sozialleistungen von der Diagnosestellung bis zum Tod. Das Öffentliche Gesundheitswesen 51, 12-16, Sonderdruck.

Gschrey-Düver, I. (submitted). Ambulante medizinische Versorgung von AIDS-Patienten. Falltypische Leistungskostenanalyse.

Gebührenordnung für Ärzte (GOÄ) (1988). Stand 01.07.1988. Deutscher Ärzte Verlag, Köln.

Hanpft, R., Reinecke, F., and Beske, F. (1988). Ausgaben für und Kosten der Diagnostik und Therapie HIV-infizierter Patienten. Paper presented at: Deutscher AIDS-Kongreß, München, 8. January.

Helm, E.B., Brodt, R., Wegner, R., Staszewski, S. et al. (1987). Spontanverlauf der HIV-Infektion. Eine Bilanz 5 Jahre nach den ersten AIDS-Erkrankungen in Frankfurt/M. AIDS-Forschung 2, 567-572.

Johnson, A.M., Adler, M.W., and Crown, J.M. (1986). The acquired immune deficiency syndrome and epidemic of infection with human immunodeficiency virus: cost of care and prevention in an inner London district. British Medical Journal 293, 489-492.

Koock-Walewski, A. and Stille, W. (1989). Was kostet AIDS? Eine Kosten-Leistungs-Analyse stationärer Fälle. Schwer Verlag, Stuttgart.

Staszewski, S. et al. (1989). Langzeiterfahrungen mit Zidovudin in der Behandlung der HIV-Infektion. Vortrag auf der 95. Tagung der Deutschen Gesellschaft für Innere Medizin, Wiesbaden.

AIDS/HIV Costs in England: the Case of the Oxfordshire District

M. Rees

1. Introduction

Two main approaches have been used by the Department of Health's AIDS Costing Project to assess the cost of AIDS/HIV in England. These are patient costing through the use of patient records and hospital and district-wide costing, which aims to extract AIDS/HIV costs from the hospital or district global cost totals. Both methods have their advantages and disadvantages, which this paper will briefly discuss. The main part of the paper, however, consists of a short account of the use of the latter method in one English district, Oxfordshire.

2. Patient versus hospital-wide and district-wide costing

2.1 Patient costing

Patient costing has a number of advantages as an approach. It identifies details of AIDS patient treatment, including treatment given before the AIDS stage. It was found that early, pre-1986 diagnosed, AIDS patients at St Stephen's and St Mary's Hospitals in London had sometimes been treated as inpatients for apparently HIV-related conditions before AIDS diagnosis. Although the average number of inpatient days involved was small, a mean of about 4 days per patient, such treatment is easily to overlooked, because it was frequently given at hospitals other than the main AIDS treatment hospital. Patient costing gives a comprehensive picture of the progress of the disease, and enables costs to be attached to its different phases. It shows the extraordinary variety of AIDS patient treatment, that there is really no such thing as the typical or representative AIDS patient. The method can be used produce valuable AIDS patient statistics. For example it enables us to calculate the average length of stay per patient or per patient admission. The early London AIDS patients referred to had a cumulative length of inpatient HIV-related stay of about 91 days.

In spite of these advantages AIDS patient costing has significant disadvantages. The first is the confidentiality problem. AIDS doctors are not generally very willing to allow outsiders to look over AIDS patient records, and if they do, they demand careful supervision. Records cannot be taken out of the hospital, for example, and usually not away from the ward or clinic. The records of a particular patient may not be readily available, perhaps because they are being used for research by one of the doctors. AIDS patient costing is very time-consuming, as anyone who has ever seen the size of the medical records of such patients will appreciate. AIDS patients are the most complex of patients, with frequent readmissions and referrals. They will often have separate inpatient and outpatient records. The records may be disorganised and difficult to read, and may have omissions.

The information is usually obtained from the records of patients who have died, in order that a comprehensive picture of AIDS patient costs may be obtained. This may have the disadvantage that unrepresentative samples of patients are used, for if sampling is confined to deceased patients, those who survive for longer than average after AIDS diagnosis will tend to be omitted. Many studies of AIDS patient costs seem to have fallen into this trap. If, however, representativeness is ensured by sampling at AIDS diagnosis, some of the sample will survive for long periods, which means that it may not be possible to cost fully the sample until some years after diagnosis. This in turn will mean that the most of the patients in the sample will have died some years before the completion of the study, which will be very out-of-date by publication. This is important if treatment methods are changing, as is the case with AIDS.

There is also the problem of both describing and costing individual items of treatment. The costing of a referral, for example, should involve both a count of the number of units of treatment given, if economically sensible units exist, and also a costing for each unit. This may mean special investigations within the departments concerned to determine exactly what treatment is given to AIDS patients, the costs of a unit of treatment, and possibly a review of the treatment of individual patients, which may not be given fully in the main patient record.

Finally, and very importantly, the patient costing approach omits many important AIDS/HIV costs, such as infection control, teaching, research, some testing and counselling and administration. Although it might be possible in theory to attach such costs to AIDS patients, it would not really be the correct approach because many of these costs are not AIDS patient costs, and in any case could not be approached by means of the patient record.

2.2 Hospital or district-wide costing

This is, in theory and I believe in practice, the more comprehensive approach. By not focusing solely on patients it enables more accurate costings to be obtained for financial planning purposes. Such planners generally want an answer to the question, How much is AIDS/HIV costing now, and how much is it going to cost in the future? AIDS patient costing is usually a means to answering questions of this type rather than a goal in itself.

The hospital or district-wide approach does, however, have difficulties. There are problems in identifying departments, or individuals, that do AIDS/HIV work. This can be done from information given by those centrally involved in AIDS treatment, via leads like "so and so does this", or "I refer patients with this condition to that department". Yet clearly however wide a survey of this sort is undertaken, there is still the chance of omissions. We, for example, managed to leave out the work being undertaken by the Drug Dependency Unit on AIDS prevention at the Charing Cross Hospital in the Riverside district, not being aware of the unit's existence. It was not mentioned because everyone assumed that its work must have been known to us.

A considerable level of co-operation is required for the hospital or district-wide approach, because it involves interviewing very large numbers of people. Most people working on AIDS/HIV are very willing to give their time to help in studies of this sort, some hoping perhaps that somehow additional funding may be forthcoming. But here lies another difficulty, for a few of the more astute, or politically aware, doctors may see such costing exercises as part of the financial bargaining process, though fortunately examples of this are quite rare. Such is the usual attachment of the medical profession to accuracy, that it is normally possible to divine such manoeuvres from other statements made about their work. There are often, though, genuine difficulties in making sensible assessments of how much AIDS/HIV-related work is being done, and as time and motion study would be unrealistic, one must rely on personal statements about the use of time. This means that such assessments will frequently be very approximate.

3. General costing methodology problems

We can briefly focus on some of the main methodological problems. These are the issues of average versus marginal costs, of financial and non-financial costs, and of direct and indirect costs.

In many respects those funding AIDS/HIV work may be more interested in the marginal or incremental approach, for they wish to compensate hospitals for the additional work that AIDS/HIV entails. If the average cost criterion is used, hospitals and districts may be given what appears to be excessive funding for undertaking the new activity, which they have been able to accommodate within existing facilities. The overheads allowed might have been incurred anyway in the provision of their regular work.

There are many difficulties in adopting marginal cost criteria, however, not the least the instability of such costs over time. As time goes on marginal cost will tend to rise to meet average cost, because in the long run all costs may be regarded as variable. When the marginal approach is adopted a cost may be attached to activities arbitrarily, depending on the order in which those activities were set up. Usually the later an activity starts the less "overhead" it will have to bear, and so the less it will cost under marginal criteria. For such reasons in practice the average cost approach is the more satisfactory.

The second issue is whether the cost involved appears as part of the accounts. Take the case of a doctor who has found that he is starting to treat large numbers of AIDS patients. As he was employed before the AIDS problem started the financial implications of this may not appear in the accounts. But the cost may be borne by those other patients, whom he is now unable to see, or by the doctor himself because he is having to work harder. Harder work may be seen as a free good by the funding authority, but in extreme circumstances it can give rise to 'burn out' and other problems. There is also, naturally, the possibility that the additional patients are served through more efficient working practices, but my own view is that, in the National Health Service, there is now little slack, or X-inefficiency, as some economists grandiosely like to call it. Most of the people involved with AIDS work hard, sometimes even too hard.

AIDS time has generally been costed by estimating proportion of total paid time in a week or month spent by a member of staff on AIDS/HIV work, and multiplying by the yearly gross cost of that member of staff to obtain an estimate of the annual cost. The alternative approach, of costing hours worked at the formal hourly wage rate plus on-cost, has also been used, especially with staff who are not centrally involved with AIDS/HIV treatment. The two methods will give different results if the hours actually worked by staff differ from the hours that they are officially assumed to work. If actual hours exceed official hours, the formal cost per hour approach will give higher costs than the proportion of time approach.

The final issue discussed in this section is that of so-called direct and indirect costs. No attempt has been made to identify costs of the indirect type - the value of the people who are dying, man hours of work lost by the patients, etc. - for these costs are outside the scope of the project, which is concerned solely with health service costs and their financial implications.

4. District costing in England - districts being costed

Three of the 190 or so English districts have been selected for detailed costing.

Riverside

This is an inner London district with the largest number of AIDS cases in the UK. It contains two main teaching hospitals, the Westminster Hospital and Charing Cross Hospital, and also one of the two largest AIDS hospitals in the UK, St Stephen's Hospital. St Stephen's is about to close in order to rebuild, but although the inpatient work is to be transferred to the Westminster Hospital pro tem, much of the day patient and outpatient work is scheduled to remain on the St Stephen's site. Riverside was costed in 1987/8.

Oxfordshire

This district is centred on Oxford. So far there are only a small number of AIDS cases, but the district has the largest haemophilia centre in the UK, with about 10% of all UK haemophiliacs. The district has made considerable efforts in AIDS prevention and education. It is also a teaching district and highly involved in AIDS/HIV research. Oxfordshire was costed in 1988/9.

Brighton

This district has about the largest AIDS problem in England and Wales of any district outside London. The reason for this is the proximity of Brighton to the capital, and its popularity with homosexuals. It also has a substantial drug problem. The costing of the district has just started, following agreement with the district authorities. It will be costed at 1988/9 price levels.

5. Particular costing problems in Oxfordshire

To illustrate the district-wide costing approach, the case of Oxfordshire has been selected.

There are special difficulties in the costing of AIDS/HIV in this district, most of which arise because of the particular nature of AIDS/HIV treatment in haemophiliacs.

Additional Factor VIII costs

Haemophiliacs are given Factor VIII as a blood clotting agent, and indeed it was their need for this that caused many haemophiliacs to become infected with HIV. About 130 HIV-positive haemophiliacs are treated by the Oxford Haemophilia Centre, although half of these actually live outside the Oxford Region. HIV infection does not of course cause haemophilia, but if haemophiliacs become infected with HIV they make exceptional demands on the health care system, because their HIV must be monitored intensively in relation to the underlying haemophilia condition. They frequently have severe social and emotional problems, and may also increase the administrative load for various reasons. Non-infected haemophiliacs are now monitored less frequently, because the Haemophilia Centre has had to divert time from them to those who are HIV positive. The haemophiliac AIDS patients, of which in January 1989 there were 7 at the Oxford Haemophilia Centre, also take a great deal of time and effort.

One special problem is the substantial increases in the cost of Factor VIII over the last four years, because of the need to heat-treat the blood to destroy the virus, because slightly more now has to be used for the same clotting effect, and because additional amounts are now given to HIV positives in order to avoid bleeds. Further, and this is the main reason for Factor VIII cost increases, the price has risen considerably, not only because of the cost of heat treatment but also because of a world-wide blood shortage.

Chronic hepatitis in HIV-positive patients

A number of haemophiliacs suffer from chronic hepatitis, which is treated at the Liver Unit at the John Radcliffe Hospital. It is a contentious issue as to whether this should be regarded as HIV related, although all the patients so suffering in Oxford over the past few years have been HIV positive. These patients, however, are very similar to AIDS patients, and they have picked up their hepatitis from contaminated blood. Their hepatitis-related condition and eventual death would result in a "saving" in AIDS costs if these costs were not included. The costs of these patients have therefore been included in the study.

Surgery on haemophiliacs

Haemophiliacs sometimes require surgery, after bleeding into the joints. Most of such surgery is on HIV-positive patients, because the more severely affected haemophiliacs were given greater quantities of Factor VIII than those less severely affected, and so were more likely to become infected with HIV. Only the additional costs associated with HIV infection were taken into account in the study.

Additional abortion costs

Abortions in Oxford have risen from about 100 to 170 a month over the last year. The increase is in young, under 25, unmarried women. Opinion in the district is that this is an unanticipated consequence of the strenuous AIDS prevention effort at the national and at the district/city level. Young women are coming off the pill because of fear of HIV infection, and condoms are a less reliable means of contraception. The costs of these abortions have not been included in the totals below, but might have been.

6. Estimated AIDS/HIV costs in Oxfordshire in 1988/9

These costs are given in Table 1. Total district revenue expenditure in Oxfordshire in 1988/9 will be about £133 millions. Estimated district AIDS/HIV revenue expenditure is nearly £1.6 millions, or about 1.2% of total district expenditure. This total is nearly double previous estimates. The difference is because of the average cost method, which includes overheads, and because of the more accurate identification of costs.

Table 1. Estimated AIDS/HIV costs in the Oxfordshire District by hospital unit (1988/9)

Hospital	Main HIV function	Estimated expenditure £000s	Expenditure in %
Radcliffe Infirmary	HIV outpatients	234	13.1
Churchill Hospital	Haemophilia, AIDS inpatients	996	55.9
John Radcliffe Hosp.	Pathology, some AIDS outpatients	208	11.7
Warneford Hospital	Psychiatry	94	5.3
Littlemore	Drug abuse	90	5.0
Nuffield Orthopaedic	Operations, dentistry	74	4.2
Other	Miscellaneous	86	4.8
Total		£1,782	100.0

Note: Totals include some non-NHS expenditure.

Over half the costs are incurred at the Churchill Hospital, which contains the Haemophilia Centre and the AIDS Inpatient Ward. A further 25% are incurred at the Radcliffe Infirmary and the John Radcliffe Hospital, which contain most of the HIV outpatient work and the pathology, respectively.

Table 2 gives the same cost total broken down by client/activity group. These divisions contain elements of arbitrariness but probably give a reasonable overall picture. It is particularly interesting that in Oxfordshire only about 16% of total costs is incurred in the treatment of AIDS patients alone. Hence a costing that focused on these patients

Table 2. Estimated AIDS/HIV costs in Oxfordshire by client group and activity (1988/9)

Client/activity group	Expenditure £000s	Expenditure in %
Haemophiliac AIDS	98	5.5
Haemophiliac HIV	191	10.7
Additional Factor VIII	453	25.4
Other AIDS	206	11.6
Other HIV	86	4.8
Drug misuse	98	5.5
Infection control	123	6.9
Counselling/testing/admin	276	15.5
Research/teaching	251	14.1
Totals	£1,782	100.0

Table 3. Unit cost per year results for Oxfordshire

1.	Haemophiliac AIDS patients, excluding F VIII	£14,000
2.	Other AIDS patients	£17,000
3.	All HIV + haemophiliacs inc. AIDS exc. F VIII	£2,800
4.	Non-treatment costs per head of population, exc. research	£1

would have missed 84% of total AIDS/HIV costs. Oxfordshire is doubtless an unusual district in this respect; in Riverside, which is similar in size to the Oxfordshire district but with over 6 times the numbers of AIDS patients at the time of costing, nearly 60% of total costs were calculated as related to AIDS patient work.

Haemophiliac costs, excluding research and teaching, but including haemophiliac counselling etc., are 42% of total costs. An interesting percentage, 7%, is that for infection control. Oxfordshire has made stringent efforts in this direction over the past two or three years.

Unit costs are given in Table 3. Unit costs per year for non-haemophiliac AIDS patients are about £17,000. It is based on only 12 patients, but is very similar to the figure for Riverside for 1987/8, which was based on 120 AIDS patients. The non-factor costs of haemophiliac AIDS patients is slightly lower, at about £14,000. Although AIDS patients seem to live on average less than 18 months, the mean cost of an AIDS patient in the UK from diagnosis to death is probably at least 1.5 times the £17,000 figure, because currently patients are weighted towards the initial, and hence less treatment intensive, part of the disease. AIDS patient numbers are growing, which means that more recently diagnosed patients are entering than deceased patients are leaving.

It is also worth noting that the non-treatment costs, excluding research, in Oxfordshire work out at about £1 per head of population in the district. These costs are incurred on providing HIV drug misuse services, infection control, counselling, administration and prevention. If such services were provided nationally to Oxfordshire per capita levels the cost would be about £50 millions.

7. Conclusions

The method of district-wide costing gives comprehensive estimates of AIDS/HIV costs in single districts and is probably to be preferred to AIDS patient costing using patient records. Many of the district-wide costs are not associated with AIDS patient, and even HIV-positive patient, treatment. Although the results from a single district cannot be generalised readily to other districts, it is hoped that the results from a number of districts will give a reasonable picture of the overall situation. But even the results from this single district indicate that AIDS/HIV costs can be considerably higher than previously thought.

The Regional Costs of AIDS in Spain

J. Ginestal Gómez

This paper has, as its main target, a short-term forecast of hospital resources needed for AIDS patients. For this we shall use the data available up to April 1989. The bulk of the problem consists in using, as efficiently as possible, the few data that are so far available, as this is the first work on that subject made in the Basque Country (and in Spain).

Work on the problem at stake is relevant for two reasons: First it can give a good idea to health authorities of the resources used by AIDS at present (and probably in the near future). Second, a forecast of physical resources needed in the short run, with a fixed supply of hospital beds, can be at least as important as money costs.

It is only with such information that the near future can be planned. This, however, does not imply an agreement with the "status quo" of care pattern; it only implies the likely impact of that "status quo" in terms of physical resources. Therefore the trade-offs betwen different group of illnesses can be assessed properly. Moreover, a rough attempt to evaluate those resources in terms of money is offered. But, due to lack of relevant data, the estimation of costs can only be an approximation.

The paper will be divided into several sections. The first section will give a brief description of AIDS in the Basque Country, as of March 1989. Some simple forecasts will be made in the second section and in the third a very rough cost study will be found. The final section will deal with some resources forecast.

1. Overview

AIDS is a difficult problem as it involves habits of an affected/at risk population. Therefore, the spread of the HIV is not decreasing at a rate one would expect once the ways of transmission are known. This is particularly the case for those areas in which the main focus of infection are drug abusers. Such a situation is the one faced in the Basque Country.

At a first glance, it is 74.3% of the 362 AIDS cases (registered as of April 1989) that correspond to the i.v. drug users group. However, if we include all those cases related to that group (i.e. people infected by drug abusers or drug abusers with another risk activity), the figure would approach 82%. Regarding age and sex, patterns are very similar to other countries: 79.28% of the cases are male, and their average age is 26.9 years.

The trend followed by the infection does not follow the same pattern for every risk group. As should be expected, drug abusers (and related groups) are growing faster than the remaining groups, the growth rate of which is, in fact, declining.

Survival time has been steadily growing over the past years; this is mainly due to two factors. First, illness is diagnosed earlier and, second, the treatment with AZT is progressing. Considering the last cohorts only and assuming that the median equals the mean (Fig. 1), the average survival time is now around 15 months. A proper survival analysis has not been carried because of the small sample. Regrettably, this problem will only take a short time to disappear.

2. Projections

As we have mentioned before, our target is to set a framework to study hospital resources as referred to AIDS. Therefore projections become a key issue if one is to calculate the likely impact of AIDS on hospital resource allocation.

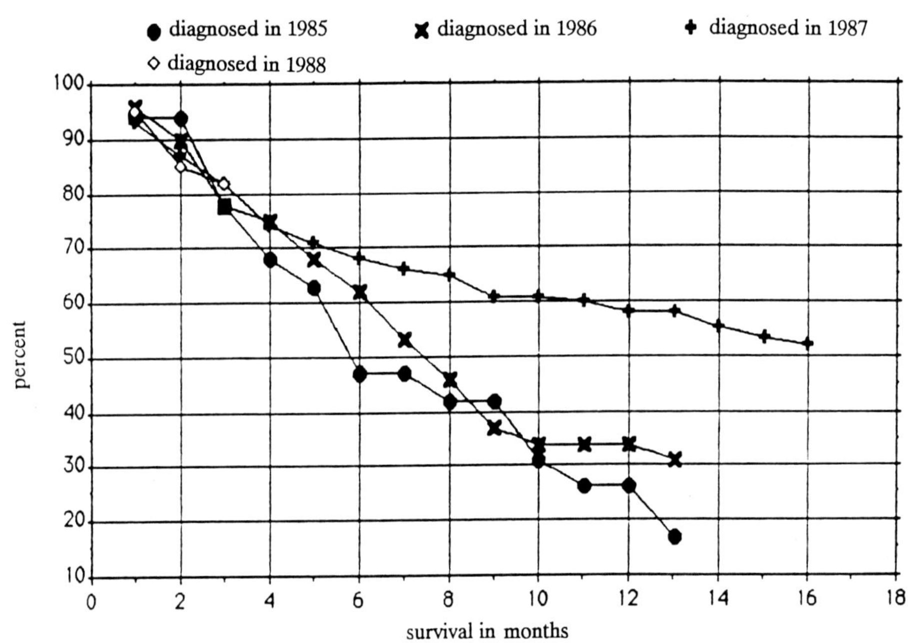

Fig. 1. Survival curve of AIDS cases

At this stage, we have not considered complex mathematical and statistical models. This is for two reasons: First, there is a lack of suitable data both in quantity and quality; secondly, those models have performed relatively poorly at predicting. Although more complex models are more suited to interpret and contrast theories, experience points to the fact that simple models are far more accurate in short-run predictions. Hence, we will only show here an exercise for very simple regression models, which are basically nothing but "trend finders", i.e. by regressing the number of cases against time (under different functional forms), one tries to capture the underlying trend, at least in the short-run. We have tried several models, and the best performance has been shown by the simplest models, particularly linear and log-linear ones. These results have been interpreted as a confirmation of our initial hypothesis, namely that we are at the begining of the explosive period.

Two considerations have to be made, however: First, since it is hoped that the trend will eventually change, these figures will have to revised periodically; in addition we will try more complete models, those which weight observations according to their location in time, to adapt the model of changes in the trend (MA), and those which incorporate changes in the pattern (logistic family). However, up to now, the performance of the alternatives mentioned has been relatively poor (probably indicating a consistent pattern). Second, patterns are quite different for different risk groups, as was indicated above; so we will have to keep record of isolated groups, especially drug abusers[1].

Data are in themselves a problem, particularly because of lags in recording. In our case, the last three observations cannot be considered as they will change substantially in the years to come. There are some techniques to deal with this problem by correcting these data to the likely final figures. However, previous information has been consistently substituted by the updated one, so that the actual records only retain the last figure. Hence, it is impossible to estimate the lag pattern. A serious implication of that lack of information is the need to predict (!) the past. For our exercise we have included fifteen observations only (from March 1985 to September 1988), although the last observation was March 1989.

We have to stress that, although some luck has to be taken into account, previous documents have predicted the figures for June 1988 and September 1988 quite accurately. Results for the linear and explosive model (semi-logarithmic) are presented below because of their good performance. Quarterly evolution of cases is shown as well (Table 1).

1) Results for isolated groups are available at request.

Table 1. The quarterly evolution of the AIDS cases

	Quarter	Cases observed	predicted ln (1+x)	predicted (linear trend)
1	1	4	-	-
2	2	6	-	-
3	3	4	-	-
4	4	13	-	-
5	5	9	-	-
6	6	11	-	-
7	7	13	-	-
8	8	16	-	-
9	9	20	-	-
10	10	21	-	-
11	11	21	-	-
12	12	24	-	-
13	13	31	-	-
14	14	28	-	-
15	15	-	40	31
16	16	-	46	33
17	17	-	53	35
18	18	-	61	37
19	19	-	70	39
20	20	-	80	41

3. Cost considerations

The exercise in this section corresponds to hospital costs for 1987 only. These costs are calculated, as we shall see, in a very rough way and only for full AIDS patients. Any-how, such an exercise is a relevant one to delimit the necessary information, apart from being an approximation to the real costs. Of course, its being a rough measure is due to the lack of data; so the main point of the exercise was not only to decide what data should be collected but also how. This point is not a trivial one since lack of data is due to a negative predisposition by hospitals and physicians.

At first we will set the main direct costs involved. Such costs accrue at:
- Hospitals (inpatient)
- Outpatient facilities
- Primary care facilities
- Other services (psychiatric, social, etc.)
- Community and family care

To calculate the full total, one would need a flow chart (see Fig. 2) of patterns of care, which would tell us, for different types of people, the average frequencies of attendancy at the different medical facilities. Once these frequencies are converted into units, the problem is to calculate the cost of each unit.

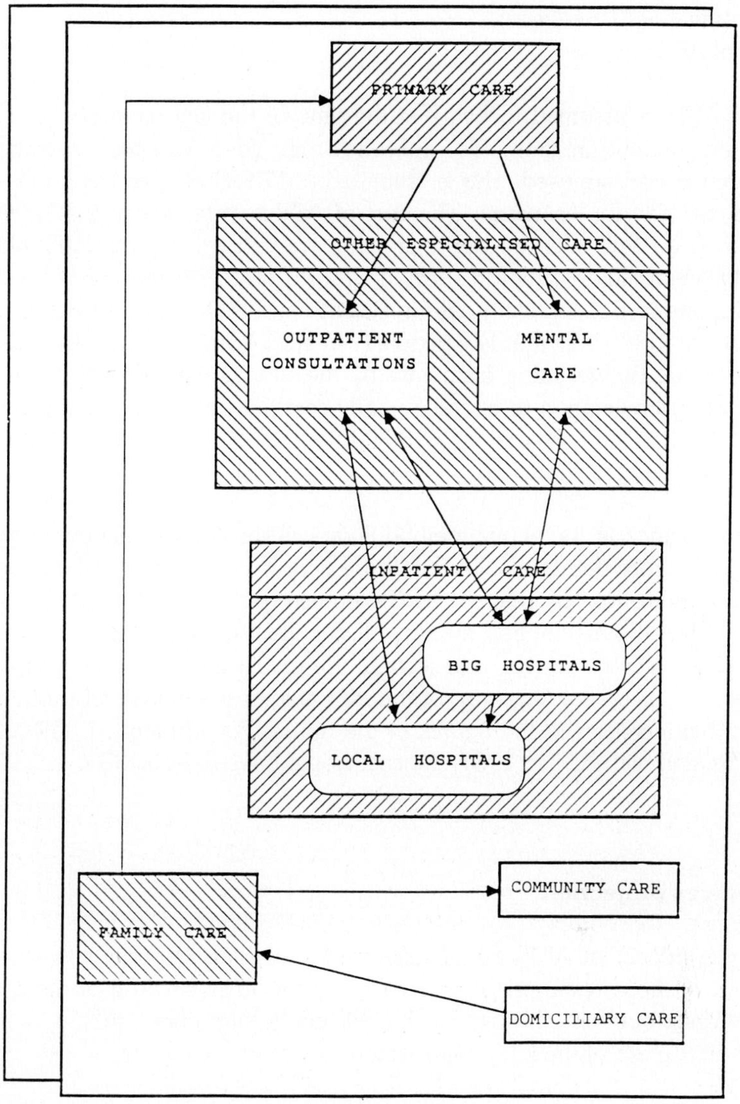

Fig. 2. Patterns of care

At present, given the available data, this exercise is not possible at all. Therefore we have calculated, for one year (1987), inpatient cost only, taking data available. This could be taken as a bottom limit for costs. Our data refer to two hospitals (Aránzazu and Basurto), the only ones with (few) available records. The record contains the following information:

- Number of inpatient spells
- Number of inpatient days each time

- Patients with AZT treatment
- Costs of AZT.

Full blown AIDS is assumed to begin at the time of the first inpatient spell, which is probably an underestimation. To approach the costs roughly, average current expenditure per bed are used. This is estimated at 17,920 pts per day for Basurto and 20,824 pts per day for Aránzazu. The cost of AZT is estimated at 1,300,000 pts per patient per year. With such an approximation we can calculate 17,100,000 pts and 21,150,000 pts of AIDS costs for 1987 in Basurto and Aránzazu respectively. These costs correspond to 811 inpatient days in Basurto and 890 days in Aránzazu. We have to take account for the fact that few people (2 in each hospital) were being treated with AZT at that time. By weighting each case by the survival period within that year, we can have an approximation to average yearly cost per patient. Once the weighting is performed, such a cost results in 2,736,000 pts in Basurto and 2,500,000 pts in Aránzazu per patient per year.

Even a short glance at the above methodology will show the weakness of the results. However, until more data are collected, those figures provide hospital managers with, at least, an indication of real costs. Two main points are distorting the results downwards. First the assumption that an AIDS patient consumes the same amount of resources as an average patient, and second, the small number of patients treated with AZT. Moreover, given the big share of the AZT cost in the individual's total cost, one can expect big increases of the figures in the future. For instance, if 30% of patients had been treated with AZT in 1987, the cost would have risen by 38% or 31% in each hospital.

4. Resources projection

To know the impact of AIDS on hospital resources is as important as to know the money costs of those resources. Again many caveats arise because of the quality and quantity of data, but then, this approach is still better than pure intuition, and it would give us a better grasp of the information needed .

The data used are the ones of the projections in the second section, of the expected survival (15 months as previously stated) and of average use of facilities per year in outpatient as well as inpatient visits. For outpatient visits, the mean in the Basque Country is 4.5 (calculated from treatment protocols and confirmed as an average use). For days of hospital bed occupation, our sample shows 5, 5, 12, 12 and 14 days for each term of survival as average. Now it only remains to apply the survival time both to the known cases and to future (projected) cases to obtain a projection of the likely future resources used by AIDS patients.

The results are shown in Fig. 3a and 3b; Fig. 3b shows the results for a 10% decrease in the average inpatient and outpatient care per patient. In Fig. 3a, 2,000 bed days are predicted to be occupied by AIDS patients in the Basque Country in the first quarter of 1990. Similarly, near 1,000 outpatient consultations will be required in that period. Notice that these figures double those for the last quarter of 1988 (the first predicted quarter). A straightforward conclusion would be the necessity to shift away the bulk of AIDS care from hospitals, lest these become completely congested. Apart from that, most qualified opinions point to the fact that alternative care would improve the patients' well-being anyway.

5. Conclusions

This is the overall work we are trying to complete. The need is not only to update averages and projections but to make them more accurate. To do the latter we would need better data. To achieve the former, the use of scenarios and more suitable statistical techniques seem to be the obvious path. This too, however, depends crucially on data.

This framework is to be taken as a flexible one, for more data and more satisfactory methodology will have to be implemented within it, and changes in the AIDS patterns are to be expected. These changes refer not only to epidemiological trends but also to

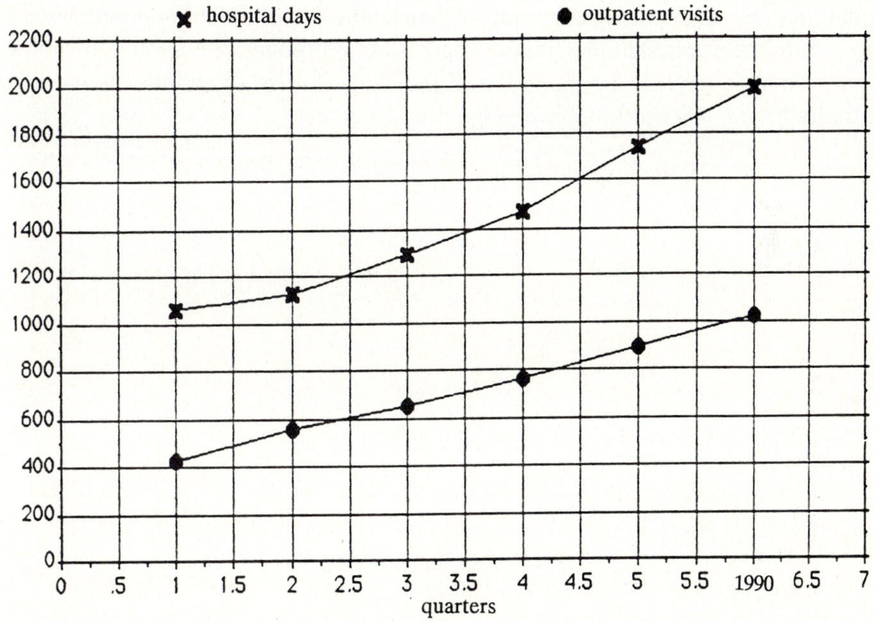

Fig. 3a. Predicting hospital days and outpatient visits; standard

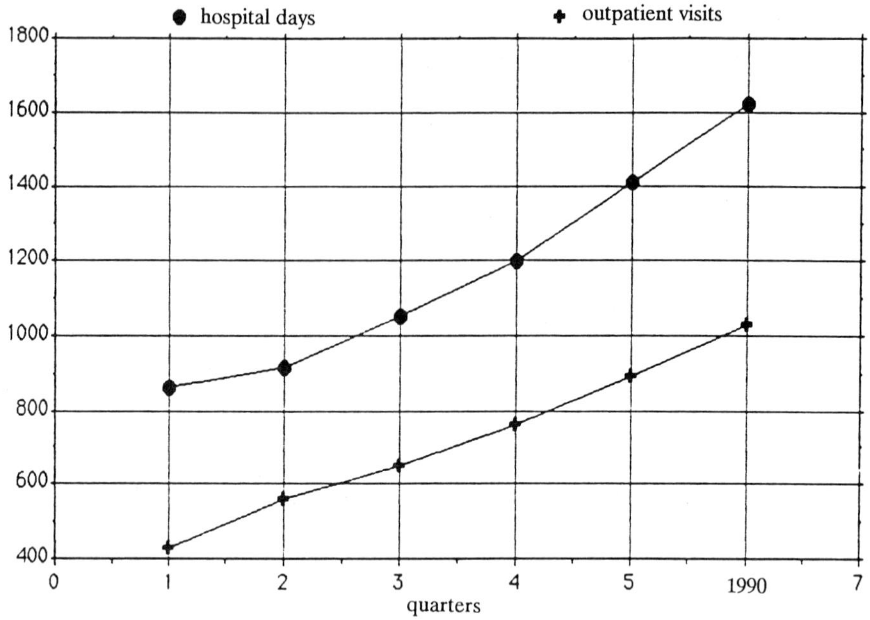

Fig. 3b. Predicting hospital days and outpatient visits; 10% decrease in inpatient and outpatient care

care patterns. The epidemiological trends will make the use of the more adaptative and complete statistical forecasting techniques necessary. Moreover, the evolution of those trends (as we have already mentioned) and the likely change of attitudes towards the illness in the future, will presumably change the care pattern.

Indicators and Trends of Direct and Indirect Costs of AIDS on a National Level: Results from Switzerland

M.R.H. Pedergnana

1. Introduction

1.1 Problem

The epidemic of acquired immune deficiency syndrome (AIDS) will be severe in Switzerland. Although there has been a swift and comprehensive nationwide prevention programme since February 1987, which slowed down the new infection rate, the Federal Office of Public Health (FOPH) in Switzerland estimates from a wide variety of epidemiological data that between 20,000 and 30,000 persons are infected with the human immunodeficiency virus (HIV) (FAC and FOPH, 1989, 7). Cumulative estimates range from 9,000 to 15,000 persons with AIDS (PWAs) until the end of 1995 (FAC and FOPH, 1989, 7; Pedergnana et al., 1988, 42-47). Since the beginning of the AIDS epidemic, there have been 702 PWAs reported up to December 31, 1988 (FAC and FOPH, 1989, 18).

Are there enough resources (hospital beds, hospital personnel, etc.) to cope with between 5,000 and 10,000 PWAs in 1995? Who will pay the cost? Can Swiss health care insurers afford to pay (their share of) the costs for treating PWAs? Does AIDS threaten the solvency of Swiss life insurers? How high will the direct and indirect costs be? How large is the projected social burden of illness and premature death due to AIDS and HIV infection relative to other diseases? How much will AIDS influence overall medical care expenditures across the nation until 1995?

In this study, the questions outlined above are investigated by combining epidemiological projections with data from a multi-center medical care cost study and with data from various other studies. Furthermore, we inquire whether factors other than inpatient treatment are of prime importance for medical care costs.

Switzerland has for many reasons a unique, decentralized health care system. All acute care beds are in purely state- or community-run nonprofit hospitals, whose capacities are approved by the majority of voters in a given state or community. Hospitals provide expensive and sophisticated care. Public financing of inpatient care via taxes and low per diem reimbursements for federally subsidized health insurance plans are further characteristics in a country where more than 98% of the population are members of the so-called social (and nonprofit) health care insurance co-operatives.[1)]

The main problem is that, due to the lack of effective incentives, health care expenditures have been rising with an average growth rate of 10% for the last 25 years. Economists seriously doubt whether the efficiency and effectiveness of the health care system has been improving during the same period (Sommer and Gutzwiller, 1986).[2)] In such a system, AIDS is an additional factor intensifying the current illness of the Swiss health care system.

1.2 Objective, assumptions and procedure

This paper presents the results of a comprehensive, two-year-long study on the influences of AIDS on the Swiss health care system. We try to summarize trends and indicators of direct and indirect costs of AIDS in Switzerland in the near future. As a time-horizon, we have chosen the end of 1995 because the economic impact of AIDS in Switzerland has become fairly predictable for the next six years.

We have tried to consider changes in diagnostic and therapeutic technology and experience, and based our study on four assumptions. As do many experts, we too believe that, first, there will be no drug available to cure AIDS or to prevent an HIV infected person from developing AIDS until at least the mid-1990s. Second, we expect a prolonged life expectancy from diagnosis to death of PWAs. Third, we assume that no vaccine against HIV infection will be on the market until 1995. Fourth, we assume that FOPH's estimate of 20,000 to 30,000 HIV infected persons in Switzerland is correct.

The purpose of the second section is to give up-to-date epidemiological information and indications of the possible outcome of the AIDS epidemic until 1995. In the third section, we will have a look at the cost dimension to present an order of magnitude of the economic impact of AIDS on the Swiss health care system, and we glance at those who have to bear the costs.

2. Epidemiological aspects of AIDS in Switzerland

We present the descriptive epidemiology of AIDS and HIV infection in Switzerland based on data up to December 31, 1988. All data are from the FOPH, which is responsible for national AIDS surveillance and epidemiology as well as prevention and education programmes on a national level.

---

1) Health Maintenance Organizations (HMOs), Preferred Provider Organizations (PPOs), Diagnosis Related Groups (DRGs) and other alternative insurance models are all forbidden in Switzerland.

2) Medical care is more likely to produce improvements in so-called subjective components of health rather than improvements in morbidity and mortality rates. In Switzerland, one typically buys more caring, but little additional curing.

2.1 HIV epidemic in Switzerland

As a result of several investigations and evaluations, and based on 10,279 confirmed seropositive tests (34.4% in the Canton Zurich, 17.5% in the Canton Geneva), the FOPH estimates that 15% or 15,000 of the estimated number of homosexual or bisexual male population and 50% or 7,500 of the estimated number of IV drug users are HIV infected. While the new infection rate has practically come to a standstill among homo- and bisexual men, the FOPH believes that HIV is still spreading among IV drug users (FAC and FOPH, 1989, 14-25).

2.2 AIDS epidemic in Switzerland

Not surprisingly, given the data on the HIV epidemic, the number of newly diagnosed AIDS cases has increased substantially since 1982 (see Fig. 1). Table 1 describes the patient groups of AIDS cases, indicating a large majority of homo- and bisexual men,

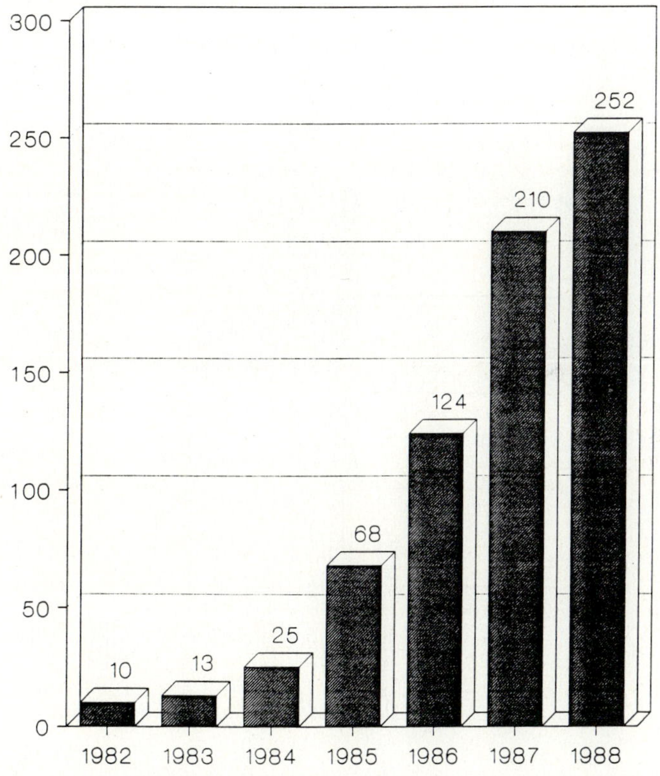

Fig. 1. AIDS cases per year of diagnosis in Switzerland

Table 1. Reported AIDS cases in Switzerland

Homo- or bisexual men	384	(54.7%)
IV drug user (m: 131; f: 65)	196	(27.9%)
Heterosexuals in contact with HIV infected people (m: 31; f: 32)	63	(9.0%)
Children, hemophiliacs, transfusion and others (m: 35; f: 24)	59	(8.4%)
Total on December 31, 1988	702	

and a rapidly increasing proportion of IV drug users. Fig. 2 shows the 702 AIDS cases (33.6% in the Canton Zurich, 13.0% in the Canton Geneva) by sex and age. 71% of the AIDS cases are in the range of 15 - 44 years (FAC and FOPH, 1989, 14-25). Though we cannot draw stringent conclusions for the whole population, it is interesting (and relevant for indirect costs) that among PWAs, men are older than women, mainly because homosexual men are older than IV drug users.

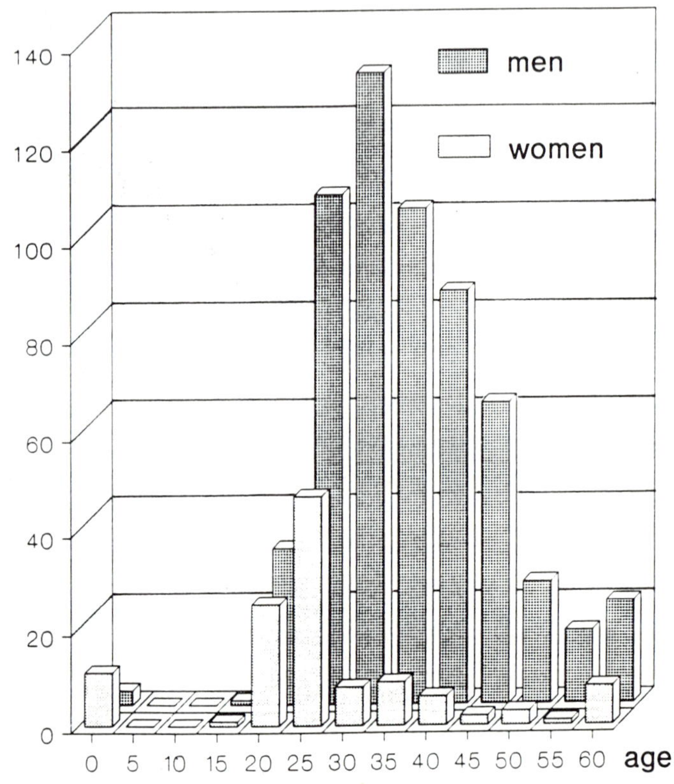

Fig. 2. Age distribution of AIDS cases by sex in Switzerland

2.3 Forecasts

Every forecast is made uncertain by unknown factors (number of HIV infected people, time of infection, incubation time). Nevertheless, estimates of the likely progress of the epidemic are necessary because there must be thorough planning of care for those infected, those with manifestations and those dying.

The further development of the HIV epidemic is uncertain, but the relatively low number of confirmed seropositive test results (835) (FAC and FOPH, 1989, 18) in 1988 gives hope that the nationwide, concerted, vigorous and sustained STOP AIDS preventive campaign has been very effective so far. FOPH epidemiologists estimate with sophisticated statistical and epidemiological modeling that cumulatively between 13,000 and 15,000 PWAs have to be expected at the end of 1995 (FOPH, 1988, 539-542). Earlier estimates (Pedergnana et al., 1988, 33-51) range from 9,000 (optimistic case) to 15,000 (pessimistic case), with the probable estimate of 12,000 PWAs. In order to estimate the impact of AIDS on health care institutions, we have to be more precise and take into account a slowly increasing average life expectancy of a PWA from currently 15 months to 24 (pessimistic), 36 (probable) and 48 (optimistic) months by 1995 (Pedergnana et al., 1988, 40-42). These three estimates were combined with three differently increasing life expectancy rates, but in this paper we will concentrate on what we consider the most probable estimate of all: we expect 6,800 living PWAs (2,500 diagnosed in 1995, and 4,300 diagnosed earlier) at the end of 1995 (Fig. 3).

To assess the direct and indirect costs per year, it was necessary to divide all PWAs into three patient groups:

Group 1: Those who were newly diagnosed and did not die;

Group 2: Those diagnosed in a prior year who lived all 12 months;

Group 3: Those who died during the year (we applied the same methodology as the one described in Scitovsky et al., 1986, I-1).

Group 4: was drawn for better understanding of the first half of the probably S-like epidemic of cumulative AIDS cases (Fig. 3).

Some Swiss epidemiologists believe that the HIV epidemic is reduced to the original risk groups (male homosexuals and IV drug users) and has not affected the heterosexual population. They question the current estimates of the FOPH that there are 20,000 to 30,000 HIV infected people and criticize the prevention program that started in 1987 and was first addressed to the broad heterosexual population instead of high-risk groups (Pedergnana et al., 1988, 98). We believe that according to today's knowledge, such doubts can be justified. But we should also take into account and prepare for the worst possible case.

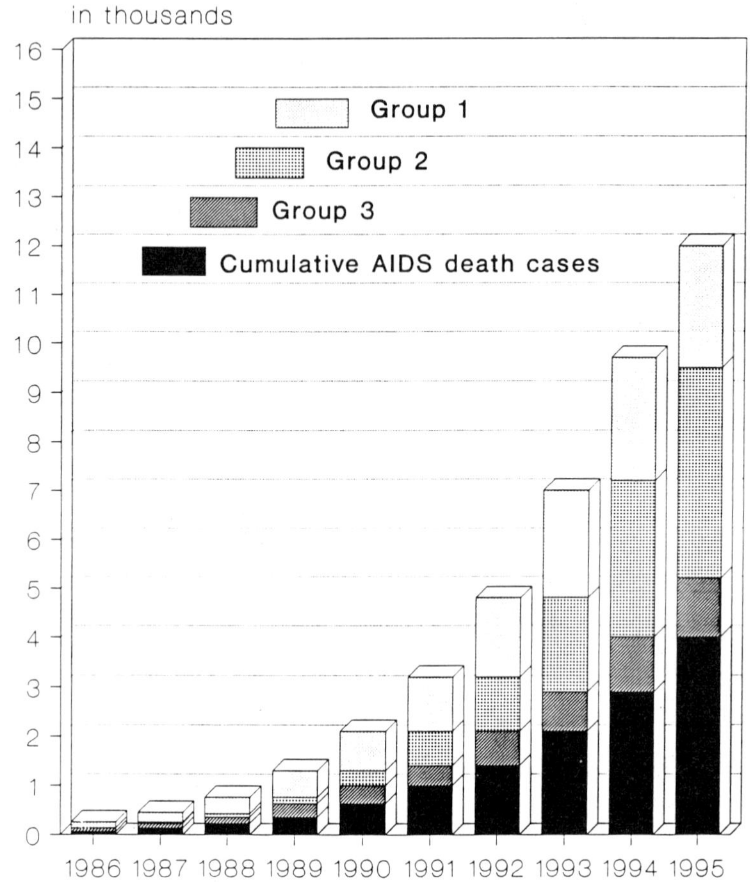

Fig. 3. Best estimate of AIDS epidemic in Switzerland

3. The cost dimension

Total costs of AIDS comprise direct, indirect, and intangible costs. The latter are costs not measured in money: We think in this context of the grave psychic load and the personal grief of all people concerned with AIDS. There was especially great concern about high direct costs. The indirect costs of this fatal disease, however, are many times greater, because 75% of all PWAs in Switzerland are between 20 and 50 years old and belong to a highly productive age group that had enjoyed low morbidity and mortality rates up to now.

The major impediment to data collections and cost analyses (all estimates are in 1988 constant Sfrs.) concerning the AIDS epidemic in Switzerland was a strong skepticism towards health economics. Nevertheless, we are now able to give fairly exact data on direct costs of the HIV epidemic and rather good indicators of indirect costs for 1986 through 1988.

3.1 Direct costs

Direct costs are the costs of health and social care including both personal care and nonpersonal services like screening of blood donations, voluntary serostatus testing, prevention and information programmes, health education, staff training, research and various support services. Our estimates are prevalence-based, because they proved to be very useful for hospital and federal budget planning (compare Scitovsky et al., 1986, IV-1). Unlike in incidence-based estimates where all medical care costs are attributed to the year in which the patient was diagnosed, with the prevalence-based approach we estimate the costs (and need for resources) for a given year. This is especially important when estimates are made for a still young disease where diagnostic and therapeutic experience is growing fast, and life expectancy from diagnosis to death is very likely to increase significantly within a few years.

3.1.1 Personal treatment costs

An investigation carried out at three University hospitals in Switzerland (Zurich, Basel, and Lausanne; all of them having outpatient departments) showed that patterns of health service use and treatment costs of PWAs are similar. 104 PWAs or about 30% of all PWAs who had been treated between 1982 and 1988 and who had died before summer 1988 were selected for costing research (Table 2). In a retrospective analysis, detailed data on inpatient and outpatient treatment were abstracted from the medical

Table 2. Personal health care costs of people with AIDS in Switzerland (in 1988 Sfrs.)

Hospital	n	Inpatient days	Range	Cost per day	Station. care cost	Ambul. care cost	Lifetime costs
CHUV[a]	26	63.5	6-156	722	46,200	1,600	74,000
UHB[b]	18	59.4	6-187	900	53,500	5,700**	59,200*
USZ_1[c]	44	57.0	3-293	753	42,900	15,000**	57,900*
USZ_2[d]	16	39.9	1-119	753	30,000	27,400**	57,400*
Total	104	56.5	1-293	772	43,600	11,900	74,000

Source: a Griffiths et al. (1988)
b Rufli et al. (1989)
c AIDS-Kommission des Kantons Zürich (1988)
d Amberg and Pedergnana (1989)

* These costs are not lifetime costs since only the medical history of the patients' main hospital could be considered. They include no institutional care in other acute hospitals, psychiatric clinics, nursing homes or hospices.

** Only ambulatory care provided by the outpatient departments of UHB and USZ were considered.

records of each patient and costed, using 1988 tariff scales intended in principle to cover full current (hospital budget) running costs. Capital costs and amortization costs are included; drugs were costed at hospital prices (20% below market prices). In all analyses, costs incurred following a confirmed full-blown AIDS diagnosis (following CDC definition) were considered. The majority of the patients analyzed were diagnosed in the years 1985 and 1986 (range 1982-1987). There were no substantial methodologic differences among the four studies.

A prevailing trend in these data could not be found. The average number of days per case has stayed fairly stable since the start of the epidemic. Institutional utilization and inpatient costs per case did not drop significantly.

Estimated lifetime costs of PWAs in Switzerland are 74,000 Sfrs., including ambulatory care, inpatient acute care, chronic care in hospices and custodial facilities (e.g. for dementia) and the various forms of extensive outpatient support. The data do not consider time costs of the patients. The value of the services provided by family members, friends and others in support of the person's basic activities of daily living is also not included. Though unpaid, these services nevertheless represent a real consumption of resources, and hence a real cost.

The CHUV study is the only one in Switzerland analyzing the whole medical history of AIDS patients. The 26 PWAs spent an average of 92.9 days in institutional care (range 23-226 days):
63.5 days in the CHUV (range 6-156 days),
9.0 days in other acute hospitals (range 0-113 days),
13.7 days in psychiatric clinics (range 0-156 days), and
6.7 days in nursing homes (range 0-61 days).

At 722 Swiss francs per day - just one patient was treated in an intensive care unit - total inpatient costs amounted to an average of 67,000 Swiss francs. According to the authors, it seems reasonable to suppose that the total costs of all medical and home care, from diagnosis to death (lifetime costs), of PWAs treated at the CHUV as their main, but not only hospital, were 74,000 Sfrs (Griffiths et al., 1988, 4).

The CHUV study further showed that 50% of PWAs were living alone (6 lived with their family, and 7 were married or lived with another person). It was estimated that PWAs were hospitalized "for social reasons" in 35% of all days spent in institutions, i.e. patient days in acute inpatient care facilities did not require the technical services of the institutions concerned, but the lower level of support they required was not available or was refused at home (Griffiths et al., 1988, 2).

There are no substantial differences in the average number of days of hospitalization, except for those 16 patients with adult Kaposi's sarcoma at USZ who required fewer inpatient days but, on the other hand, a lot more outpatient care (AIDS-Kommission des Kantons Zürich, 1988, 10).[3)]

Compared with the University hospitals in Lausanne and Basel, outpatient care in Zurich is substantially higher. This is partly due to some medical research projects on the effects of alpha-interferon and zidovudine. But most interesting is that, though treatment patterns differ within Switzerland, the effect on total treatment costs of the patients' main hospital remains small. From a perspective of institutional costs or resource allocation and utilization associated with PWAs, it is important to focus not simply on inpatient care but also on outpatient treatment. This is especially true because we can expect improvements in outpatient care of PWAs as medical personnel and institutions are still learning how to treat them. The availability of outpatient treatment in Zurich (studies USZ_1 and USZ_2) has improved rapidly in the last three years as community care and home support have extended their health services field to PWAs. From this point of view, it is unlikely for inpatient care to become more dominant in the future of PWAs within the Canton Zurich, and, on the long run, within Switzerland. It is rather likely that outpatient care is being further substituted for inpatient care. Care alternatives merit a lot more attention than they have received until now.

Some of the most expensive treatment patterns[4)] can be considered experimental because the disease is still new and few standards have emerged. On the whole, however, the four analyses are revealing remarkably little variation in average daily hospital charges. The average of 772 Sfrs. per inpatient day appears to be typical. Compared with other patients, PWAs do not account for higher per-day-costs within University hospitals. At USZ overall level, PWAs cost even 100 Sfrs. per inpatient day less than the average patient (Amberg and Pedergnana, 1989, 7).

One particularly noteworthy aspect of these data is that PWAs' health care insurers covered only 50.5% or 61.1% of all inpatient costs and 18.5% or 57.1% of all outpatient costs at USZ (Amberg and Pedergnana, 1989, 8) and at UHB (Pedergnana, 1989, 14-16). The remaining uncovered costs (excluding the fixed part like overhead charges, capital costs and costs covered by others due to various reasons) mainly led to an increase in the hospital budget deficit which is covered indirectly by the Canton's taxpayers.

If new therapeutic treatment or drugs are developed with the result that PWAs live longer, then lifetime costs will not necessarily increase. As time passes, increased

3) On average, PWAs had 26 ambulatory consultations at USZ per year, or an average consultation rate of 45.5 per patient (range 0-85). A retrospective study at USZ_2 further showed that persons with lymphadenopathy syndrome had 8, and with AIDS related complex 16 consultations per year.

4) e.g. one PWA who spent 6 days in an intensive care unit got treatment for 51,400 Sfrs.; another PWA spent 293 days in a university hospital and cost 220,000 Sfrs.

training and experience of physicians and nurses should lead to lower per patient costs and to earlier discharge. The efficacy of therapeutic measures will obviously increase. Thus we believe that average lifetime costs of PWAs in Switzerland will remain at 74,000 Sfrs.

Personal medical care costs for all PWAs in a given year are estimated to increase from 8 million Sfrs. in 1986 and 12 million Sfrs. in 1988 to 60 million Sfrs. by 1991 and 225 million Sfrs. in 1995 (FAC and FOPH, 1989, 68).

Finally, but of prime importance, it has to be pointed out that we analyzed the average total costs and not the marginal or extra costs of treating an additional (AIDS) patient. To get the marginal costs, we would have to subtract all fixed costs, e.g. the costs for an empty hospital bed. It must be emphasized that marginal costs are between 20% and 25% lower than the average total costs. This is especially true as long as new nursing facilities (existing acute hospitals have an average occupancy rate of 80%) do not become necessary. No separate facility fully dedicated to AIDS care has been opened yet in Switzerland.

Marginal costs have to considered when new treatment strategies are planned. A substitution of hospital care by community-based services is generally favorable, but it is not always cheaper. We are strong opponents of unpaid personal health services (Aids Regionalhilfestellen, Pro Familia, Samariterbund and so on) that substitutes for long-term institutional care, the way Swiss health care insurers favor it. Many Swiss cities started to order nonprofit health care organizations to take care of PWAs and pay them, but because treatment at home still depends heavily on the continued participation of unpaid volunteers, it might not be easily copied abroad. These costs are often ignored, since they do not have to be covered in health agencies' budgets, and because there are usually few data from which to estimate them. However, their omission can lead to suboptimization in choosing care strategies. For example, a community care-oriented strategy is almost certainly cheaper than a hospital-based one. However, it may be considerably less economic than it seems at first once the costs of unpaid services are added and may also place a heavy cost burden on families and other unpaid sources of care.

Further analysis, especially in the fields of alternative courses of action, is required. There are no studies which provide a valuable, active management support for the benefit of decision-makers in the health care system. A simulation model which is geared to Switzerland should evaluate the efficiency and effectiveness of different interventions and its impact on the health care system and also on various third-party payers.

3.1.2 The impact of AIDS on Swiss hospitals

The impact of AIDS on Swiss hospitals has been overestimated in the past. Only an estimated 0.01% of all inpatient days in acute care hospitals in 1988 can be traced back to PWAs.

35 of all 45,600 acute beds in Switzerland would have been enough for all inpatient care of PWAs according to our estimate of 13,000 acute hospital days needed in 1988 (Fig. 4). Even in 1995, the estimate of 165,000 hospital days translates into a requirement of only 450 acute beds or just 1.0% of all acute beds. Furthermore, the estimate of 55,000 days in psychiatric clinics for PWAs with severe neurologic and psychological manifestations additionally requires 150 beds or 1.0% of all their bed capacity in 1995. This explains why, at an average occupancy rate of well below the optimal rate of 85% for acute care hospitals, there is no need for supplementary

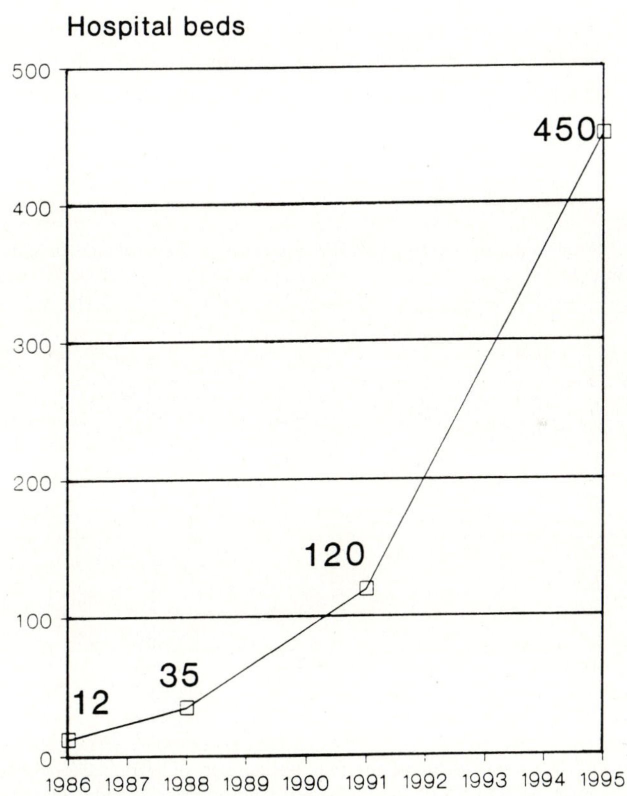

Fig. 4. Need of beds for patients with AIDS in acute care hospitals in Switzerland

hospital facilities for PWAs. AIDS is not a problem of hospital capacity but undoubtedly accents the severe lack of health care personnel in Switzerland (FAC and FOPH, 1989, 71).

3.1.3 Prevention, information and education

AIDS has been institutionalized in the political arena fairly quickly. It was recognized as a problem rather early, and first of all, a broadly representative ad hoc Federal AIDS Commission (FAC) with 25 members was established in 1984. In the meantime, the FAC has been supplemented by a Federal Commission to Control AIDS Research and by an Interdepartmental Working Group for Questions Related to AIDS. On the state level, there are another 13 AIDS Commissions, and on the community level, there are numerous working groups. A comprehensive, sustained, successful and internationally acknowledged national STOP AIDS Program was launched in February 1987. Public awareness of the dangers of AIDS has considerably increased.

The FOPH further focused on health education, a key to AIDS prevention and control. Including all expenditures for training of hospital personnel, the FOPH spent 20.1 million Sfrs. on all preventive measures from 1986 to 1988 and was assisted by Cantonal measures (Table 3).

Table 3. Estimated direct costs of AIDS and HIV infection in Switzerland (in million Sfrs.) (from FAC/FOPH, 1989, 68)

	1986	1987	1988
Personal medical care costs	6.0	8.0	12.0
Information, prevention	1.5	8.6	10.0
Blood donor screening	7.0	7.0	7.0
Blood HIV testing	6.0	12.5	12.5
Research	2.0	4.5	10.0
Other direct costs*	1.5	5.8	8.5
Total	24.0	46.6	60.0
Payers:			
- Federal Government	2.5	13.2	19.3
- State & local governments	4.3	6.2	9.1
- Health care insurers	3.0	4.0	6.0
- Other payers	12.9	20.8	22.0

* Including Switzerland's personal, technical and financial support of WHO's Global Program on AIDS; Swiss have implemented national AIDS prevention programs in Iran, Uganda, Ruanda, Morocco etc.

3.1.4 Compulsory screening of blood donations

Since the introduction of HIV antibody screening in November 1985, around 650,000 blood donations are tested each year. It was certainly worthwhile, because no new transfusions associated with HIV infections have been reported since November 1985. Today blood transfusions appear to be as safe as before the emergence of the AIDS epidemic (Frey-Wettstein et al., 1988, 149-153).

But the costs for the screening of all blood donations including the costs of replacement of blood[5)], both covered primarily by the Swiss Red Cross which had to increase its price for blood products by 10 Sfrs. or 16% to 70 Sfrs. per unit in November 1985, amount to 7.0 million Sfrs. yearly (FAC and FOPH, 1989, 72).

3.1.5 Voluntary HIV antibody testing

There were around 250,000 HIV antibody tests taken in the past two years for various individual reasons. Pre-test and post-test counselling associated with serologic testing cost between 30 and 80 Sfrs. (50 Sfrs. on average) amounting to total costs of 12.5 million Sfrs. (FAC and FOPH, 1989, 72). Most tests were taken by general practitioners and then tested in private laboratories. Laboratory support for confirmation tests and serostatus diagnosis is given by the FOPH National Center for Retroviruses and by five University laboratories.

3.1.6 Research expenses

Research expenses have been increasing rapidly in the last three years (Table 3). There have been various sources of public (mainly FOPH) and private institutions which supported research mainly at Departments of Medicine at the five universities in Switzerland.

3.1.7 Development of direct costs

Non-personal costs for prevention, research, blood screening and testing exceeded personal medical care costs by a factor of 5 in 1988 (Table 3). This is going to change very soon as non-personal costs are not expected to rise a lot above their current level. If we look at the payers, the biggest burden is carried directly by federal, cantonal and local governments and indirectly by the unaffected employed society, e.g. through the marginally decreasing (or less increasing) production and consumption process and through marginal premium or taxation increases.

---

5) Self-deferral of donors belonging to high-risk groups was instituted (before and after donations) in November 1985.

There is some concern that the AIDS epidemic places a financial burden on Swiss health care insurers, since 1% of the population has a special private insurance plan and more than 98% are covered by the standard governmentally subsidized health care insurance plan (Pedergnana et al., 1988, 76).[6] From the point of view of hospital deficits, it is necessary to know that the Swiss health care system typically has two categories of patients: those in private wards (one bed rooms), and those in public wards (up to eight beds to a room). Patients in private wards typically have a superior health care insurance plan. Their insurers are supposed to come up with all expenses at the hospital. Patients in public wards have a standard health care insurance coverage. Their insurers pay a digressive per diem reimbursement for each inpatient day, depending on length of stay, number of beds in the room, cantonal (provincial) domicile and citizenship, but regardless of all diagnostic and therapeutic measures taken.[7] As a matter of fact, an additional patient in public wards adds marginally to the hospital deficit which is covered directly by the Finance Department of the canton (state) and indirectly by the canton's taxpayers. The normal patient in a public ward or his health care insurer as the regular third-party payer typically covers only 50% of the real overall medical care costs. This rate is not significantly higher or lower for PWAs.

Yearly expenditures of all 400 Swiss health care insurers amounted to more than 8 billion Sfrs. in 1988 and have risen annually by 10% for the last 30 years. Relating the increase of their 1988 expenditures of around 800 million Sfrs. to the PWAs' treatment costs of 6 million Sfrs., it seems fairly clear that the current and future burden for Swiss health care insurers is relatively low and certainly manageable (FAC and FOPH, 1989, 68).

With 60 million Sfrs. or 0.3% of total medical care expenditures in 1988, we cannot say that AIDS has led to a major resource reallocation within the Swiss health care system. Even with increasing direct costs due to AIDS, the health care costs of rheumatism (Pedroni and Zweifel, 1986) and alcohol consumption (including costs of automobile accidents due to alcohol: Leu and Lutz, 1977), if they do not decrease immensely, will be far higher in 1995 (Fig. 5; data on other illnesses or diseases in Switzerland is not available).

---

6) There has been no case of an uninsured or underinsured PWA up to December 31, 1988. Besides that, self-pay (out-of-pocket expenses) is strictly limited in the Swiss health care system.

7) e.g. at the UHB University Hospital Basel, inpatients or their health care insurers of Swiss citizens from Basel (Canton Basel as their residence) have to pay 260 Sfrs. per day for the first 30 inpatient days in public wards. After 90 and 180 inpatient days of the same patient in the same calender year, the per diem reimbursement falls to 145 and 115 Sfrs. respectively, or between 10% and 20% of the patient's daily medical care costs, regardless of what diagnostic or therapeutic measures are taken at the hospital. The figures differ from canton to canton, and from hospital to hospital.

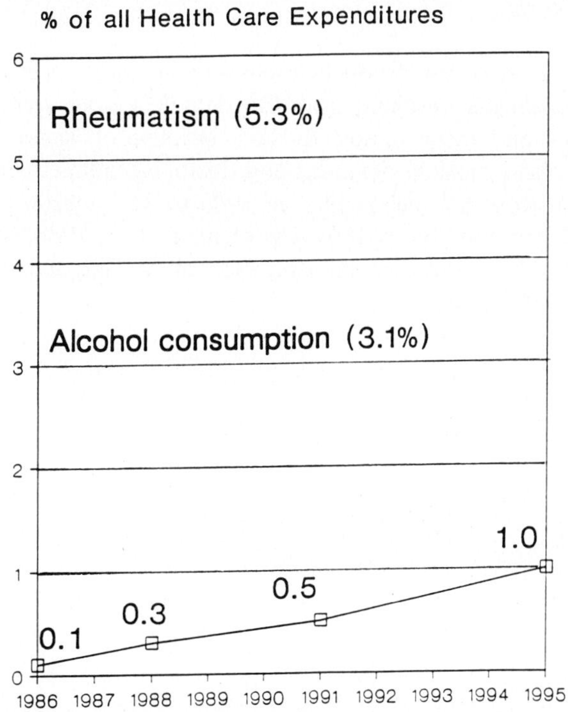

Fig. 5. Estimated direct costs of AIDS, alcohol consumption and rheumatism in % of all health care expenditures in Switzerland

3.2 Indirect costs

The indirect costs of AIDS and HIV infection involve measuring and somehow weighing the life years lost due to illness and premature death. Although these costs have tended to be ignored by Swiss health authorities, AIDS as a fatal disease represents a substantial loss of future productivity. As other studies have suggested, these costs are five times higher than direct costs due to AIDS (Pedergnana, 1988; Scitovsky et al., 1986).

Enough has been written on how to value the premature loss of life years and on the importance of indirect costs (Mishan, 1971; Landefeld and Seskin, 1982; Rice and Hodgson, 1982; Jones-Lee, 1985; Drummond et al., 1987). We applied the human capital approach for both morbidity and mortality costs despite the appeal of the willingness-to-pay approach on theoretical grounds. Without going into further details (Pedergnana et al., 1988), we want to present our findings for Switzerland.

3.2.1 Morbidity costs

Morbidity costs consist of the productivity losses to society, as measured by wages, salaries and supplements, resulting from the days lost from work among currently employed persons and those unable to work because of illness. Assuming a 50% working ability[8)] between AIDS diagnosis and death, we estimate morbidity costs due to AIDS will grow from 6.7 million Sfrs. in 1988 to 31.7 million Sfrs. in 1991, and eventually to 129.9 million Sfrs. in 1995 (Pedergnana et al., 1988, 67), or far less than the morbidity costs due to tobacco smoking, alcohol drinking and rheumatism (Fig. 6) (FAC and FOPH, 1989, 73).

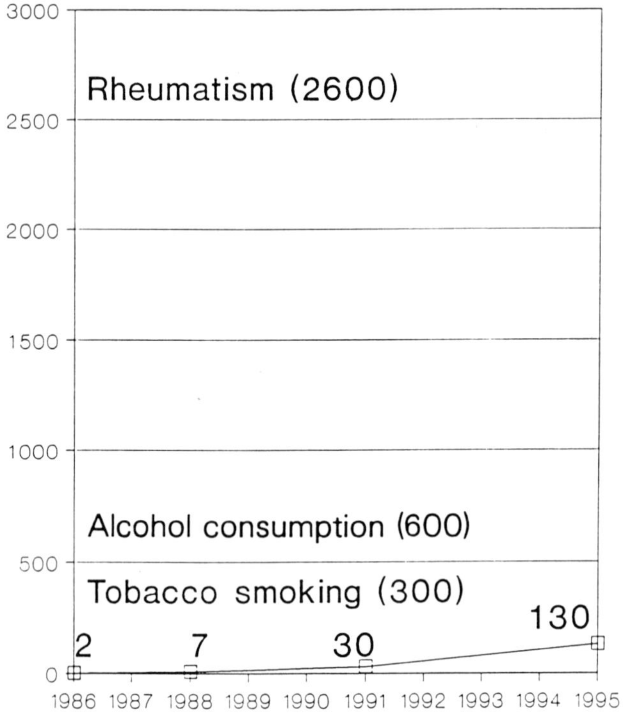

Fig. 6. Estimated morbidity costs of AIDS and HIV infection and other illnesses in Switzerland (in 1988 million Sfrs.)

8) The awareness of the infection by the patient's employer or colleagues can have repercussions on the employment of such a patient, even if the infected is perfectly able to perform his duties on a full-time basis.

3.2.2 Mortality costs

Mortality costs are the discounted present (4%) values of wages, salaries and supplements, and the imputed values of housekeeping services lost following the premature death of persons who would have otherwise been productively employed or keeping house.

Table 4 shows an increasing number of potential life years (between 1 and 70) lost due to AIDS. In 1987, 3,000 or 1.1% of all life years lost were due to AIDS and HIV infection. The rate of premature deaths due to AIDS is going to increase dramatically. An estimate, based on average life expectancy per sex and age minus 10% because of the large number of IV drug users, shows an increase from 4,800 life years lost in 1988 to 46,600 life years lost in 1995 (Fig. 7).

These estimates may question the solvency of Swiss life insurers. However, the actual and potential impact of AIDS on Swiss private health care and life insurances has been grossly overestimated. Until the end of 1988, we estimated cumulative losses and expenses due to AIDS and HIV infection at less than 20 million Sfrs., which is practically nothing related to total (ordinary and group) life insurance premiums of more than 12 billion Sfrs. each year.[9] Although we expect a rise of AIDS related expenses for life insurers, we estimate that the impact will not rise above 0.3% of overall premiums before 1995 (Pedergnana et al., 1988, 76). The solvency of Swiss life insurers is and will not be threatened by AIDS. Male and female applicants of a life insurance coverage of 100,000 Sfrs. or above have to take the HIV antibody test to

Table 4. Potential life years lost due to AIDS and other death causes in Switzerland in 1980, 1986 and 1987 (Bundesamt für Statistik, Abteilung Gesundheitsstatistik)

Death causes	Year								
	1980			1986			1987		
	Men	Women	Total	Men	Women	Total	Men	Women	Total
AIDS	37	0	37	2,000	187	2,187	2,367	594	2,961
Tuberculosis	432	150	582	357	65	422	265	112	377
Stomach cancer	2,292	1,297	3,589	2,052	1,087	3,139	2,057	1,180	3,237
Lung cancer	11,175	1,890	13,065	11,727	2,165	13,892	10,725	2,457	13,182
Diabetes mellitus	1,292	1,435	2,727	1,680	1,060	2,740	1,587	910	2,497
Coronary diseases	31,564	9,050	40,614	29,977	7,757	37,734	28,764	7,194	35,958
Traffic accidents	26,819	7,531	34,350	24,397	6,241	30,638	21,838	5,735	27,573
Suicide	27,012	10,730	37,742	25,185	9,115	34,300	25,992	8,362	34,354
All death causes	186,794	92,914	279,708	177,325	86,866	264,191	178,858	83,281	262,139

9) It is not surprising that the Swiss Life Insurance Association (VPL) decided to collect AIDS related claims data, but not to publish the results.

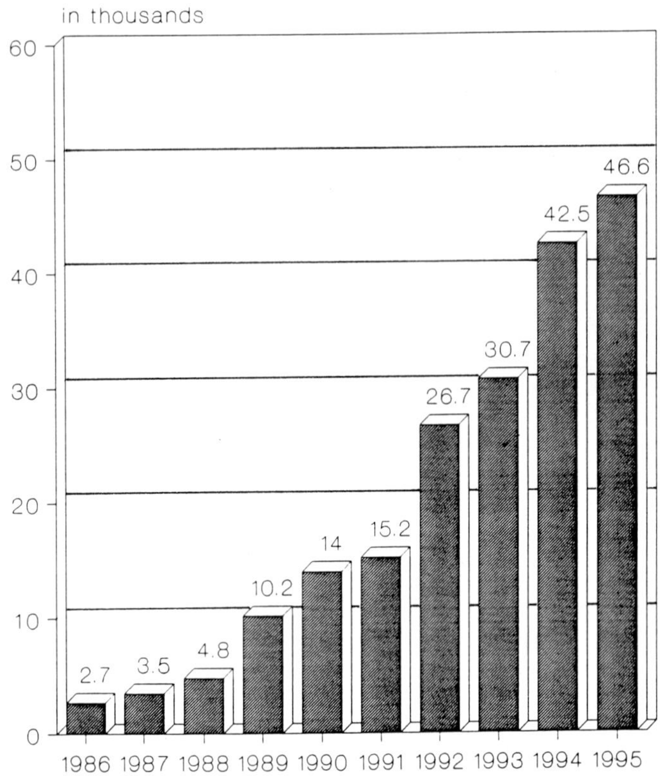

Fig. 7. Estimated life years lost due to AIDS in Switzerland (Pedergnana et al., 1988, 72)

further reduce the insurer's exposure to AIDS related costs. Until now, there have been no signs that strong antiselection took place in Switzerland[10)], but precise figures about seropositive applicants have never been published.

Estimated mortality costs show an increase from 80 million Sfrs. in 1986 to 400 million Sfrs. in 1991, and to 1,200 million Sfrs. in 1995, and will by then reach the current level of mortality costs due to alcohol drinking (Fig. 8) (Pedergnana et al., 1988, 67).

3.3 Intangible costs

The intangible costs cannot be expressed in terms of money owing to measurement difficulties, but the cost of psychical and physical pain, discomfort, anxiety, impairment, disability, handicap, etc. are going to intensify with expected illness and death rates in the future. We also mean the so-called third epidemic of economic,

10) Information provided by A. Chuffart, Swiss Re in Zurich, Switzerland, in October 1988.

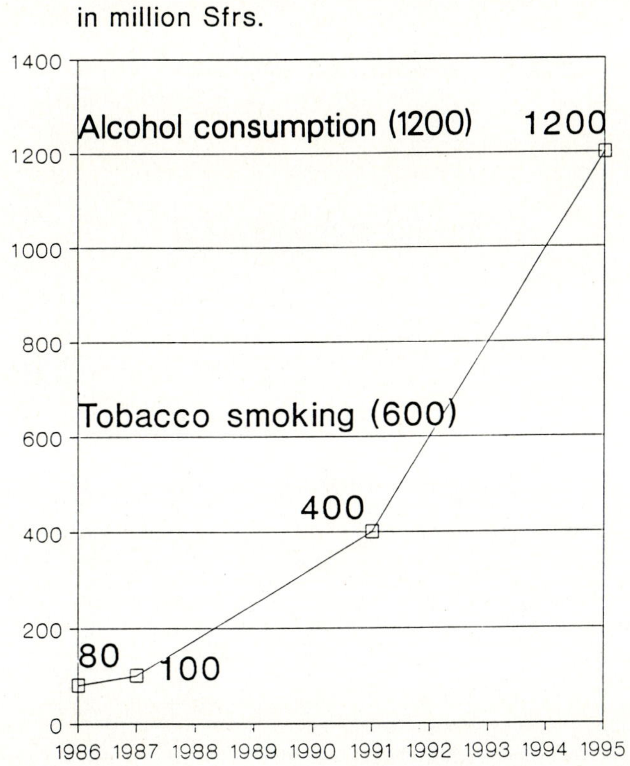

Fig. 8. Estimated mortality costs due to AIDS and HIV infection in Switzerland (in 1988 million Sfrs.)

social, political and cultural reaction to AIDS and HIV infection, which follows relentlessly the HIV and AIDS epidemic. The influence on morals, habits, attitudes and prejudices is indisputable, but the question is: How much does society have to pay for it?

3.4. Social costs

As a consequence of the chapters outlined above, social costs due to AIDS and HIV infection are estimated to rise from 0.11 billion Sfrs. in 1986 to 1.6 billion Sfrs. in 1995 (Fig. 9), especially because of the high death toll among the economically and socially most productive age groups. All estimates are reliable in so far as we can foresee that AIDS is not a major threat to the Swiss health care system. Nevertheless we have to undertake measures to cope with the AIDS epidemic in the most efficient way, not wasting scarce (health care) resources.

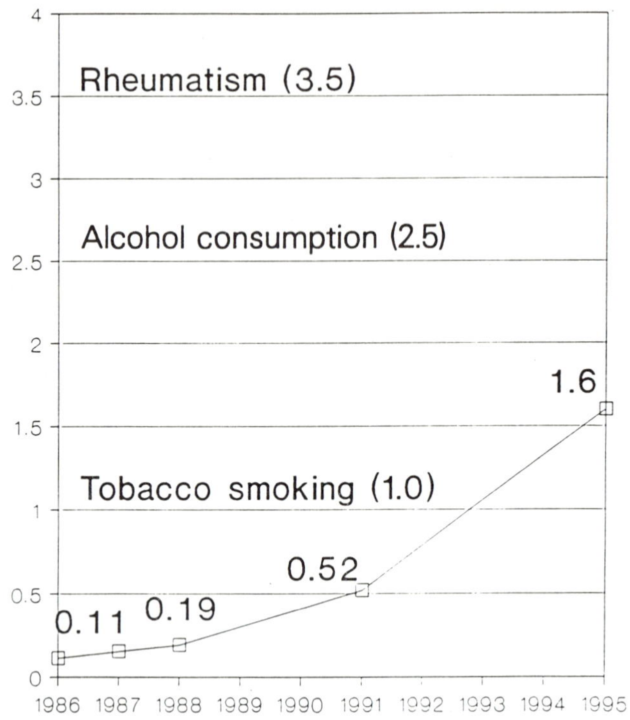

Fig. 9. Social costs of AIDS, tobacco smoking, alcohol drinking and rheumatism in Switzerland (in billion Sfrs.)

4. Summary

Indicators and trends show that the economic impact of AIDS on the Swiss health care system will increase rapidly within the next six years. Prevalence-based estimates of total direct and indirect costs of AIDS in Switzerland show an expected increase from 110 million Sfrs. in 1986 to 1.6 billion Sfrs. in 1995.

To assess the likely future impact of the cumulatively estimated 12,000 PWAs in Switzerland, we combined epidemiological data with cost studies.

The direct costs of AIDS in Switzerland (nursing care, research, screening, information etc.) added up to 60 million Sfrs. in 1988, equaling 0.3% of total health care costs. The direct costs are estimated to rise to 255 million Sfrs. or 1.0% of total health care expenditures by 1995, even though a 17-fold increase compared with the 702 AIDS cases thus far has to be expected. AIDS therefore is probably not responsible for either the "explosive" increase of Swiss health care expenditures or a major resource reallocation. AIDS will influence the total consumption of medical care resources in Switzerland only marginally.

Because of the deadliness of the disease, the indirect costs of AIDS (value of lost productivity and future earnings due to illness and premature death, affecting predominantly younger people) are about five times greater than the direct costs.

The average lifetime costs of a PWA are estimated at 74,000 Sfrs. On average 50% of all inpatient and outpatient costs are covered by the PWA's health care insurer. The remaining costs are carried by governmental institutions. Swiss health care insurers had to carry a much smaller load than was originally expected. We can even say that the costs of health care and life insurers in Switzerland have been negligible so far. The solvency of Swiss health care and life insurers is not threatened due to AIDS related claims until 1995.

The social costs of AIDS in 1995 will exceed the social costs of tobacco smoking but, though considerable, will still be far less than the social costs of rheumatism and alcohol consumption.

References

AIDS-Kommission des Kantons Zürich (ed.) (1988). AIDS-Bericht 1988, Situations-Analyse, Konzepte und Massnahmen. Zürich.

Amberg, W. and Pedergnana, M. (1989). Inpatient and outpatient treatment costs of AIDS patients at the university hospital of Zürich, Switzerland. Working paper, March.

Drummond, M.F., Stoddart, G.L., and Torrance, G.W. (1987). Methods for the economic evaluation of health care programmes. Oxford University Press, Oxford.

FAC (Federal AIDS Commission) Eidgenössische Kommission für Aidsfragen und FOPH (Federal Office of Public Health) Bundesamt für Gesundheitswesen (eds.) (1989). AIDS in der Schweiz. Die Epidemie, die Folgen, die Massnahmen. A Report to the Federal Council and to the Members of the Parliament, February.

FOPH (Federal Office of Public Health) Medizinische Abteilung (1988). Projektionen der AIDS-Ausbreitung in der Schweiz. Bulletin des Bundesamtes für Gesundheitswesen 42, 539-542.

Frey-Wettstein, M., Leder, A., and Schütze, M. (1988). HIV-Übertragung durch Bluttransfusionen: eine Studie des Blutspendedienstes SRK. Schweizer medizinische Wochenschrift 118, 149-153.

Griffiths, A., Chave, J.Ph. , and Corbaz, M.H. (1988). Health service use and treatment costs of patients with stage IV HIV infection at the centre hospitalier universitaire Vaudois, Switzerland. Unpublished manuscript, November .

Jones-Lee, M.W. (1985). The value of life and safety: a survey of recent developments. The Geneva Papers on Risk and Insurance 10(36), 141-173.

Landefeld, J.S. and Seskin, E.P. (1982). The economic value of life: linking theory to practice. American Journal of Public Health 72(6), 555-566.

Leu, R. and Lutz, P (1977). Ökonomische Aspekte des Alkoholkonsums in der Schweiz. Zürich 1977.

Mishan, E.J. (1971). Evaluation of life and limb: a theoretical approach. Journal of Political Economy 79, July/August, 687-705.

Pedergnana, M. (1988). Morbidität und Mortalität als indirekte Kosten von AIDS: Möglichkeiten und Grenzen ihrer Messung im Lichte der Prognosen über die Ausbreitung von AIDS bis 1995. Diploma Thesis, University of St. Gall, Switzerland, April.

Pedergnana, M. (1989). AIDS und die Kosten. Schweizer Krankenkassen-Zeitung 81(1/2), 14-16.

Pedergnana, M., Schmid, H., and von Wartburg, W.P (1988). AIDS - Zur Entwicklung in der Schweiz.Hans Huber, Bern, Stuttgart and Toronto.

Pedroni, G. and Zweifel, P. (1986). Die sozialen Kosten von Rheuma in der Schweiz. Pharma Information, Basel.

Rice, D.P. and Hodgson, T.A. (1982). The value of human life revisited. American Journal of Public Health 72(6), 536-538.

Rufli, Th. , Pedergnana, M., and Gürke, T. (1989). Medical care costs of patients with AIDS at the university hospital of Basel, Switzerland. Unpublished manuscript, February.

Scitovsky, A.A., Rice, D.R., Showstack, J., and Lee, P.R. (1986). Estimating the direct and indirect economic costs of acquired immune deficiency syndrome, 1985, 1986, and 1990. Prepared for The Centers for Disease Control, Task Order 282-85-0061 no.2, March .

Sommer, J.H. and Gutzwiller, F. (1986). Wirtschaftlichkeit und Wirksamkeit im schweizerischen Gesundheitswesen. Ergebnisse des Nationalen Forschungsprogrammes Nr. 8, Bern, Stuttgart and Toronto.

Costs of AIDS in a Developing Area: Indirect and Direct Costs of AIDS in Puerto Rico

D.S. Shepard

Despite the fact that over half of the world's officially reported cases of AIDS were diagnosed in the United States, the burden of AIDS affects the developing countries even more than the industrialized ones. A number of developing countries, particularly in Africa and the Caribbean, face a devastating combination of a high incidence of AIDS, strained health systems, and stagnating economies. In a model similar to the work of Over, Bertozzi and Chin (1989), this paper presents a framework to measure the total economic impact of AIDS in a developing area and applies this framework to the island of Puerto Rico and its capital city of San Juan. The measurement of economic impact is needed to determine the magnitude of the problem of HIV infection, to rank that problem in relation to other health needs, and to guide prevention and control efforts.

Categories of costs of HIV

The costs of HIV infection can be categorized according to the sector of the economy and the type of person affected (Table 1). The economic sectors distinguish the health sector from all other sectors. Persons affected are both the individuals infected with HIV and their families, and uninfected persons. The category of costs which has been most examined is the costs of persons with AIDS to the health sector. These costs, termed the direct costs in the health economics literature, measure the costs of treatment of HIV and its complications. The next most examined category is the indirect cost - the loss outside the health sector from persons infected. Indirect costs are the value of foregone economic output, which is often measured by lost earnings.

The elements in the lower part of Table 1 include public costs for surveillance, prevention, research, and screening - costs generally borne by persons not infected. Costs in the final category - uninfected persons outside the health sector - are more difficult to quantify and have been less studied. They consist of secondary impacts in such areas as: international travel and migration, tourism, quality of life, and anxiety.

Table 1. Categories of costs of HIV

Person affected	Sector affected	
	Health	Other
Persons infected with HIV and their families	Direct costs (treatment)	Indirect costs (foregone economic output)
Uninfected persons	Public costs (e.g. surveillance, prevention, research, screening)	Secondary impacts (e.g tourism)

Measuring the costs of AIDS to people infected

The direct cost of AIDS per case is measured as the product of the average cost of treatment per year times the number of years of survival with AIDS. The treatment cost per year obviously depends on the setting: inpatient hospital care is most expensive.

The indirect costs of AIDS is the sum of mortality and morbidity components. The mortality component is measured as the number of discounted "prime" years of life lost times the output per year that otherwise would have been attained. Prime life years are the adult period of life during which economic contribution would normally be greatest, defined here as the span from ages 15 through 64. The number of discounted life years lost is the discounted remaining life expectancy of prime years at the age of death. Remaining years were discounted to reflect the fact that years in the distant future are less valued than years in the immediate future.

The number of prime life years lost was calculated by considering the distribution of age at diagnosis of AIDS cases. The age at death was assumed to be 18 months beyond the age at diagnosis. For each adult age category, the remaining prime discounted life expectancy up to age 65 was calculated based on life tables.

The author summed for each prime year beyond the age 5 the product of the probability of survival multiplied by a discount factor. Then he calculated a weighted average of these sums based on the proportion of AIDS cases with death in each age category. For pediatric cases, the number of discounted years lost is the present value of each of the prime years (ages 15 to 64) times the conditional probability of survival to each of those years. The conditional probability is conditional on survival to age 5, the approximate age of death of pediatric cases. The morbidity cost per year is the number of years of illness times the lost output for each year of illness.

Costs of research and prevention while not included in this report are the value of the resources expended (generally by public or non-profit agencies) for that purpose.

Although the requisite data are difficult to obtain, it is possible to outline a methodology for estimating secondary impacts. Theoretically, secondary impacts of AIDS on quality of life could be valued through willingness-to-pay surveys. For example, to reduce the risk of sexual transmission, some public education campaigns counsel monogamy or abstinence(!) in sexual relations. In some listeners, the advice will evoke anxiety but no change in behavior. Others in the audience may deliberately change their lifestyles to be more conservative in their sexual relationships. Among both groups, the threat of AIDS probably reduces their quality of life. A thorough analysis, however, would need to consider possible beneficial effects of enhancing existing relationships and reducing the risk of other sexually transmitted diseases.

AIDS may restrict or discourage international travel. Residents from a country with a high prevalence of AIDS may find their entry to other countries impeded. Business travelers or tourists may avoid certain destinations out of fear of AIDS. In the former case, the loss from denied travel is the difference between the expected value to the traveler of a potential international trip and the expected cost of that trip. In the latter case, the loss to the destination country is the difference between the expected value of the goods and services that would have been consumed by the overseas visitors (including exports arranged during such visits), and the resource costs of providing those goods and services.

Numbers of AIDS cases to date are based on official surveillance data. In this study, numbers of cases are analyzed based on date of diagnosis, rather than date of reporting. This approach minimizes bias due to varying lags in reporting of cases to surveillance authorities. As reporting of cases appears to have been incomplete in the first years of the epidemic, the apparent explosive growth prior to 1984 may overstate actual growth rates.

Future estimates of the costs of AIDS were developed on two alternative projections on the number of cases: (1) the number of cases will continue to grow at the same rate as they have in the most recent past; and (2) the rate of growth in the number of cases will moderate, as it has been doing over several years. For assumption (1), a linear projection, the author calculated the growth rate from 1987 to 1988 and assumed that same rate would continue through 1992. Thus only the most recent two years (1987 through 1988) were used. This is termed a linear projection because the logarithm of the number of cases was calculated as a linear function of time. For assumption (2), a quadratic projection, the natural logarithm of the number of cases was regressed on both the year and the square of the year. Data from the last five years (1984 through 1988) were used. Although other researchers (e.g. Over et al, 1988) have estimated costs of persons infected with HIV, this analysis begins with numbers of AIDS cases, as an infected person incurs relatively few costs before he develops AIDS.

Estimates of direct costs for Puerto Rico

Research underway in Puerto Rico provides estimates of most of the cost components. Among direct costs, the costs of inpatient care are most important (Table 2). Average inpatient costs over a patient's lifetime range from $9,653 to $25,000 depending on the health system managing the patient's care. The lowest cost was achieved by the San Juan AIDS Institute. It is the private institute to which the Health Department of the Municipality of San Juan contracted the management of AIDS care for patients for which it was responsible beginning January 1, 1988. It replaced the system of ad hoc care by the San Juan Municipal. Through appropriate economic incentives (a specified annual level of payment) and better management, the average length of stay for an AIDS related admission averaged 11.3 days under the San Juan AIDS Institute, compared to 21.5 days under the pre-existing municipal hospital system.

Blue Cross of Puerto Rico (apparently typical of other private insurance systems) was the most expensive reimbursement system, at $25,000 per year. As these systems are similar to the health insurance systems in the mainland U.S., it shares those strengths and weaknesses. On the one hand, they provide partial financial access to the best care available on the island of Puerto Rico. Blue Cross insurance pays for most of the cost of private medical care and anti-viral drugs, such as zidovudine (AZT), for its subscribers. On the other hand, these systems provide neither incentives nor procedures for controlling costs.

The lifetime cost of outpatient care for a person with AIDS ranges from $1680 to $29,000 (Table 3). The lower amount applies to care delivered through an efficient private clinic, without the anti-viral drug AZT. The higher cost includes $800 per month for AZT. The lifetime cost of other modes of care (home, extended, and hospice care) averages only $526 per person with AIDS (Table 4). Although the importance of these types of care is increasingly being recognized, they were used by only a minority of patients in 1988, the base year for these data.

Table 2. Cost of inpatient care

Setting	Length of stay (days)	Cost per day ($)	Episodes per pt. per year	Cost per pt. per year ($)	Years alive after Dx	Lifetime cost per pt. ($)
San Juan AIDS Institute	11.3	341	1.67	6,435	1.5	9,653
Private hospital; no AZT	16.4	387	1.67	10,599	1.5	15,899
Municipal hospital	21.5	354	1.67	12,710	1.5	19,065
Private hospital; with AZT	16.4	417	1.67	11,421	2.0	22,842
Blue cross of P.R.; AZT*	NA	NA	NA	NA	2.0	25,000

* Assumes half of total cost is for inpatient care

Table 3. Cost of outpatient care

Setting	Visits per pt. per year	Cost per visit	Cost per pt. per year	Years alive after Dx	Lifetime cost per pt.
San Juan AIDS Institute	4.4	255	1,120	1.5	1,680
Private doctor; no AZT	11.2	116	1,300	1.5	1,950
Private doctor; with AZT	15.6	929	14,500	2.0	29,000

Table 4. Cost of other types of care

Setting	Units	Quantity	Cost per unit ($)	Lifetime cost per pt. ($)	% of pts. receiving	Expected lifetime cost per pt. ($)
Home care	Visits	6	127	762	10%	76
Extended	Days	15	150	2250	4%	90
Hospice	Days	30	200	6000	6%	360
Total						526

The overall lifetime direct cost of care per person with AIDS is the sum of costs of care in inpatient, ambulatory, and other modes. Among groups of patients studied within San Juan, this sum ranged from $11,773 for patients treated by the San Juan AIDS Institute to $51,842 for private patients receiving AZT (Table 5). No comparable data have yet been compiled for the island of Puerto Rico as a whole.

As a working assumption, the author assumes that the cost of public patients in Puerto Rico is comparable to costs of the San Juan AIDS Institute. In the past, the absence of case management and well structured outpatient care probably increases use of expensive inpatient care. But other patients may have not received much care. For the

Table 5. Lifetime cost of care per patient ($)

Setting	Assumed Share	Input care	Output care	Other care	Total care
San Juan AIDS Institute	70%	9,653	1,120	526	10,773
Private; no AZT		15,889	1,950		17,839
Municipal hospital		19,065			19,065
Blue cross	30%	25,000	NA	NA	50,000
Private; with AZT		22,842	29,000		51,842
Weighted average	100%				22,541

future, however, AIDS officials throughout the island are scrutinizing the results from the San Juan AIDS Institute and seeking to develop models to replicate its benefits. Also, it is assumed that the cost of private patients taking AZT in San Juan is representative of private patients throughout the island.

In both San Juan and Puerto Rico as a whole, approximately 70 percent of patients are medically indigent. The remaining 30 percent are generally insured with employment based insurance which will allow a person with AIDS to obtain AZT. Thus, the overall direct cost of AIDS is a weighted average of the costs in the public and private sectors, weighted by the relative share in each sector. This overall average is $22,541 per year.

Indirect costs for Puerto Rico

The bulk of indirect costs from AIDS are losses from illness and death during the prime period of life. Table 6 shows the number of discounted prime years lost from premature mortality in adults. The adjusted percentages are based on 1988 surveillance data from the Municipality of San Juan, which follow a pattern similar to the official surveillance data for the entire island. The number of life years lost from morbidity is based on a disability level of 50 percent. Each pediatric case leads to a smaller loss in discounted life years than an adult case. Although the absolute loss in life years is less for a pediatric case, the life years are more heavily discounted. There is no morbidity loss in a pediatric case because the morbidity occurs prior to the prime period. Table 7 shows the overall number of years lost per case.

Determining the economic value of each of these lost years is a difficult problem in Puerto Rico, as in many developing areas, because only a small share of the population is employed in a formally recognized job (Table 8). Only 70 percent of Puerto Rico's 3.3 million persons are over age 15, and only about half of those are in the labor force (i.e, working or looking for work). Among those in the labor force, the

Table 6. Prime life years lost from mortality per adult case

Age category	Mid-point	Age at death	Prime adj. %	Disc. expect. prime years lost	Lost (at 5%)
13-19	16	17.5	0.7	45.2	16.8
20-29	25	26.5	24.6	36.6	15.7
30-39	35	36.5	52.0	27.0	13.8
40-49	45	46.5	17.9	17.5	10.8
50+	55	56.5	4.9	8.2	6.2
Weighted average				26.8	13.36

Table 7. Discounted prime life years lost per AIDS case

Source	Adult	Pediatric
Mortality	13.36	9.88
Morbidity	0.74	0.00
Total	14.10	9.88

Table 8. Puerto Rico: selected labor market data, 1986

Group	Number (1000s)	Percent
Total population	3276	100.0
Age 16 and over	2303	70.3
In labor force	986	30.1
Employed	809	24.7
Working 35 hours or more	579	17.7
Unemployment rate		18.9

Sources: Government of PR

unemployment rate is 18 percent. Furthermore, even among those working, some may be involuntarily working part time. So overall, only about one out of six Puerto Ricans is working in a formal job during a given week.

Studies on the cost of illness in the United States value lost time primarily based on the average wage of people employed. That computation would be inappropriate, however, where only a small share of the population is formally employed. Although a literature search could not find any macro-economic studies of the shadow wage of labor, Puerto Rican economists consider the minimum wage on the island ($3.70 per hour) as a good estimate. Taking unemployment into account, the economic value of a year of prime life is then $5,700 (35 hours per week x 48 weeks x $3.70, less 18 percent). This amount reflects all productive activities - market employment, running a business, caring for children and other dependents, etc.

In Puerto Rico, the majority of persons with AIDS were intravenous (IV) drug users at the time they acquired the infection. According to official surveillance data, IV drug use was the only risk factor for 57 percent of adult or adolescent cases, and was a joint risk factor in another 11 percent of cases in persons who were both homo- or bisexual and an IV drug users.

Some critics would argue that the economic activity for these persons has no economic value, or indeed, that it is negative. This paper does not follow this reasoning. First, the designation of IV drug use the risk factor for AIDS indicates a condition at the time of infection. The latency period until diagnosis averages some 7 years and a user may well have successfully quit such use in the interim. Although only about a quarter of treatment attempts successfully maintain abstinence for at least a year (Hunt, Barnett, and Branch, 1971), the cumulative effect of multiple attempts over seven years is undoubtedly greater. Waiting lists to enter drug treatment programs testify to the desire by many IV drug users to break their habit.

The present value of the indirect costs of an AIDS case is thus $80,000 (13.29 years times $5,700 per year) for an adult case and $56,000 for a pediatric case. To interpret these amounts, it is helpful to compare them to the 1988 per capita GDP of $ 5,600. For an adult case, the direct costs are 4.2 times the per capita GDP; indirect costs are 14.8 times, and total costs are 19.0 times. Among the 2869 cumulative cases reported as of July 10, 1989, 981 new cases were diagnosed during 1988, and 2,761 cases had been diagnosed cumulatively through December 31, 1988. Thus, the economic cost of AIDS cases diagnosed in 1988 (the latest year with complete data), the direct cost of AIDS was $22 million, the indirect cost was $78 million, and the total was $100 million, or 0.54 percent of the GDP of Puerto Rico.

Numbers of cases

This study uses the number of officially declared AIDS cases by the Puerto Rican surveillance authorities reported as of July 10, 1989, but diagnosed as of December 31, 1988 (Latin American Center for Sexually Transmitted Diseases [CLETS], unpublished data, 1989). Fig. 1 shows the historical and projected numbers of AIDS cases through 1992. The trend projections forecast a cumulative number of AIDS cases through 1992 of 10,240 (quadratic projection) to 15,340 (linear projection). The lower estimate is based on the quadratic estimate (with a steady reduction in the rate of growth), while the higher estimate maintains the recent rate of growth.

Fig. 1 displays the costs of AIDS from persons infected based on the linear or trend projection. Fig. 2 displays these costs based on the more conservative, quadratic projection. In both figures, the lower bar denotes direct costs, and upper bar indicates indirect costs. Under the trend projection, the combined direct and indirect costs would be $541.2 million. To appreciate the magnitude of that amount for Puerto Rico, it is 2.6 percent of the present GDP of Puerto Rico or about $164 for each inhabitant of the island.

A similar linear projection was applied to the municipality of San Juan, the capital of Puerto Rico. San Juan deserves particular study because its incidence of AIDS per 100,000 population is second only to Washington, D. C. among all the metropolitan areas of the United States. Combining direct and indirect costs, the projected total for 1994 will amount to $270 for every person in the municipality. The per capita costs are relatively higher for the municipality because the AIDS cases are concentrated in a smaller population.

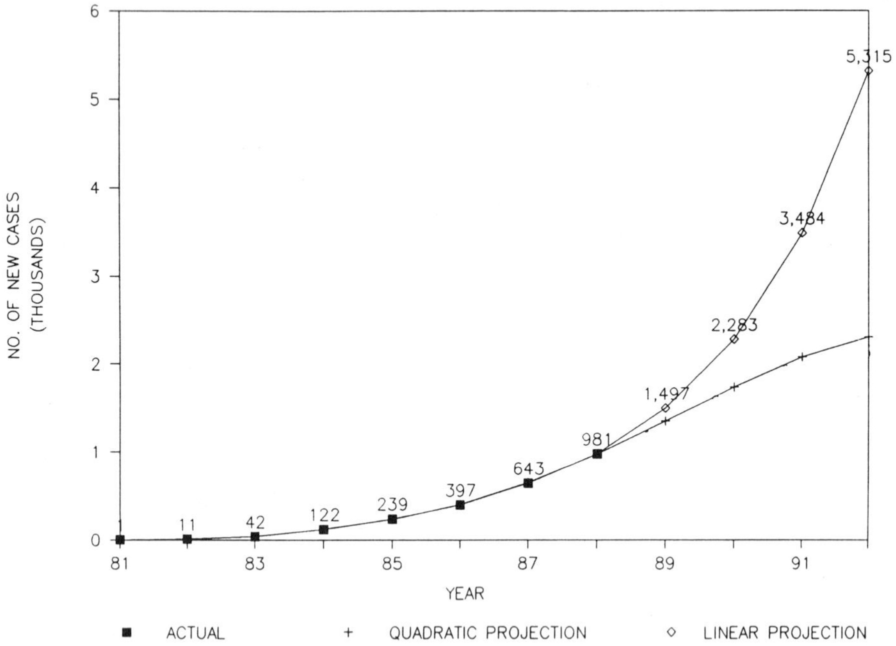

Fig. 1. Puerto Rico: numbers of AIDS cases by diagnosis year

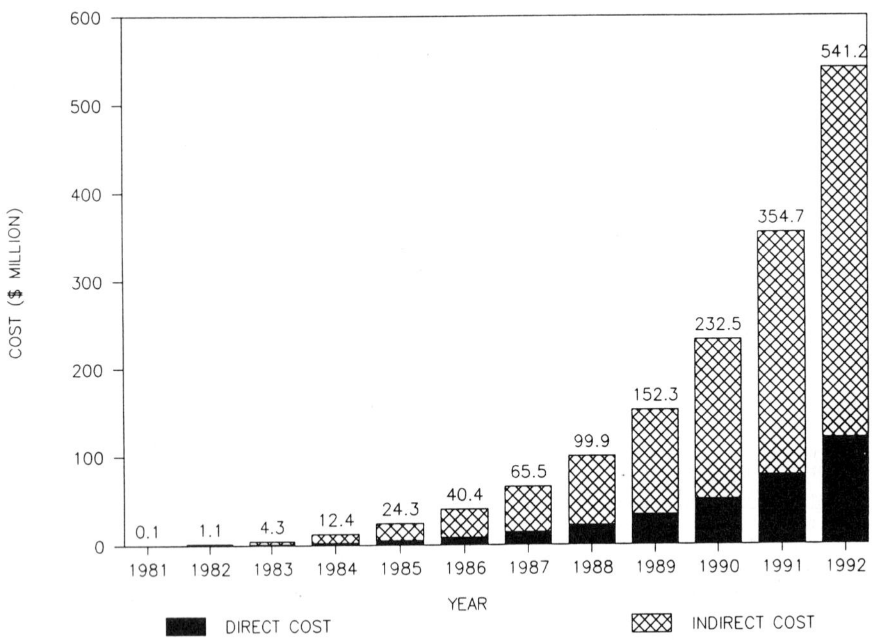

Fig. 2. Trend projection of economic costs of AIDS, Puerto Rico, 1981-1992

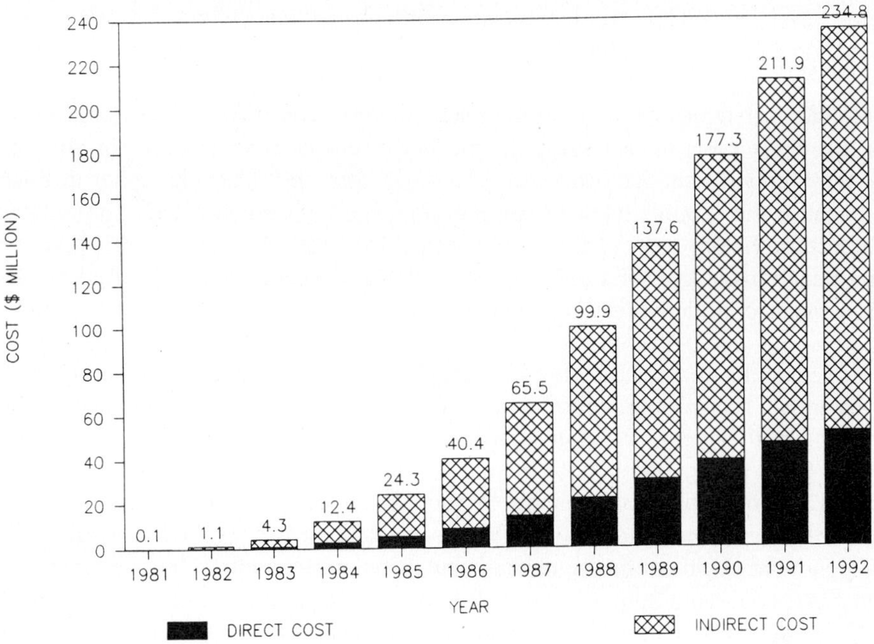

Fig. 3. Low estimate of economic costs of AIDS: Puerto Rico 1981 through 1992

Discussion and implications

The only other developing areas for which the author is aware of published studies of the costs of AIDS on a population basis are Zaire and Tanzania (Over et al, 1988). While Over et al. (1988) report primarily the cost per person infected with HIV, we can derive the cost per case of AIDS (termed "symptomatic HIV+") by dividing the cost per infected person by 0.354. This divisor is the time-adjusted proportion of infected persons which Over et al assumed would become symptomatic before dying from some other cause. The total (indirect and direct) cost per AIDS case ranges from $940 to $3230 for Zaire, and $2460 to $5320 and Tanzania. The Zaire numbers range from 15 to 54 times the per capita GDP; the Tanzania numbers range from 24 to 52 times the per capita GDP. The estimate for Puerto Rico, mentioned earlier, is 19 times the per capita GDP.

The multiples of GDP are higher for the two African countries because there HIV is transmitted primarily heterosexually and AIDS affects persons employed productively in the modern sector disproportionately. The groups primarily affected by AIDS in Puerto Rico - IV drug users and homosexuals - do not enjoy above average income. In Puerto Rico, as in the United States as a whole, the transmission of HIV follows primarily "pattern I" (homosexual and IV drugs). According to the epidemiologic patterns used by WHO, these African countries exhibit Pattern II (homosexual) transmission (Mann et al, 1988).

A final difference concerns the ratio of indirect to direct costs. The indirect costs are 3.6 times the direct costs in this study. In the two previous studies from Tanzania and Zaire, they ranged from 5 to 66 times. The direct costs are relatively higher in Puerto Rico because the island's health costs are relatively high for its GDP. This situation arises because health costs of the employed Puerto Rican population are covered by private health insurance, and costs of many others are covered by Medicaid or other public assistance, underwritten in part by the federal government of the United States.

These calculations demonstrate that the payoff to an effective educational program will be substantial. To illustrate, consider the expenditures on AIDS education in 1988 in San Juan. In that year, the municipality spent $300,000 to reduce risk behaviors, primarily by IV drug users, homosexuals. The decline in risk behaviors and new infections among male homosexuals in the United States over the last five years indicates that sustained education has been successful for this group. It is assumed that this expenditure could cut the number of new infections with HIV+ by 10 percent over the next year. As about 30 percent of HIV infections develop AIDS over four years, the educational program would cut the number of AIDS cases by about 3 percent in 1992. The present value of these savings would amount to $7 per capita. The expenditure is 70 cents per capita. Thus we would see a savings of $10 for every $1 invested. To be more precise, behavioral measures and the timing of any changes need to be considered more carefully. Nevertheless, these studies of direct and indirect cost confirm our conventional wisdom that prevention is a sound economic use of the services.

As the initial framework indicated, AIDS also imposes other types of costs. Loss of life imposes burdens beyond the economic costs derived here. Alameda and Martinez (1989) have also noted the importance of this component for Puerto Rico, but the adequate data for estimating these losses are lacking. Thus, the costs presented in this paper can be considered lower bounds of the complete costs of AIDS.

This work leads to several conclusions. The trend projections show that there are very substantial economic impacts of AIDS. For cases newly diagnosed in 1992, the costs in San Juan will be about $270 per person. For the island of Puerto Rico as a whole, the costs will be about $164, which is 2.6 percent of the gross domestic product. Because of these high costs, even a modestly successful educational program promises to have a high payoff.

Acknowledgement. The author is grateful to John Balling, Allison Brucker, Jorge Garib, Yamil Kouri, and Steven Schall for their assistance.

References

Hunt, W.A., Barnett, L.W., and Branch, L.G. (1971). Relapse rates in addiction programs. Journal of Clinical Psychology 27, 455-456.

Lozada Alameda, J. and Martinez Gonzalez, A. (1989). Economic-analysis of AIDS of Puerto Rico. Paper presented at the V International Conference on AIDS, Montreal.

Mann, J.M., Chin, J., Piot, P., and Quinn, T. (1988). The international epidemiology of AIDS. Scientific American 259(4), 82-89.

Over, M., Bertozzi, S., Chin, J., N'Galy, B., and Nyamuryekung'e, K. (1988). The direct and indirect cost of HIV infection in developing countries: the cases of Zaire and Tanzania. In: The Global Impact of AIDS (eds. A.F. Fleming, M. Carballo, D.W. FitzSimons, M.R. Bailey, and J. Mann). Alan R. Liss, Inc., New York, 123-135.

Over, M., Bertozzi, S., and Chin, J. (1989). Guidelines for rapid estimation of the direct and indirect costs of HIV infection in a developing country. Health Policy 11, 169-180.

Financial Aspects

Some Implications of AIDS for Permanent Health Insurance

A.D. Wilkie

I am an actuary from the United Kingdom. Actuaries are responsible for advising life assurance companies and pension funds about mortality rates and sickness rates.

In Britain most health services are provided by the National Health Service. Private medical care, paid for through medical expenses insurance, is relatively small, and used mainly for elective surgery, rather than for what may prove to be terminal care.

Medical expenses insurance is provided on a yearly renewable basis, that is the premium rates and policy conditions can be changed by the company at each annual renewal date. It has therefore been legally and commercially possible for the companies providing medical expenses insurance to exclude treatment for AIDS in their policies. They have therefore not been very interested in assessing the possible costs of treating those with HIV infection.

A different class of insurance business in Britain is called "Permanent Health Insurance" (PHI). This form of insurance is offered by a number of life insurance companies. It provides a monetary payment each week or each month, for so long as someone is sick - as defined by the policy conditions. For some policies the benefit starts immediately, or at least as soon as the insured person has been sick for one week. In other cases the benefit only starts after the insured has been sick for a deferred period such as 13 weeks or 26 weeks.

The longer the deferred period the more the insurance is like a benefit for total disability, rather than for sickness.

The word "permanent" in the title relates to the fact that the policy is on a permanent basis. An individual may effect a policy, perhaps at age 30, which will continue on the same guaranteed terms until age 60 or 65. The benefit of so many pounds per month is paid for by a fixed premium of so many pounds per year. The insurance company does not have the right to change the premium rates or the policy conditions. The companies are therefore very much concerned about how much claims may rise on existing policies because of AIDS.

For new policies, the companies have usually introduced an exclusion clause, either excluding payment if the insured is sick with AIDS, or excluding all benefit, and refunding premiums, if the insured is found to be HIV positive. This may avoid a future problem, but there is still the problem of the policies on the books.

The actuarial profession in Britain many years ago set up a committee (the Continuous Mortality Investigation (CMI) Committee) to investigate the mortality rates experienced by life offices, which also investigates the morbidity experience of PHI offices. I happen to be the chairman of that committee. The offices send in data, which are analysed and published, and from these data it is possible to construct standard tables, against which the experience of different offices can be measured, or which offices can use in the absence of their own experience.

During 1986 I began to develop a model to represent the spread of AIDS in the population, which would be of use to both life insurance companies and PHI companies. This model has formed the basis of Bulletins published by the AIDS Working Party of the Institute of Actuaries (AIDS Working Party, 1987a, 1987b, 1988, 1989). An important feature about a model for AIDS for these purposes is that it should be age-specific, that is, it should take into account the potentially very different experience of different age groups. Ordinary mortality and sickness rates vary very considerably with age. Mortality and sickness rates also vary considerably by sex, but so far in Britain the vast majority of AIDS cases have been among males, and much too little is known about the extent and spread of the epidemic among females for any calculations to be usefully carried out. We are therefore only considering the effect on males.

The model simplifies reality by assuming that the only spread of HIV is among homosexual males, and that all cases recorded so far have been in this group. In fact over 80% of UK AIDS cases have been among homosexuals. It is possible that in due course the separate epidemics among injecting drug users and among heterosexuals may grow to an extent which is worth considering, but at present too little is known about the rate of spread of the disease, at least among heterosexuals.

A second simplification we make is to assume that each age cohort, that is the group of people born in the same year, can be treated independently. Those born in year Y only infect others born in year Y, and there is no cross-infection between those of different ages. To the extent that sexual activity between homosexuals of different ages balances out, this is not an unreasonable simplification.

A diagram of the model we have used is shown in Fig. 1. It is quite a simple one. The population living at any one age is divided into four states which we call: Clear, At Risk, HIV Positive and Sick with AIDS. Those who are Clear have no chance of getting AIDS. Those who are At Risk do have a chance of getting AIDS, if they are infected by someone in the Positive state. Those who are Positive are infectious, but not yet sick. Those who are Sick with AIDS are treated as not contributing to new infections, and to have a high chance of dying from AIDS.

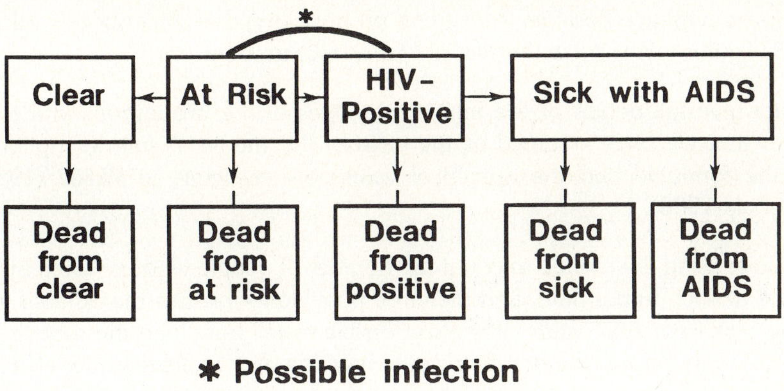

Fig. 1. A model of the spread of AIDS

Those in any of the living states may die from causes other than AIDS, and we have assumed the same mortality rates for all these states. Those who are sick from AIDS may die from normal causes or may die from AIDS. The age of the cohort is taken into account. Since each cohort is treated separately, it is possible to take account of the calendar year passed through as well. The period of time that someone has been in the Positive or Sick states is also taken into account, so that, for example, the chance of someone who is Positive developing AIDS can depend on how long he has been Positive.

Lines with arrows in the diagram represent the possible transitions between states. It will be seen that those who are At Risk may move to the Clear state. We use this to represent a change in behaviour, so that they no longer have any chance of becoming infected. Those who are At Risk may instead become Positive, and those who are Positive may become Sick.

The model does not represent varying degrees of sexual activity among those At Risk or Positive. However, we have to some extent represented the fact that highly promiscuous homosexuals are likely to have been infected first, while those with a lower degree of sexual activity may be infected later, by allowing the parameters that affect the infection intensity to reduce with calendar year.

The proportions in each state in the population at any time are controlled by a series of differential equations, which I shall not describe in detail. They are the usual equations for representing continuous transfers between states, except for the rate of new infections, which depends both on the number At Risk and on the number Positive. It is now possible in the model to represent different degrees of infectivity among those who are Positive, depending on how long they have been in that state, but in the figures I shall show this was not taken into account.

I shall not give full details of the numerical values of the proportions and transition intensities that we have assumed as the basis of the model. A full description of the model, the formulae and the numerical values are available in Wilkie (1988) and Daykin et al. (1988).

It is possible, using the model, to count the number of people who are forecast to be in each state at each future date, and therefore possible to forecast the number who will be in the Sick from AIDS state. It is also possible to tell how long these have been in this state, and therefore whether they would have an eligible claim under a PHI policy with a deferred period of so many weeks.

In the first instance the Institute of Actuaries AIDS Working Party used three models which they called A, BC and F. The essential features of the models are as follows: basis A assumed that 5% of the male population at the peak ages was At Risk, with lower proportions among older ages and younger ages. It assumed no change in behaviour, and no effect of drugs such as AZT.

Basis BC assumed two types of behavioural change, first a transfer from At Risk to Clear, at the rate of 10% a year, starting in 1987, and secondly a fall in the infection intensity, so that the doubling time of the epidemic, which began at one year, lengthened to two years by 1992.

Basis F assumed both of these behavioural changes, but assumed only 2.5% of males in the At Risk category, and assumed also that AZT would have the effect of doubling the expected lifetime of the Sick from about 1.4 years up to 1987 to 2.8 years after 1992, with a gradual change in between.

All these bases were calibrated against observed numbers of cases and deaths in the United Kingdom up to 1987. Many of the features of the model were based on experience outside Britain, particularly in the USA, but also from the Frankfurt study.

In fact the number of new cases of AIDS in 1988 in the UK was only a little up on 1987, and the number of deaths fell. These numbers were well below anything we had forecast, and we are in the process of revising our forecasts in order to try to take these new facts into account, perhaps by assuming an earlier behavioural change, perhaps by infectiousness that varies with the duration that somebody has been Positive. New forecasts for mortality have just been published in the UK (AIDS Working Party, 1989), but new forecasts for sickness have not yet been constructed.

The model simplifies reality by assuming that there is a straightforward transition from HIV Positive to Sick with AIDS. The reality is of course much more complex. We do not yet know at what stage in the development of the disease someone will have a justifiable claim under a permanent health insurance policy. We therefore carried out calculations on two assumptions - one that a period of eligible sickness only commenced when someone became Sick with AIDS and was continuous from that time onwards till death, the other that the period of sickness commenced as soon as someone became HIV positive and continued through sickness to death. The first assumption gives figures that are probably too low; the second gives figures that are almost certainly far too high. But they form useful outer limits of possibility.

We also considered two types of policy - one where benefit commences after one week of sickness - virtually immediately as far as AIDS is concerned, and the other where benefit commences only after 26 weeks of sickness. We thus have four different types of comparison, each on three sets of assumptions.

Results on the first of our assumptions are shown in Fig. 2, which shows rates of sickness by age, for someone aged 30 in 1988, which is the worst age in our model, on the assumption that benefit is only paid when someone is Sick with AIDS but is paid immediately. The rates are in weeks of sickness per year, and four lines are shown. Three of these are forecasts on bases A, BC and F, and the fourth, which has quite a different shape, shows the claim rates experienced by PHI offices in the years 1975 to 1978 on their ordinary business, as published by the CMI Committee (1984).

It can be seen to what a relatively small extent sickness claims are increased in those in their 30s and 40s. There is quite a large proportional increase at these ages, claims from AIDS being perhaps an extra 30% to 60% of the normal claims. But when we consider the sickness that is likely to develop anyway above age 50 or so, the extra claims from AIDS do not bulk very large. Since most UK policies give cover up to age 60 or 65, the addition of AIDS claims, though significant, is not likely to be disastrous for the companies.

The position would be different if claims were paid as soon as someone became HIV positive. Fig. 3 shows the results on this assumption, again for an immediate claim. The extra AIDS claims are considerably larger, but are still balanced by the normal claims above age 50.

In Fig. 4 we have a comparison on a 26-week deferred basis. That is, no claim is paid for the first 26 weeks of sickness either for AIDS or for other claims. The vertical scale is different from that of the earlier graphs. AIDS claims are relatively greater, and in Fig. 5, which shows claims on the assumption that they are paid from 26 weeks after someone becomes HIV positive, they are much larger still.

These results may not be very important for those concerned with the provision of medical care, but they show a possible approach which can be used to estimate the requirements for medical care for those who are infected with HIV or are suffering from AIDS. In order to make such forecasts one would need to have information about the medical care requirements of individuals at different states in the development of

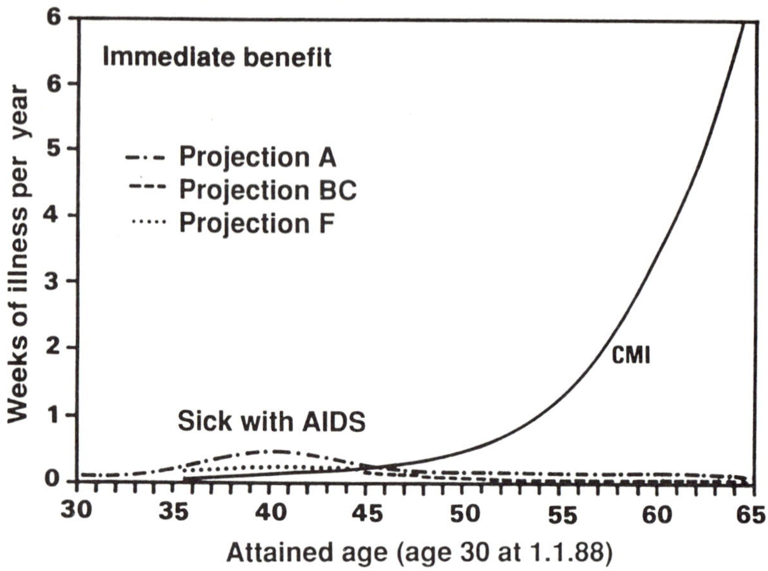

Fig. 2. Weekly monetary benefits paid immediately after the beginning of sickness, in the case of HIV/AIDS from the stage of full blown disease[1)]

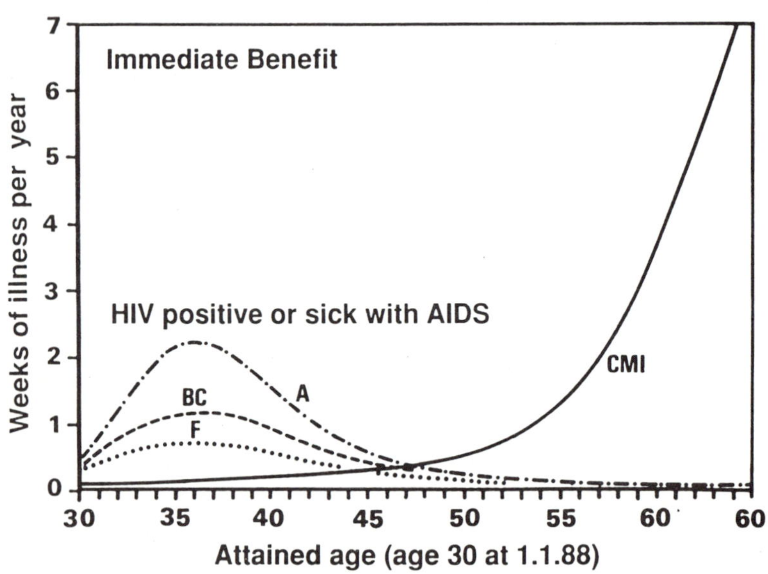

Fig. 3. Weekly monetary benefits paid immediately after the beginning of sickness, in the case of HIV/AIDS from the beginning of the infection[1)]

1) for abbreviations, see text

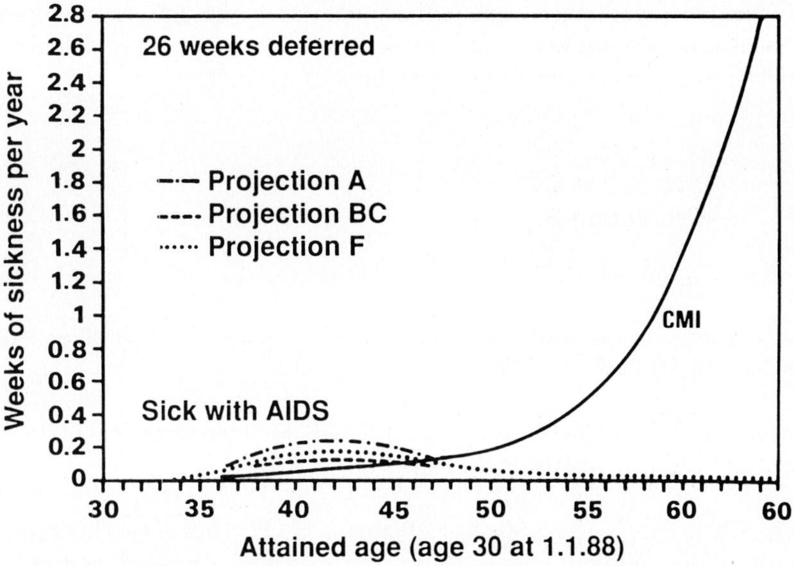

Fig. 4. Weekly monetary benefits paid only after 26 weeks of sickness, in the case of HIV/AIDS from the stage of full blown disease[1)]

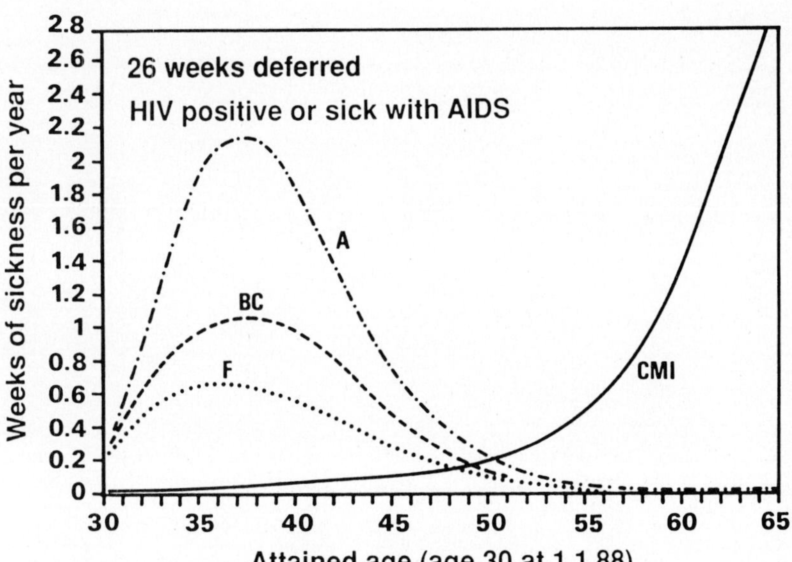

Fig. 5. Weekly monetary benefits paid only after 26 weeks of sickness, in the case of HIV/AIDS from the beginning of the infection[1)]

1) for abbreviations, see text

their illness. These may not be the same for haemophiliacs or drug users or women as for homosexual men, which is all that our model represents so far. More complicated models would be necessary to include these categories specifically.

References

AIDS Working Party of the Institute of Actuaries. Bulletins No. 1 (1987a), No. 2 (1987b), No. 3 (1988), No. 4 (1989).

CMI Committee (1984). Sickness experience 1975-78 for individual P.H.I. Policies. Continuous Mortality Investigation Reports, No 7, 1-161.

Daykin, C.D., Clark, P.N.S., Eves, M.J., Haberman, S., Le Grys, D.J., Lockyer, J., Michaelson, R.W., and Wilkie, A.D. (1988). The impact of HIV infection and AIDS on insurance in the United Kingdom. Journal of the Institute of Actuaries, 115, 727-837.

Wilkie, A.D. (1988). An actuarial model for AIDS. Journal of the Institute of Actuaries, 115, 839-853.

Scenarios and Policies

Planning for AIDS or HIV Related Services in Greece: First Steps towards Operational Schemes

M. Diomidis, A. Sissouras

Abstract

The epidemic of the acquired immune deficiency syndrome (AIDS) necessitates early planning of services and allocation of resources. This paper aims to provide preliminary information on the epidemiology of AIDS in Greece and the use of hospital resources by patients with AIDS in two Athenian hospitals. AIDS patients required on average 25 days of inpatient hospital care, each at an estimated current average lifetime cost of $ 6,880. Sociodemographic data and information on medical utilization were obtained from review of outpatient and hospital records.

The usefulness of operational research for the development of expert advisory systems and for evaluation studies (i.e. of HIV testing) is discussed and suggestions are made to study costs and financing of AIDS more systematically and to invest in preventive services throughout Greece in order to reduce the future social and financial costs of AIDS.

Introduction

It is always difficult to discuss the planning and economics of a terminal or debilitating disease because the focus of attention must be on the devastation it brings to its victims and their families. AIDS is no exception. However, a discussion which includes service planning for people with AIDS is made even more complicated by the mystery and fear that surrounds this disease. There are several characteristics of the disease that distinguish planning for AIDS from planning for other epidemics:

1. AIDS being a relatively new disease, there is absence of longitudinal studies on the transmission dynamics and the development of the disease. This causes problems of both estimating future demand for health services by client group, and defining the stages of the disease.
2. The client group is a heterogeneous mixture of people of different ages, lifestyles and stages of the disease, who therefore require a broad variety of services. Some high risk groups are reluctant to collaborate with the services they are entitled to, resulting in consequences both for their own health and the spread of the infection.

Medical treatment for the victims of AIDS, particularly when delivered on an inpatient basis, is costly. The treatment required for the systemic infections characteristic of AIDS patients tends to be lengthy and frequent. Information on average length of hospital stay for AIDS victims is sporadic and ranges from 12 to as high as 150 days. The estimated costs associated with these admissions range from $ 42,000 (Seage, 1986) to 147,000 (Hardy, 1986). In England, attempts to estimate the costs of clinical and preventive services for an inner London health district that has treated 18% of the cases in the United Kingdom, led to an average lifetime cost of $ 6,800, with an average of 50 days of inpatient hospital care (Johnson, 1986).

Although a substantial amount of research has been done on epidemiologic, immunologic and clinical aspects of AIDS, there has been little investigation into the economic aspects of the disease, and even less into the role that operational research and systems science can play in the fight against AIDS. In England, there is a growing movement to introduce operational research models to tackle the problem of planning and resource allocation, using the dynamic systems approach. In fact, an AIDS study group has been rather uniquely formed within the British O.R. society, which is generating a great deal of interest in the area. Various studies are reported (see a brief in the O.R. Newsletter, Feb. 1989 about a special conference on O.R. in AIDS) such as the work by Dr. Shahani (1988) at the University of Southampton on the development of simulation models and Tom Bowen's from the DHSS discussing the development and dissemination of a microbased model to assist Health Authorities in resource planning for service delivery. Dr. R. Hurrion of the University of Warrick introduced a microcomputer system developed as an expert advisory system for consultation by individuals, in particular nonclinical categories, as a contribution to public education.

Quality assurance for AIDS services and assistance to AIDS counselling groups are two other areas where operational research could be used in the future; but further investigation, more cooperation and exchange of information between the people involved in economics and operational research on AIDS at an international level is more than necessary in our fight against this disease.

The epidemiology of AIDS in Greece

In our country, the Ministry of Health responded very quickly to the oncoming AIDS epidemic. The first case in Greece occurred with a bisexual student from Zambia living in Athens (day of diagnosis: 25.10.83). During 1984 five more cases were identified (three bisexual, one homosexual and one heterosexual). From 1984 until 1989 the number of AIDS cases has increased dramatically. Currently, 226 AIDS cases are registered, of whom 91 have already died. The estimated number of HIV carriers runs from 8,000 to 16,000.

According to the Ministry of Health & Social Welfare (see Table 1), the percentage of haemophiliacs who received blood or blood products not screened for HIV is rather high. Since 1985, blood and blood products are screened for the presence of the virus in all blood banks of the country, according to EEC recommendations. Homosexuals comprise the second highest risk group of people infected with HIV. There is a high percentage of homosexuals among HIV carriers in the major area of Athens (12%), compared with the rest of the country (16%). Homosexuals are a well-organized group, supporting each other in cases of crisis. Hopefully, they have responded quite well to public education campaigns; currently, the incidence rate among them, at least in the capital area, is decreasing (~2%) (Ministry of Health, 1988).

The incidence of the disease among drug users in the major area of Athens is 0.5-3%. Greek drug users usually live in ghettos and they do not interact with other people. For this reason, the incidence of the disease among them is still low. Information and education of this high-risk group requires special efforts and, for a long time, has been rather difficult. This is so because many drug users are not known to the public health services and treatment units (like Ithaki, Strophi), and only a small number are regular users of specialist health or social services (e.g. Centre of Mental Health and Hot-line for drug users) (Ministry of Health 1988).

Prostitutes are also a well-organized group. Prostitution is legalized in Greece; registered prostitutes are screened and followed up every month by the AIDS Reference Centre at the School of Public Health in Athens. The incidence of AIDS in this high-risk group has not increased lately (Papaevangelou and Kallinikos, 1986). The incidence of AIDS in the general population as of August 1988 is believed to be around 0.02% according to WHO; for 1989 600-1,600 cases are expected.

Table 1. AIDS cases in high risk groups beginning 1988 in percent

High risk groups	% of AIDS cases
Homosexuals	13.6
Prostitutes	6
Call-girls	1.8
Drug-users	4.9
Foreigners	1.9
Blood donors	0.02
Blood recipients	4.3
Haemophiliacs	47.1

Source: Ministry of Health & Social Welfare

Clinical management

Infected individuals, whether asymptomatic or with more or less severe clinical manifestations of HIV infection, will need inpatient and outpatient services. Data from 30 AIDS patients treated in two Athenian hospitals are shown in Tables 2 and 3.

The average cost of an inpatient day in an Athenian teaching hospital, where these patients were treated, was $ 127 (1988 prices, Laikon Hospital, cost statements 1987-88). The average lifetime cost for patients with AIDS, managed in general medical wards, was - based on 50 days of inpatient care - $ 6,360. The total cost of 1,003 days of inpatient care amounted to $ 127,581.

The average lifetime cost of outpatient care, on the basis of 10.9 visits per case over a mean of 24 weeks, came to $ 520 (Laikon cost statements 1987). The heterogeneity of clinical problems in patients and the small sample size prevented us from analysing the hospital use by diagnostic category. Thus the total cost of life-time hospital care on the basis of current patterns amounted to $ 6,880.

While staying in the hospital, AIDS patients required many operative investigations. This is significant not because of the extra resources required in terms of staff but because of the difficulties of sterilizing the equipment, which makes it necessary to provide special equipment for the treatment of AIDS patients. Only 5% of admissions in the group studied required intensive care. This may reflect recent evidence that the outcome for patients treated in intensive care units is very poor.

A number of specific requirements arise for clinical management as the epidemic grows. Special equipment is just one of them. Many AIDS patients will require side-rooms, not necessarily because they pose an infection risk to other patients but because they are very sick or demand certain procedures that require extra precautions for health care staff.

Table 2. Length of stay per admission in two Athenian hospitals (n = 30)

Number of admissions	62 days
Mean length of stay per admission	25 days

Table 3. Lifetime length of stay per case in two Athenian hospitals (n = 15)

Mean weeks of follow-up	24
Mean bed days per case	50

The question arises of providing specialized wards. As of the beginning of 1989, we have unified in- and outpatient services in seventeen different hospitals (Teaching, District and Provincial Hospitals) around the country.

Unfortunately, the question of dental services is the one largely debated in Greece. Current guidelines advocate that HIV carriers should inform their doctors and dentists of their antibody status and that dental care should be undertaken in general dental practice, but patients found most of the times their practitioners unwilling to treat them, particularly in areas where many of HIV carriers reside, like Athens. A proposal to consider specialized dental services in certain hospitals is under discussion in the National Advisory Committee on AIDS.

Prevention in high-risk groups

The goal of prevention is to reduce the rate of spread of the virus. In the absence of a simple strategy like a vaccine, this has to rely on changes in behaviour. The role of the antibody test in this process is only one part of a long process which involves lifestyle and behavioural change. In Greece the antibody test is offered free-of-charge by seven Reference Centers around the country. Screening for the general population is offered free at two University Laboratories in Athens.

As we have estimated, during the last two years approximately 1,000 people attended the seven Reference Centers across the country and asked for testing and counselling services.

Recently, we looked at the groups attending the AIDS Reference Center at the School of Public Health in Athens. Among the people who have asked for testing and consultation there, 70% were homosexuals, 20% were bisexual men and another 10% were heterosexuals. The costs of providing the services include expenses for trained counsellors, for laboratory staff to do the antibody testing, and for kits and laboratory procedures. We anticipate the costs of an AIDS Reference Centre (they are all funded by the Ministry of Health) to be in the order of $ 73,000 this year.

Health care staff

Health care staff require regular training in "what does and what does not constitute a risk for HIV infection". This includes control of infection policies and good health and safety practices.

The major financial cost is the implementation of the guidelines of the National AIDS Advisory Committee. For the training of health professionals, workshops focusing on AIDS prevention have been promptly held. Health education material especially for health care staff has been prepared and sent to Community hospitals and Health Centres. Funding for planning guidelines and service implementation has amounted to $ 120,000.

Blood and blood products

Before 1986 we did not have any AIDS cases among haemophiliacs or patients receiving blood and blood products. During 1987, 14 cases (26.4%) of haemophiliacs with AIDS and 7 cases (13%) of patients receiving blood or blood products were reported. As of 30.9.1988, the number of haemophiliacs and transfused patients with AIDS somehow decreased: out of a total of 151 cases, there were only 4 (6.3%) of haemophiliacs and 5 (7.9%) other patients receiving blood or blood products. Since 1985 by govermental decree, all blood and blood products (domestic and imported) have been screened in all blood banks of the country for the presence of HIV. During 1987 only 0.02% of blood donors, mostly homo- and bisexuals, were found to be HIV carriers. The cost to the National Blood Transfusion Service for testing kits alone is approximately $ 2 million per year (Ministry of Health, 1986).

Planning arrangements at a national level

In view of the projected increase in the number of AIDS cases and in the underlying pool of HIV infection, a National Advisory Committee of AIDS residing at the Ministry of Health was formed in 1983. The task of this committee is to plan for the development of inpatient and outpatient services and to allocate appropriate resources. Any commitment of resources, though, will depend on both the current and future size of the epidemic and on the geographical distribution of the problem, while planning strategies need to be considered at National, Regional and District levels. Resource needs for clinical care are, for the time being, centered on Athens since over 80% of the AIDS cases have been reported in the capital area. Resources for preventive strategies must be considered nationwide if the spread of the virus is to be reduced. Districts and regions outside Athens may not see the control of the HIV epidemic as a current priority, though by the time they see their first case of AIDS, it is likely that they will already have a significant problem on their hands.

For 1988 the Ministry of Health has committed $ 145,000 specifically to AIDS. For 1989 the earmarked money for AIDS will amount to $ 1,180,000. This money will go to five general areas:

- Clinical management of infected individuals
- Advice and prevention for high-risk groups
- Protection and education of health care staff
- Safety of blood and blood products
- Education and prevention for the general population

Public health education campaign

Public Health Education Campaigns have two purposes. The first is to allay the kind of hysteria which has been part of much of the media coverage, focusing on fear of acquiring the virus from cups and door handles. The second purpose is to provide information and guidelines to those at high risk who will not be health service attenders. The recent Public Health Education Campaign in Greece has a cost of approximately $ 470,500.

We should, however, not underestimate the contribution of the voluntary and private sector in leading initiatives on health information and providing imaginative strategies for risk reduction both within and outside the health service.

According to our opinion, the message for AIDS prevention should be mostly provided outside health service institutions in gay pubs and clubs and at "street level" to work with drug users and prostitutes. For this purpose health care personnel, voluntary organizations and leaders of the high-risk groups should cooperate locally and nationally. Adequate funding should be invested to ensure a better flow of educational material, an evaluation of preventive programmes, a sharing of local strategies and a closer local monitoring of the HIV epidemic both within and outside high-risk groups.

Although the National Advisory Committee on AIDS has caught the prevention message it has done very little with the issue this year. The School of Public Health, Department of Sociology, in collaboration with the Ministry of Health and WHO is conducting a study to evaluate the level of knowledge, the attitudes and belief of the general population in Athens, as they have developed after the Public Health Education Campaign. Meanwhile at the University of Crete Medical School a study on the evaluation of the effectiveness of the AIDS health education campaign in Greece is under way (Philalithis et al., 1988).

Some methodological issues regarding HIV testing

Meta-analysis, decision analysis and cost-effectiveness analysis can be especially useful in the study of testing for the HIV. For example, meta-analysis can be used to synthesize the results of studies reporting the performance of the test. In prelicensure tests, the ELISA test was found to be both highly sensitive and specific (Johnson, 1987). However, this test was done under specified conditions that are not present in regular testing situations, so that the actual accuracy of the tests as used is likely to vary from these benchmark values (MMWR, 1988).
Meta-analysis can answer three questions:

1. What is the average effect of treatment?
2. Where and with whom is a treatment particularly effective or ineffective?
3. Is treatment at all feasible?

The results of the meta-analysis can be put into models for decision making based on tree diagrams. Decision analysis is useful in modelling HIV testing in three ways:

1. Calculation of post-test probability
2. Deciding whether to test or not to test
3. Comparison of tests and testing sequences.

Finally, the values from meta-analysis and decision trees can be used for a cost-benefit and a cost-effectiveness analysis.

Cost-benefit analysis compares investments in different programmes and values all outcomes, including mortality and morbidity. Cost-effectiveness analysis determines the most efficient or productive use of limited resources; for that, a monetary value of life and health to be assessed is not required (Weinstein, 1980). In the case of AIDS cost-effectiveness analysis can be used in various ways:

1. To evaluate alternative HIV testing methods including newly developed tests.
2. To estimate the distribution of the financial burden of testing among different populations and in different settings.
3. To evaluate the cost implications of currently available testing methods under different settings and for different populations.

A final point to support the usefulness of meta-analysis, decision analysis and cost-outcome analysis in HIV testing is the role of risk and uncertainty in decision-making. Clinicians have always had to make decisions without definitive information, since tests often leave the health care professionals still unsure about a diagnosis (Sox, 1986). Probability is a useful tool to quantify uncertainty; however, studies have shown that many physicians do not objectively analyse pre-conditional and post-test probabilities and use them in decision making. The general population uses objective probability estimates even less than physicians. People want to believe that a test can be 100% accurate and give them a perfect answer. Testing for HIV involves choices, none of which are perfect, a fact that is important for the public and the policy-makers to realize. Meta-analysis, decision analysis and cost-outcome analysis can make probability estimates more accurate and render the choices clearer.

In this era of cost-containment, the appeal of techniques that objectively examine the allocation of resources is undeniable. By improving our ability to predict the consequences of alternative policies and providing a framework for assessing those consequences, meta-analysis, decision analysis and cost-outcome analysis can lead us to better decisions. However, we should remember that the value of any analysis depends on how its results are translated into changes in practice (Weinstein, 1985). The irony of evaluation research is that the more we know, the harder it is to make decisions. As Oliver in the comic strip "Bloom Country" said when asked about the purpose of life: "Life is the futile passion for the pursuit of rationality."

Going back to the case of AIDS, apart of the sensitivity and specificity of the HIV antibody tests, it is more than necessary to point out that it is this service that provides practical and acceptable guidelines to reduce the risk of either acquiring or transmitting the virus, and that therefore it should be regularly used both in high-risk groups and for random anonymous testing for low-risk groups.

Comments

It is well known that individuals with AIDS require a substantial amount of health care resources. Our study population received its care at two sites, which may not be representative of other institutions. Furthermore, our sample size was limited and may not have been representative of AIDS patients as a whole.

An extension of this study to include an additional five hospitals that care for 80% of the AIDS cases in Athens is to be undertaken in the forseeable future. An evaluation of data from a variety of clinical settings with different patient characteristics will allow us to refine these preliminary findings and to clarify differences in patterns of care and different subgroups of patients. And although our paper is a descriptive one, we hope that our results provide at least baseline and preliminary data for policy-makers.

Conclusion

AIDS has become an important public health problem in Greece, and there will be some people arguing that it might absorb too many resources and too much media time, and there will be others who argue for the opposite. Resources are one thing, action is another. Both should be planned and implemented to have a positive outcome for the control of the AIDS epidemic in our country.

References

Hardy, A.M., Rauch, K., et al. (1986). The economic impact of the first 10,000 cases of AIDS in the United States. Journal of the American Medical Association 255, 209-11.

Hatzidimitriou, K., et al. (1988). The frequency of HIV, HBV, and syphilis antibodies in Greek blood donors. XX Congress of the International Society of Blood Transfusion in association with the British Blood Transfusion Society.

Johnson, S.E. (1987). Use of a commercial Elisa test for the diagnosis of infection by the AIDS virus, in a patient population. Diagnostic Microbiology Infections Disease 6, 267-271.

Johnson, A., et al. (1986). The acquired immune deficiency syndrome and epidemic of infection with human immonodeficiency virus: costs of care and prevention in an inner London district. British Medical Journal 293, 489-492.

MMWR update (1988). Serologic testing for antibody to human immunodeficiency virus. MMWR 36(52), 833-845.

Ministry of Health (1988). AIDS monthly report. Athens.

Mandalaki, T. et al. (1986). HTLV-III antibodies in Greek haemophiliac patients. Iatziki 50, 167-170.

Papaevangelou, G. and Kallinikos, G. (1986). AIDS: International and Greek experience on AIDS. Athens Min. Med. Greca 12, 339.

Papaevangelou, G. (1985). Recent evidence of the AIDS problem in Greece. Iatriki 48, 69.

Philalitis, A.E., Georgoulias, V., Tsilivakos, V., Vlachonikalis, I., and Fioretos, M. (1988). Evaluation of the effectiveness of the AIDS health education campaign in Greece. Paper presented at the IV International Conference on AIDS, Stockholm.

Seage, R. et al. (1986). Medical care costs of AIDS in Massachousetts. Journal of the American Medical Association 256(22), December.

Shahani, A. et al. (1988). Modelling the natural history of AIDS as a social process. 1988 Mason Conference: Focus on AIDS, Oxford, September.

Sox, M.C. (1986). Probability theory in the use of diagnostic tests. Annals of Internal Medicine 104, 60-66.

Stephanou, T. (1986). Governmental assistance to AIDS victims. Ministry of Health, Division of Public Health, Iatziki 50, 263-266.

Weinstein, M.C. and Finenberg, H.V. (1980). Clinical decision analysis. Philadelphia: WB Saunders, Co.

Weinstein, M.C. and Stasou, W. (1985). Foundation of cost effectiveness analysis for health and medical practices. NESM 196(13), 716-721.

WHO (1988). WHO Country Report. August.

Epidemiological Models and Socioeconomic Information: Methodological Aspects of AIDS/HIV Scenario Analysis

J.C. Jager, M.J. Postma, F.M. van den Boom, D.P. Reinking, J.C.C. Borleffs, S.H. Heisterkamp, J.A.M. van Druten, E.J. Ruitenberg

1. Introduction

A rapidly growing, multidisciplinary body of literature on the spread of the human immunodeficiency virus (HIV), which causes the acquired immunodeficiency syndrome (AIDS), is available. Among the fields involved, virology, immunology, epidemiology and clinical studies prevail. In recent research attention is also paid to mathematical models for HIV transmission and the economic and sociocultural aspects of the epidemic. In this paper we discuss the incorporation of these three components into AIDS research directed to scenario analysis. Scenario analysis is a technique of surveying the future by means of scenarios. Application of relevant techniques aim to support decision making in public health problems.

We present some general features of scenario analysis, followed by an outline of the current state of AIDS research using epidemiological models. The phases where one meets methodological problems on the way from basic research to scenario analysis in support of public health policy making are indicated. We present a conceptual framework for scenario analysis of the social, cultural and economic impact of AIDS. Our ongoing research projects are reviewed to illustrate their potential contribution to the establishment of AIDS scenarios.

2. Scenario analysis

Scenario analysis emerged during the early 1950s as a technique applied to military problems in Santa Monica at the Rand Corporation. In this respect we could mention the name of Kahn, "the father of the scenario technique". Since then scenario analysis has become the vogue in other fields as well (Organisation for Economic Co-operation and Development, 1979; International Institute for Applied System Analysis, 1980). Nowadays public health is a major field for applications. This is the case in the Netherlands (e.g. Steering Committee on Future Health Scenarios, 1985, 1986, 1987, 1988). Scenario analysis is a technique to scout the future society by means of scenarios.

A scenario is a description of a possible path, governed by a series of developments, leading from the prevailing state of a part of society to a future state, with the goal to gain insight into the mechanisms that determine the path, the future state and the possibilities of influencing these mechanism (Hoogeveen and Brouwer, 1989). An important publication on future studies (Kahn and Wiener, 1967) defines a scenario as a hypothetical sequence constructed for the purpose of focussing attention on causal processes and decision points. The latter definition stresses mainly the strategic aspects of scenarios.

It is useful to classify scenarios as exploratory and strategic (target setting) (Pannenborg, 1985; Brenner, 1986). An exploratory scenario could be defined as an outline of a natural or expected course of events. They explore the future assuming particular developments that might occur. The so-called zero scenario is an exploratory scenario. It describes a future in which all developments continue their current course. It is an extrapolation of trends that already exist in society. It might be a prediction, given unaltered policy. With respect to AIDS we might imagine a zero scenario as a description of the path of the incidence of AIDS cases or HIV infected patients in a surrounding in which no new developments (behaviour change; therapeutics; vaccine) or prevention activities occur. The other family of scenarios that makes up the class of exploratory scenarios is the what-if scenario. These scenarios explore a future in which certain, clearly defined, new developments occur. An exploration of a future with a vaccine that renders resistance against HIV is a what-if scenario. Fig. 1 presents, schematically, exploratory scenarios. We find ourselves on the left, in the present. Via different paths different future states are arrived at on the right. One path could represent the zero scenario, the others different what-if scenarios.

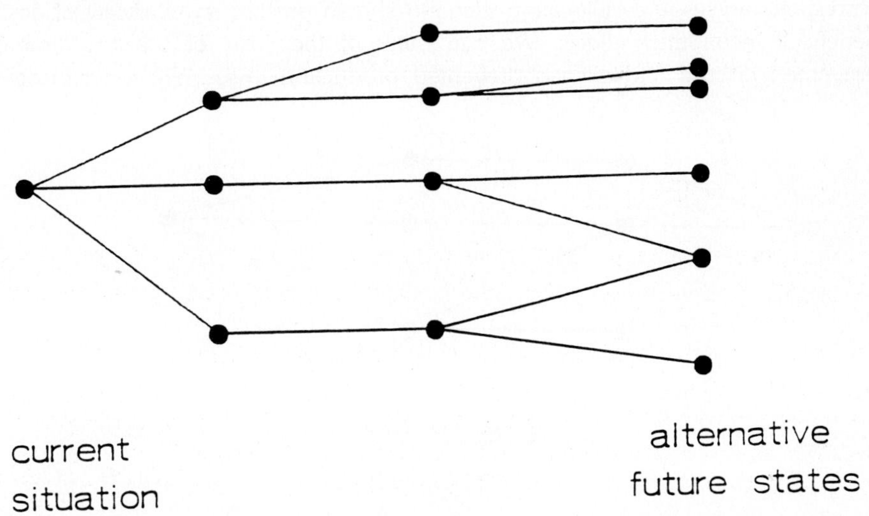

Fig. 1. Exploratory scenarios

A second type of scenario is the family of the strategic scenarios. In these we aim at reaching a desired goal. A definition that applies here is a hypothetical sequence of events, constructed for the purpose of focussing attention on causal processes and decision points. This type of scenario shows the strategy, the causal sequence of efforts to cope with a problem in society, and the effects of the strategy. The effects, nevertheless, can only be recognized by comparing the strategic scenario with the natural course of events, which is described in the zero scenario. In the absence of a zero scenario a strategic scenario has to be compared with another scenario as a reference. In this case it is difficult to evaluate realistic effects implied by the relevant scenario, so strategic scenarios cannot exist in isolation.

With respect to the AIDS epidemic we could imagine a strategic scenario e.g. as a chosen programme that blocks needle exchange amongst intravenous drug users and the effect of the blocking on the epidemic, leading to the desired future state. Fig. 2 exhibits strategic scenarios. We find ourselves on the left again, in the present. A desirable future state of society is defined. This future state can be reached via a number of strategies.

In Brenner (1986) a third type of scenario is recognized. This category comprises the resource allocation scenarios, which delineate the resource implications of strategic scenarios. The strategic scenario shows the implication of a strategy, the corresponding resource allocation scenario gives insight into the feasibility of the strategy in an economic sense. The strategic scenario might be extended with a cost-benefit or cost-utility analysis for this purpose.

Let us return to the strategic scenario with blocking needle exchange. The corresponding resource allocation scenario should present an overview of costs and beneficial (economic) effects. We can think of the costs of the programme and prevented disease and alleged prevented production losses. We have presented a

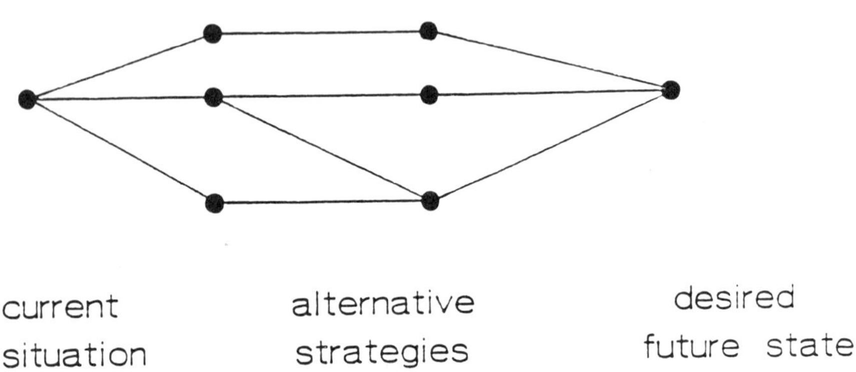

Fig. 2. Strategic scenarios

hierarchy of scenarios. Resource allocation has to be based on strategic scenarios, and strategic in turn cannot function without exploratory scenarios. The exploratory scenario assesses the magnitude of the problem, the strategic scenario provides a way to cope with the problem, and the resource allocation scenario checks the feasibility of the latter.

The resource allocation scenario lays emphasis on the implications for the economy of a strategic scenario. We could, however, also think of scenarios that deal with epidemiological, social, demographical or cultural aspects. With respect to social aspects one can think e.g. of the impact of the epidemic on quality of life as experienced by patients, stigmatization and discrimination of groups at risk and legal measures taken.
In principle we have a categorization into two types of scenarios: exploratory and strategic (see Table 1). A parallel categorization is based on the aspects that the scenario pays most attention to, e.g. economic, epidemiological, social, demographic or cultural impact.

3. Position of epidemiological models in AIDS/HIV scenario analysis

This section indicates the role and position of epidemiological models in current quantitative research on the spread of HIV aimed at the support of public health policy making (prevention, health care planning). Referring to our own work carried out under the auspices of the Ministry of Welfare, Public Health and Cultural Affairs in the Netherlands we present an outline of the present state of this research, and we will try to define further research priorities. Fig. 3 shows the position of disciplines and research activities involved. This scheme might be helpful in a discussion of (1) results of research already obtained and (2) remaining problems.

The integrated application of data collection, statistical data analysis and mathematical modelling takes a central position (Fig. 4). Many mathematical models have already been developed, and we refer the reader to the several reviews now available (Her

Table 1. Categorization of scenarios

Scenarios		Aspects
exploratory	zero what-if	epidemiological social demographic cultural economic
strategic		(e.g. resource allocation)

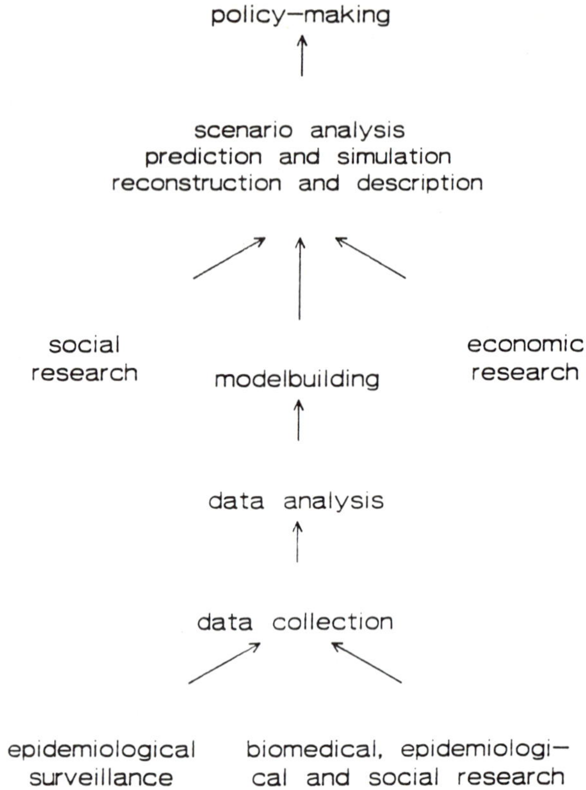

Fig. 3. Overview concerning the position of disciplines and research activities involved in the quantitative analysis of the AIDS epidemic. Surveillance and basic research render the epidemiological data that are collected. After and together with data analysis model building is commenced. The aims of model building are, while integrating social and economic research, first, description and reconstruction, next, prediction and simulation and finally, scenario analysis. The last one is primarily undertaken to support policy making.

Majesty's Stationary Office, 1987, 1988; Jager and Ruitenberg, 1988; Statistics in Medicine, 1989). AIDS modelling represents a new area for research, motivated by the complexity (several linked risk groups, heterogeneity in behaviour involved in virus transmission, geographical differences) of the still extending epidemic. The present mathematical models may crudely be divided into two main groups: statistical and population dynamic models.

Table 2 summarizes the main characteristics, the general aims and the ensuing scenarios of these two groups of models. The main difference between the two groups is found in the nature of the models. The population dynamic models explicitly take into account the transmission mechanism that rules the course of the epidemic (Bailey and Estreicher, 1987; Anderson, 1988; Dietz, 1988; Isham, 1988). The statistical

Table 2. AIDS/HIV mathematical models and scenarios

* Statistical models	empirical	- description - short-term prediction	- zero scenario
* Population dynamic models	mechanistic simple	- description - reconstruction - long-term prediction - parameter estimation - sensitivity analysis - simulation	- all types of scenarios
	mechanistic complex	- generating hypotheses - incorporation of heterogeneity - sensitivity analysis - simulation	- zero excluded

models are empirical. They are based on statistical methods applied to AIDS incidence data (Morgan and Curran, 1986; Downs et al., 1987; Healy and Tillet, 1988; Her Majesty's Stationary Office, 1988; Brookmeyer and Damiano, 1989). The use of statistical (empirical) models mainly remains restricted to the description of the course of the epidemic and only allows extrapolation for a short period (e.g. 2 years). Their application can lead to zero scenarios. The so-called simple mechanistic models might be useful over a much broader range of analysis - including reconstruction, prediction, simulation and scenario analysis. If the relevant mechanistic model is of a rather complex nature, validation by data becomes difficult - their main use is the generation of hypotheses - and the assessment of a zero scenario is excluded.

Statistical models

Now we turn to statistical modelling (Table 2). We have paid much attention to the path from epidemiological surveillance to modelling (Fig. 3) to make maximal use of the data collection on AIDS cases (carried out by the State Supervision of Public Health, Division of Infectious Diseases, Rijswijk, the Netherlands). In collaboration with the WHO Collaborating Centre on AIDS, Paris, a procedure has been developed for the statistical analysis of reported AIDS incidence, the first epidemiological data which have become available since 1984 (Downs et al., 1987, 1988; Heisterkamp et al., 1988a, 1988b). By means of a maximum likelihood method the actual numbers of diagnosed AIDS cases are adjusted for the well-known phenomenon of reporting delay. The formal statistical method is summarised in Heisterkamp et al. (in press). The present application of the method makes use of the exponential model. However, it is possible to apply the method with all kinds of parametric functions. This enables the link of this empirical method to mechanistic models.

Fig. 4 shows the results of the applications to AIDS incidence reported in the Netherlands up until January 1, 1989. Extrapolation of a fitted exponential model provides predicted numbers of new AIDS cases. The prediction might be connected with economic information and alternative economic developments resulting in economic scenarios for the short-term. The method might also be applied to AIDS cases which come from a specified risk group and/or geographical area (e.g. predictions for the city of Amsterdam).

The usefulness of the method can be increased further by the incorporation of the distribution of the incubation time (see e.g. Brookmeyer and Damiano, 1989, for the intended approach) and of other relevant HIV infection stages (CDC classes). Then it becomes possible to predict prevalences for these stages, including the final stage preceding death. The latter requires the incorporation of mortality data. These intended elaborations will be profitable for short-term projections and economic scenarios. A further perspective is the combined use of this method with a mechanistic model, which could lead to strategic scenario building, projection and scenarios that exceed the short-term range.

Hardy et al. (1986) and Scitovsky and Rice (1987) estimated the economic impact of AIDS in the USA, by means of empirical projections. Application of our empirical model in a similar approach leads to exploratory economic scenarios for the Netherlands. We might think of economic scenarios based on alternative assumptions, e.g. concerning substitution of inpatient by outpatient care. However, data that are suited for combination with the empirical models that render incidence figures are not yet available. The economic information (see below under Recording system for hospital care) that is available namely seems, at the moment, most suited for combination with prevalence figures. Prevalence figures can be obtained from the incidence figures when information on mortality and progression becomes available.

Population dynamic model

Our mechanistic modelling started with the development of a model for HIV transmission within the group of homo/bisexual men - a simple model - and was extended to a multigroup transmission - though more complex - model (van Druten et al., 1988; van Druten et al., 1989; van Druten et al., submitted). The basic frame of the multigroup model is presented in Fig. 5. Only the main modes of transmission are considered, viz. unprotected anal, vaginal intercourse and needle sharing. The HIV/AIDS epidemic is a composite of several overlapping and linked epidemics, each

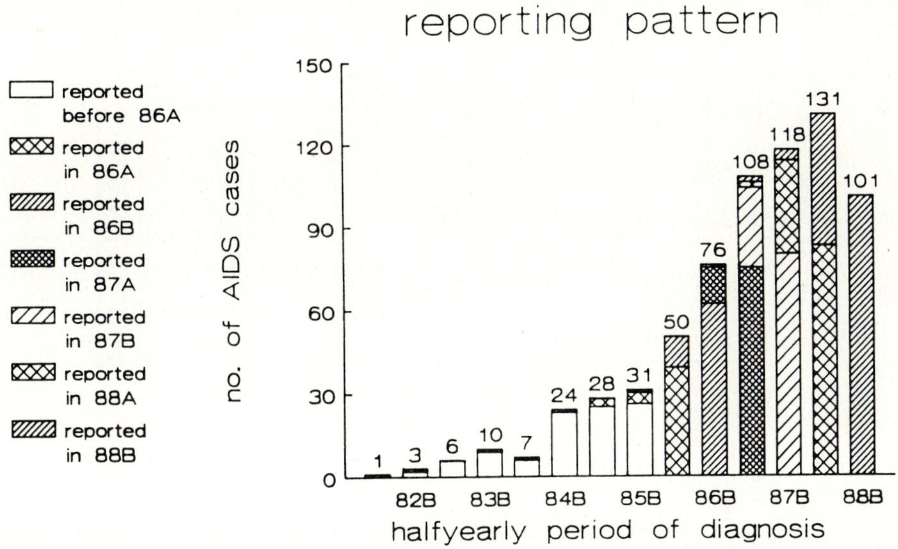

4a.

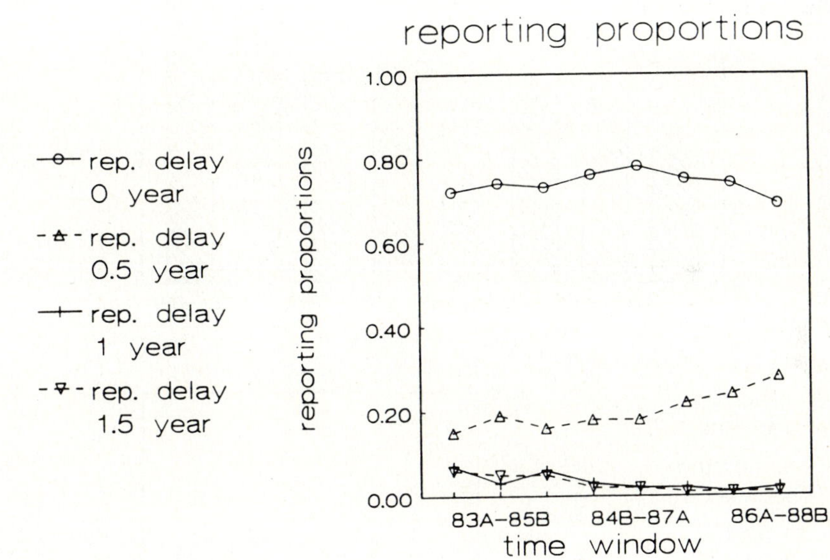

4b.

Fig. 4. The reporting pattern in the Netherlands is exhibited in **a** (Source: Bijkerk, 1989); the phenomenon of reporting delay is obvious. In **b** it is shown that reporting proportions are fairly stable over time. Some other European countries possess a less stable reporting pattern. The number of AIDS cases per half-year period, adjusted for reporting delay is given in **c**. An essential magnitude in describing the epidemic is the doubling time (see **d**); one exponential curve (characterized by a constant doubling time) could never achieve a satisfactory fit. Therefore the use of time windows has become the vogue. Predictions and confidence limits based on the most recent time window (consisting of six half-yearly periods including the last half year of 1988) are presented in **e**.

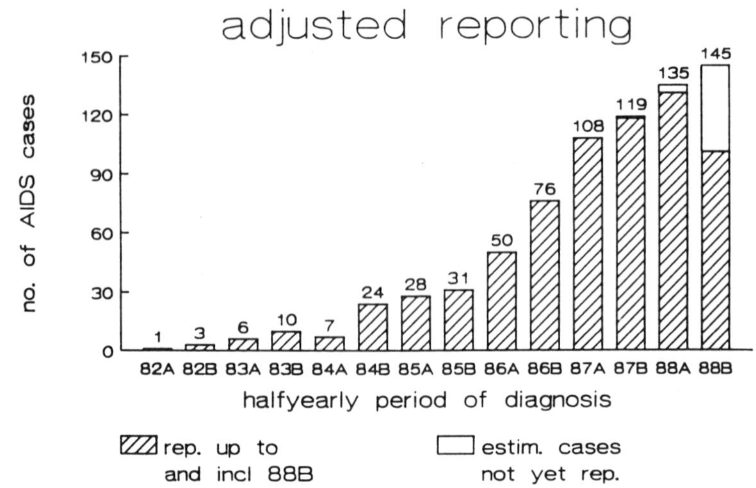
adjusted reporting
no. of AIDS cases
150
120
90
60
30
0
1
3
6
10
7
24
28
31
50
76
108
119
135
145
82A 82B 83A 83B 84A 84B 85A 85B 86A 86B 87A 87B 88A 88B
halfyearly period of diagnosis
rep. up to and incl 88B
estim. cases not yet rep.

4c.

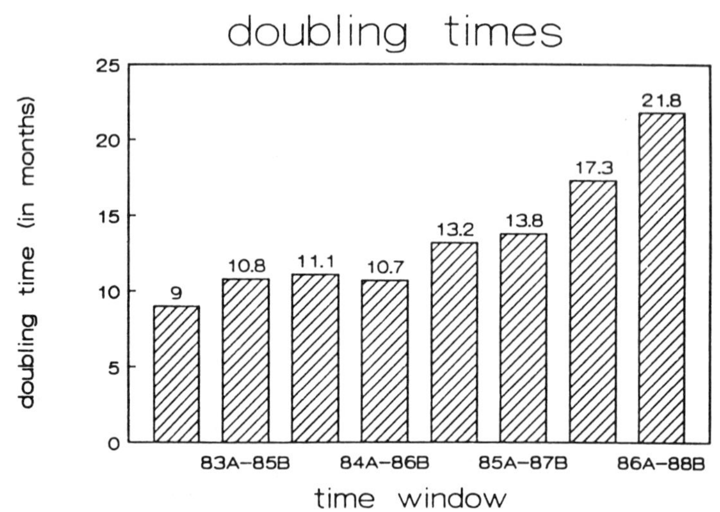
doubling times
doubling time (in months)
25
20
15
10
5
0
9
10.8
11.1
10.7
13.2
13.8
17.3
21.8
83A–85B
84A–86B
85A–87B
86A–88B
time window

4d.

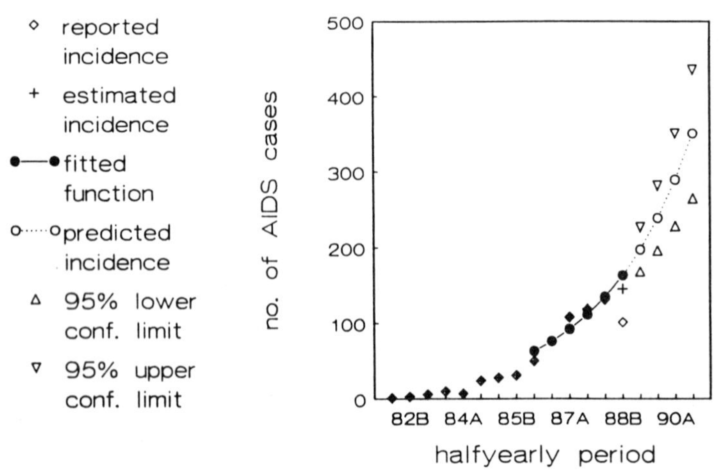
reported incidence
estimated incidence
fitted function
predicted incidence
95% lower conf. limit
95% upper conf. limit
no. of AIDS cases
500
400
300
200
100
0
82B 84A 85B 87A 88B 90A
halfyearly period

4e.

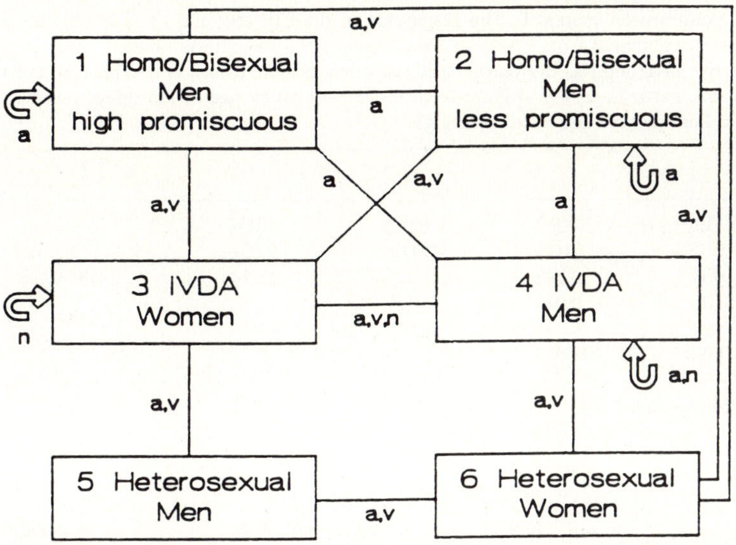

Fig. 5. The AIDS epidemic is the resultant of a number of overlapping epidemics in different risk groups. This figure shows possible contacts (with the risk of virus transmission) between and within risk groups. The three transmission modes in this model are unprotected anal (a), vaginal (v) intercourse and needle sharing (n).

with its own dynamics and time course. A major objective of the model concerns the way from the biomedical, epidemiological and social (sexual behaviour, needle sharing) information to modelling (see Fig. 3) of the epidemic in the major risk groups.

The model is designed to clarify which basic data are needed. It provides a link between basic information from biomedical, social and epidemiological studies and the mathematical formulation of the model (see Fig. 3) in the form of a transmission matrix. Table 3 presents a numerical example of this matrix. The formula in Fig. 6 specifies in a simplified way the information needed to attach figures to the matrix and to run the model. With this method of presenting formulas we aim at making models more easy to understand for non-mathematicians. We illustrate here the computation of the value 0.05 in the second row, first column (Table 3), which is the transmission potential from highly promiscuous homo-/bisexual males (group 1) to less promiscuous homo-/bisexual males (group 2). Transmission takes place only via unprotected anal intercourse. So in the summation in Fig. 6 vaginal intercourse and needle sharing need not be considered for this particular matrix element. The proportion of group 2 which has partners in group 1 is 0.1. The number of new partners in group 1 of an individual in group 2 is 25 per year. The probability of infection per partnership is 0.02. Multiplication of these three figures renders 0.05, the matrix element. The reader is referred to van Druten et al. (1988) for a detailed mathematical description and motivation of the model.

Table 3. The transmission matrix T. The magnitude in the i th row and the j th column reflects the annual transmission potential from j to i; we could refer to this magnitude times the size of group i and divided by the size of group j as the yearly basic reproduction rate from j in i. Where no entry has been made transmission between or within is theoretically impossible by one of the three transmission routes (vaginal and anal intercourse and needle sharing).

	1	2	3	4	5	6
1	1.5	0.2	0.025	0.004	-	0.0035
2	0.05	0.5	0.0016	0.001	-	0.0014
3	0.17	0.043	0.25	0.34	0.18	-
4	0.013	0.011	0.30	0.29	-	0.0087
5	-	-	0.0027	-	-	0.10
6	0.0014	0.0023	-	0.001	0.40	-

Source: van Druten et al., 1989

$$t_{ij} = \Sigma_{a,\,v,\,n} \left\{ \begin{array}{l} \text{proportion of} \\ \text{individuals in} \\ \text{group i who} \\ \text{have partners} \\ \text{in group j} \end{array} \right\} \times \left\{ \begin{array}{l} \text{number of new} \\ \text{partners in j per} \\ \text{year of an indi-} \\ \text{vidual in i with} \\ \text{partners in j} \end{array} \right\} \times \left\{ \begin{array}{l} \text{probability of in-} \\ \text{fection from infec-} \\ \text{tive person in j to} \\ \text{susceptible in i} \\ \text{per partnership} \end{array} \right\}$$

Fig. 6. The entries in the transmission matrix in words. The capital sigma stands for a summation over the three transmission modes a, v and n (see legend Fig. 5)

Furthermore, this model can be used to perform theoretical experiments (see Table 2, e.g. sensitivity analysis and simulation). For instance we can study the effects of various intervention (prevention) strategies like blocking the transmission of the virus in groups of intravenous drug users which occurs via needle sharing or blocking the transmission between or within other main risk groups. The model is useful for the assessment of all types of scenarios. If sufficient data are available, application could lead to zero scenarios, as a reference to what-if scenarios.

Recording system for hospital care

To enable the connection of mathematical models and (causal backgrounds of) hospital costs for HIV infected patients, a recording system has been developed. Jager et al. (1988) presented four other objectives of the system.

- Development of a method for monitoring and describing costs, related to hospital care and treatment of AIDS and HIV infected patients
- Assessment of a quantitative basis for the set-up of efficient AIDS services in hospitals: classification and recording system for observed variables concerning treatment and care, and corresponding database structure
- Development of a survey to measure the quality of life

- Monitoring, prediction and simulation of costs related to the course of disease, according to CDC classification

Table 4 summarizes the items which are being observed continuously on all HIV patients in the University Hospital Utrecht. In total about 350 variables are observed. The recording is operational for a period of more than two years, and the data for the first 1½ years are analyzed (Borleffs and Jager, 1989). Cost estimates are obtained for all activities involved in care and treatment.

Table 5 presents a summary of costs. Extension of the recording system in time and place (other hospitals) increases the scope of such results. The continuous registration enables the detection of fluctuations and trends. The detailed level of recording allows the detection and definition of disease stages relevant from a social and/or economic viewpoint.

It should be realized that hospital costs are not the only relevant costs (see e.g. Kahn, 1988; Drummond and Davies, 1988). Other cost categories are related to care (social services, (ambulatory) mental health care, primary health care and home care) and more general impacts of AIDS on society (research, prevention, education, life years lost, production losses, quality of life aspects). We noticed the lack of a universally accepted terminology for the classification of costs. The development of such a terminology can help to clarify which cost categories are relevant in our attempt to connect social and economic research with epidemiological modelling. In addition such a classification can support targeted data collection.

Table 4. Components of database system on treatment, care and costs, designed by AZU and RIVM

Demographic data	date of birth, residence, ...
Risk group -general	sexual orientation, IV drug use, occupation, ...
Risk group -specific	number of male/female partners, number of years of IV drug use, activity in prostitution, ...
Relevant medical listing	sexual transmitted diseases, hepatitis B, ...
CDC classification	
Clinical parameters	fever, weight loss, recent infection, dyspnoea, fitness, ...
Characteristics of care	admissions, consulations, artificial ventilation, ...
Treatment	medication, blood transfusion, ...
Diagnostic procedures	endoscopies, pulmonary function studies, haematological, immunological and biochemical tests, diagnostic imaging, biopsies, serological and microbiological studies, ...
Cost per item	
Quality of life	social background, medical state, distress, well-being activities of daily life, prognosis, ...(fixed questionnaire every 4 months)

Table 5. Costs (in- and outpatient) for treatment and care of 40 HIV infected patients under observation in the University Hospital Utrecht between January 1, 1987 and July 1, 1988 (amounts are given in Dutch guilders). Total costs and the mean per patient per year of observation are given.

	Number of patients	Mean period under observation in years	Total costs (1.5 years)	Mean costs/ patient in year
CDC II	13	0.504	33.524	5.115
CDC III	12	0.999	43.525	3.629
CDC IV	18	0.534	387.229	40.267
Total	40*	0.704	464.277	16.486

Source: Borleffs and Jager (1989)

* Three patients progressed through several CDC stages during the observation period.

Finally, we would like to draw attention to two points concerning the allocation of funds for health care. First, relevant with respect to this allocation might be the application of analogous database systems to other diseases, so that comparisons between them become possible. Second, besides the economic side of the problem the study also incorporates the social aspects of the quality of life of patients. Results on this point are expected in the next publication of the study. A customary procedure in allocating funds is relating the quality of life gained and the costs to do so. The reader might consult Rees and Roberts (1988), who reflect on and criticise this procedure in the special case of AIDS and infectious diseases in general.

AIDS scenarios

Based on the initiative of the World Health Organization and the Steering Committee on Future Health Care Scenarios, the Netherlands, we recently started an AIDS scenario study on the social and economic impact of AIDS on society. A conceptual model for this study has been designed (Fig. 7). The intended scenario project should give insight not only into the course of the epidemic but also into future effects on society. So, three aspects are suggested for a simultaneous study: epidemiological modelling linked with social-scientific and economic information.

The point of departure is that it is useful to distinguish groups at risk. So the model (Fig. 7) will be filled in for multiple groups: homo-/bisexuals intravenous drug users, IVDU prostitutes, prostitutes, health care personnel, etc. For each group the level of risk is influenced by the engagement in high-risk behaviour, the existence of high-risk situations in the surroundings and the prevalence of the infection. Risk may lead to infection and transmission. These processes together with the progression (the flow through the CDC classes after infection) may be represented in epidemiological models.

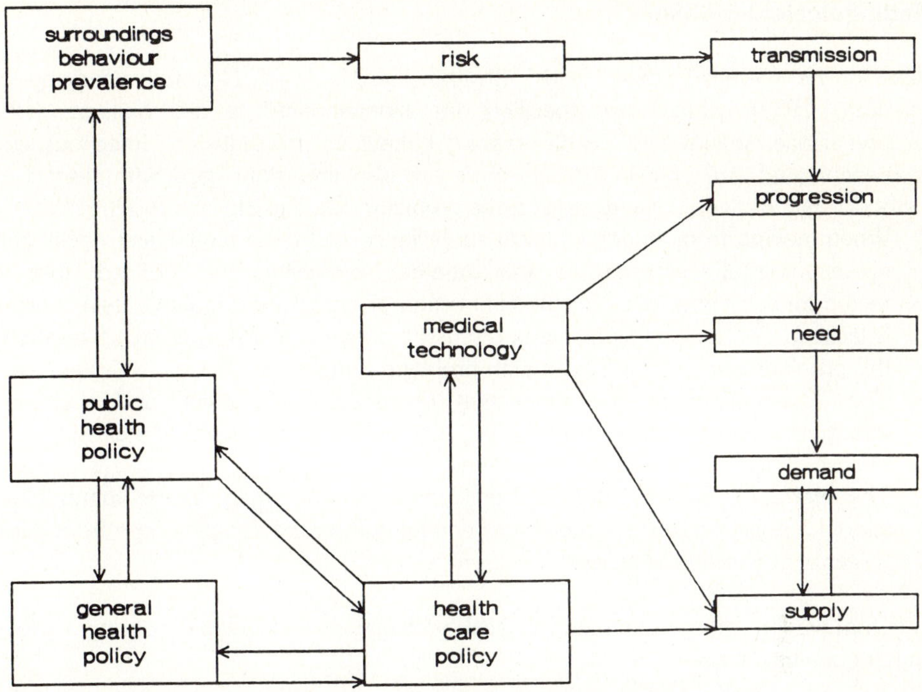

Fig. 7. A conceptual model for the Dutch scenario project on the sociocultural and economical impact of AIDS on society.

The medical technology includes all efforts to improve care for and treatment of HIV infected individuals. Also the search for a vaccine might be placed here. Next to and closely related to medical technology is the health care policy, one of the three components that influences health care. It covers all efforts in the areas of guidance, support, care and treatment of HIV infected individuals. So the funding of supply of care, regulations and instruction for health care workers are situated here. We might say that the health care policy is directed towards fulfilling the task that faces society, to provide care for HIV infected persons. Public health policy is concerned with the containment of the disease (prevention, education). General health policy, finally, represents all laws and regulations in relevant fields.

The economy in the scheme is placed at the bottom right. Medical technology shows the limit of what is possible. Together with the prevalence in the different CDC classes it establishes the objective need. Supply and need of course settle demand.
As far as we know the development of AIDS scenarios is still in its infancy. We refer the reader to Leidl (1988,1989).

Methodological problems

Next to the so-called 'data needs' (Institute of Medicine, National Academy of Sciences, 1988) which are specified by mathematical model builders (HIV seroprevalence, sexual and needle sharing behaviour, transmission, infectiousness, progression and size of risk groups), there are also important gaps with respect to methodology. We would like to stress three problems (see Fig. 3).

- When moving from epidemiological surveillance and basic biomedical, social and epidemiological research to mathematical modelling we noticed that a methodological apparatus for the connection of models and multiple data sources is lacking. The transmission matrix discussed above is a first approach for solving this problem, but statistical estimation problems remain.
- The development of the connection of models with social and economic information requires theoretical studies, such as the development of a classification of costs which play a role in the epidemic.
- The interface between models and policy making shows many shortcomings. How should a policy maker use the results emerging from the complex path from basic research to scenario analysis?

The formulation of these methodological problems has developed during various international meetings.

International collaboration

The present studies on modelling contribute to the Concerted Action (CA) on Statistical Analysis and Mathematical Modelling of AIDS of the European Communities. The National Institute of Public Health and Environmental Protection of the Netherlands is charged with this CA. Recently the proceedings of the first workshop (December 1986) appeared (Jager and Ruitenberg, 1988). For the second workshop (July 1988) a report is available. In an upcoming workshop (December 1989) attention will be asked for the above-mentioned problems: connection of models with economic, social and cultural information and modelling in support of policy making.

Proceedings from similar other recent meetings on mathematical modelling have appeared (special issues Journal of the Royal Statistical Society, 1988; Statistics in Medicine, 1989; Institute of Medicine, 1987). At the request of the World Health Organization the Dutch Steering Committee on Future Health Care Scenarios (STG) is preparing an international scenario project on the impact of AIDS on society in cooperation with The Netherlands Institute of Mental Health (NcGv) and the National Institute of Public Health and Environmental Protection (RIVM). Guidelines for the setup of this study are available on request.

4. Summary and conclusions

This paper presents a discussion on methodological aspects of research which forms a basis for reliable AIDS scenario analysis in support of policy making concerning prevention and health care planning. The integrative role of mathematical modelling is considered. Assessment of AIDS scenarios requires information from many research areas: basic biomedical and epidemiological research, social and economic research. The position of these disciplines around a skeleton of epidemiological modelling has been outlined. Types of models, their aims (possibilities) and types of related scenarios are described and illustrated by ongoing projects.

The way from basic research on HIV and AIDS to scenarios, concerning the social and economic impact of HIV infections, is complicated. The success of scenario building will depend on the development of sound methodologic links between the disciplines involved. We have mentioned the most important requirements:

- Development of a structured data collection suited for model building, e.g. the specification of a 'transmission matrix' and a recording system for hospital care and treatment
- Identification of links between models and social and economic information, e.g. classifications of costs and specification of relevant HIV stages (observation of distributions leading to prevalence models starting with incidence models)
- Development of the interface between modelling and policy making

A preliminary conceptual model as a basis for the establishment of socioeconomic scenarios is formulated.

We have considered AIDS research with the ultimate aim of predicting the future course of the epidemic and the building of scenarios. This should motivate careful attention to theoretical/methodological activities that support the execution of research, viz. (1) stating of the problem and (2) the objectives, (3) planning the data collection. These points deserve further study.

Acknowledgements. This work benefited from a grant of the European Commission in support of the Concerted Action on the Statistical Analysis and Mathematical Modelling of AIDS of the Epidemiology Subgroup of the EC Research Working Party on AIDS. In addition, this contribution was supported by the Steering Committee on Future Health Care Scenarios (the Netherlands). We thank Ir.R.T.Hoogeveen, Dr.R.Leidl and Drs.M.J.J.C.Poos for valuable comments.

References

Anderson, R.M. (1988). The epidemiology of HIV infection: variable incubation plus infectious periods and heterogenity in sexual activity. Journal of the Royal Statistical Society, A, 151, 66-98.

Bailey, N.I.J. and Estreicher, J. (1987). Epidemic description and public health control with special reference to influenza and AIDS. In: Proceedings of the 1st World Congress Bernouilli Society, 2. VNU Science Press.

Bijkerk, H. (1989). AIDS 1982-1988. Nederlands Tijdschrift voor Geneeskunde 133(10), 523-525.

Borleffs, J.C.C. and Jager, J.C. (1989). Registratie en kostenschatting van klinische en poliklinische werkzaamheden voor patiënten met HIV-infectie. Nederlands Tijdschrift voor Geneeskunde 133(15), 767-772.

Brenner, M.H. (1986). Scenarios, decision making and strategic planning: a framework. In: Scenarios and other methods to support long term health planning; theory and practice (eds. J.J. Brouwer and R.F. Schreuder). Proceedings and Outcome of a STG/WHO workshop Noordwijk, The Netherlands, 14-16 October 1986.

Brookmeyer, R. and Damiano, H. (1989). Statistics methods for short-term projections of AIDS incidence. Statistics in Medicine 8(1), 23-44.

Dietz, K. (1988). The dynamics of spread of HIV infection in the heterosexual population. In: Statistical analysis and mathematical modelling of AIDS (eds. J.C. Jager and E.J. Ruitenberg). Oxford University Press, Oxford.

Downs, A.M., Ancelle, R.A., Jager, J.C., Heisterkamp, S.H., Druten, J.A.M. van, Ruitenberg, E.J., and Brunet, J.B. (1988). The statistical estimation, from routine surveillance data, of past, present and future trends in AIDS incidence in Europe. In: Statistical analysis and mathematical modelling of AIDS (eds. J.C. Jager and E.J. Ruitenberg). Oxford University Press, Oxford, 1-16.

Downs, A.M., Ancelle, R.A., Jager, J.C., and Brunet, J.B. (1987). AIDS in Europe: Current trends and short-term prediction estimated, from routine surveillance data, January 1981-June 1986. AIDS 1, 53-57.

Drummond, M.F. and Davies, L.M. (1988). Treating AIDS: the economic issues. Health Policy 10, 1-19.

Druten, J.A.M. van, Boo, Th. de, Reintjes, A.G.M., Jager, J.C., Heisterkamp, S.H., Coutinho, R.A., Bos, J.M., and Ruitenberg, E.J. (1988). Reconstruction and prediction of spread of HIV infection in populations of homosexual men. In: Statistical analysis and mathematical modelling of AIDS (eds. J.C. Jager and E.J. Ruitenberg). Oxford University Press, Oxford, 52-76.

Druten, J.A.M. van, Jager, J.C., and Heisterkamp, S.H. (in press). HIV infection dynamics in linked risk groups. Journal of the American Statistical Association.

Druten, J.A.M. van, Jager, J.C., Heisterkamp, S.H., Poos, M.J.J.C., Coutinho, R.A., Dijkgraaf, M.G.M., Reintjes, A.G.M., and Ruitenberg, E.J. (submitted). HIV infection: a dynamic and constant size multigroup transmission model. Statistics in Medicine.

Hardy, A., Ranch, K. et al. (1986). The economic impact of the first 10,000 cases of acquired immunodeficiency syndrome in United States. Journal of American Medical Association 255, 209-211.

Healy, M.J.R. and Tillet, H.E. (1988). Short-term extrapolation of the AIDS epidemic. Journal of the Royal Statistical Society A, 151.

Heisterkamp, S.H., Jager, J.C., Downs, A.M., Druten, J.A.M. van, and Ruitenberg, E.J. (1988a). Statistical estimation of AIDS incidence from surveillance data and the link with modelling of trends. In: Statistical analysis and mathematical modelling of AIDS (eds. J.C. Jager and E.J. Ruitenberg). Oxford University Press, Oxford, 17-25.

Heisterkamp, S.H., Jager, J.C., Downs, A.M., Druten, J.A.M. van, and Ruitenberg, E.J. (1988b). The use of Genstat in the estimation of expected numbers of AIDS cases adjusted for reporting delays. Genstat Newsletter 21, 4-18.

Heisterkamp, S.H., Jager, J.C., Downs, A.M., Druten, J.A.M. van, and Ruitenberg, E.J. (in press). Correcting reported AIDS incidence: a statistical approach. Statistics in Medicine.

Her Majesty's Stationary Office (1987). Future Trends in AIDS.

Her Majesty's Stationary Office (1988). Department of a Health Working Group. Short-term prediction of HIV infection and AIDS in England and Wales. HMSO, London.

Hoogeveen, R.T. and Brouwer, J.J. (1989). Scenarios in de volksgezondheid: inleiding in de methodiek van de STG. (in press).

International Institute for Applied Systems Analysis (1980). Energy in a finite world. Laxenburg.

Institute of Medicine (1987). Approaches to modelling disease spread and impact. Report of a workshop on mathematical modelling of the spread of human immunodeficiency virus and demographic impact of acquired immune deficiency syndrome. October 15-17.

Institute of Medicine, National Academy of Sciences (1988). Confronting AIDS, Update 1988. National Academy Press, Washington D.C.

Isham, V. (1988). Mathematical modelling of the transmission dynamics of HIV infection and AIDS, a Review. Journal of the Royal Statistical Society special issue.

Jager, J.C., Borleffs, J.C.C., Geels, R.M.A., Heisterkamp, S.H., Jong, J.T.L. and, Ruitenberg, E.J. (1988). A method for monitoring hospital costs related to AIDS and HIV-infection. IV international Conference on AIDS. Stockholm (Abstracts 9521).

Jager, J.C. and Ruitenberg, E.J. (eds.) (1988). Statistical analysis and mathematical modelling of AIDS. Oxford University Press, Oxford.

Jager, J.C. and Postma, M.J. (1989). De AIDS epidemie: prognoses en economische gevolgen. In: Dilemmas bij AIDS (eds. H. Vuysje and R.A. Coutinho). (in press).

Journal of the Royal Statistical Society, special issue (1988). A 151, 3-136.

Kahn, H., and Wiener, A. (1967). The year 2000. New York.

Kahn, J. (1988). The economic impact of AIDS: models for the future, a working paper. McGill Centre for Medicine, Ethics and Law.

Leidl, R. (1988). Ökonomische Aspekte. In: AIDS und HIV-Infectionen. Diagnostik, Klinik, Behandlung. Handbuch und Atlas für Klinik und Praxis (ed. H. Jäger). Ecomed, München-Landsberg.

Leidl, R. (1989). Model-based scenarios to describe economic impacts of AIDS: the role of case-mix. In this volume.

Organisation for Economic Cooperation and Development (1979). Facing the future. Paris.

Morgan, W.M. and Curran, J.W. (1986). Acquired immunodeficiency syndrome: current and future trends. Public Health Report 101, 459-465.

Pannenborg, Ch. O. (1985). Scenarios as a method for probing and planning the future of health care. A paper for the international meeting on the future of health and health systems in the industrialized societies, Bellagio, May 27th-31th. The Hague.

Rees, M. and Roberts, B. (1988). Quality adjusted life years (QALYs) and the cost of AIDS patients. IV International Conference on AIDS, Stockholm (Abstracts 9586).

Statistics in Medicine (1989). Special issue on statistical and mathematical modelling of the AIDS epidemic (ed. R. Brookmeyer). Statistics in Medicine, 8, 1.

Steering Committee on Future Health Scenarios (1985). Growing old in the future. Rijswijk, The Netherlands.

Steering Committee on Future Health Scenarios (1986). The heart of the future/the future of the heart. 1. Scenario Report, Rijswijk, The Netherlands.

Steering Committee on Future Health Scenarios (1987). Anticipating and assessing health care technology. Rijswijk, The Netherlands.

Steering Committee on Future Health Scenarios (1988). Cancer in The Netherlands. Rijswijk, The Netherlands.

Model-Based Scenarios to Describe Economic Impacts of AIDS: The Role of Case-Mix

R. Leidl

1. Assessing future economic impacts of AIDS: a deterministic scenario approach

Considerations about the possible future of AIDS and its economic impacts are often struck by considerable uncertainty of data, both for assumptions (like the number of people infected) and for results (like the total expenditures for care last year). Theoretical background and consequently functional properties of epidemiologic as well as impact elements are not yet (well) understood. Time series to be used for an empirical specification of functions are often too short to derive reliable results. Stochastic approaches show tremendously increasing confidence intervals. Most of these problems already apply to individual elements of predicting economic impacts (like the number of people infected), let alone interrelated aspects (like the number of people infected, treatment patterns and transition probabilities).

At the moment, the modelling of the economic impact of AIDS seems characterized by a number of interrelated, unknown and not yet testable functions. To promote some understanding of the problem and its possible developments, it seems useful to start with rather simple models. From such a basis, variables can be extended and functions incorporated step by step, covering more details and replacing sections that are better understood theoretically or empirically, at later stages. With this background, scenarios based on a deterministic simulation methodology and on extensive sensitivity analyses are proposed to describe possible, alternative futures. Rather than predicting exact points or ranges for indicators, the understanding of the dynamics of epidemiologic developments and economic impacts under different assumptions is considered as the main purpose of this approach.

Basically, an epidemiologic model is here combined with economic impact functions (Leidl, 1988). The scenario methodology introduced is looked upon as one tool to describe, in a transparent way, the starting points, impact functions and consequences of AIDS. By integrating different empirical backgrounds, it can be adapted to different populations and country contexts. It can be applied in three ways:

- Testing the consistency of different assumptions with empirical results obtainable for the past
- Predicting futures by a type of "if - then" reasoning, with comprehensive sensitivity analyses

- Analyzing the effects of interventions, like the impact of prevention programmes on economic consequences, or medical advances like drug therapies or vaccination programmes.

This paper will deal with the first two of these issues (for the third, see Leidl, 1989). It introduces the model to be applied, then investigates the impact of different cost assumptions, among them the effects of case-specific costing. Finally, for alternative epidemiologic scenarios possible futures are described for a case-mix indicator, which is supposed to be meaningful both in medical terms and in terms of resource use.

2. The epidemiologic model and the economic consequences

The epidemiologic development of HIV infection and the resulting diseases in a population is described by an infection function and, starting for each infected person at the time of seroconversion, a "development of the disease" model. These two components are formulated for a high- and a normal-risk group in a population. Thus the epidemiology of HIV, pre-AIDS stages and AIDS is described by a highly aggregated model, taking into account the objective of linking impact functions with the yearly prevalences in each of the stages.

The infection function is a logistic one. It displays an exponential type of growth in the very beginning, and, proportionally to the share of people already infected, turns and approaches an assumed satiation limit. The function is described in detail in the Appendix. It has been chosen for its theoretical plausibility, because it can be tuned to fit observed data, and because of its flexibility during processing. Effects like behavioural change can be operationalised in changes of one parameter, i.e. the growth rate of infection.

The development of the disease in the model used here is defined by the probabilities of progression from HIV to ARC (AIDS-related complex, taken as a label for pre-AIDS symptomatic stages) or to AIDS for 16 periods. Actual parameters were derived from epidemiological studies as far as available (i.e. data for 10 years; see also Appendix).

Both epidemiologic elements, the spread of the infection and the onset of the natural history of the disease model for the cohort infected, taken together can generate yearly prevalences of cases in each stage. Economic impact functions, formulated per case type, can then be linked with these period prevalences to produce total impact indicators.

The operationalisation of the economic consequences is summarized for direct costs in two sectors of care and for one indicator of indirect cost (Table 1).

Table 1. Indicators for economic consequences

Information needed	Impact indicators	
Hospital care		
- Days per year per case (AIDS) - Days per year per case (ARC) - Daily inpatient rate	Beds needed: Direct cost:	cases * days/310.25 (occupancy norm: 85%) total days * daily rate
Outpatient care		
- Cost per year per case (AIDS) - Cost per year per case (ARC)	Direct cost:	cases * cost
Social burden		
- Age of patients at time of death - Age-specific life expectancy	Indirect burden:	cases * mean years lost (mortality only)

For the purpose of clarity and simplicity, the further discussion will however focus on direct cost of care indicators only, i.e. indicators for health care expenditures, which are especially relevant for health insurers.

Both the epidemiologic and the economic part of the model have to be filled empirically. For epidemiology, this is accomplished by using study data on the natural history of the disease, and by retrospectively fitting assumptions for the two risk groups so that the resulting AIDS cases will match the number of AIDS cases reported officially. This also produces figures for the still unknown numbers of cases in pre-AIDS stages.

The economic data may be taken from cost studies. The implications of some of their variation is discussed in the next section, where possible fits for the epidemiologic development and the results of German cost studies are used to add empirical weight to the model. With alternative assumptions therefrom, the effects of different cost assumptions in describing the past are explored.

3. The sensitivity of total expenditures with respect to type of epidemic, level of cost, patterns of care and case-specific resource needs

In the following applications of the model, the basis of empirical reference is the Federal Republic of Germany. As described, the number of AIDS cases reported officially is used to "tune" the model to a population (about 60 million) and a spread of

AIDS matching the one in the FRG (1669 cases at the end of 1987 for the time being, which will have to be revised for reporting lags later). In the economic part, cost studies are used to define possible values for assumptions as well as some upper and lower limits (Hanpft et al., 1988; Reinecke et al., 1988; Koock-Walewski et al., 1988; Koock-Walewski and Stille, 1989). The available studies use classifications of cases in three stages: HIV cases, LAS/ARC cases as types of symptomatic disease and AIDS cases as the full-blown type. For the purpose of this paper, it is assumed that case definitions in both the epidemiologic and the economic part sufficiently overlap to be linked with each other.

First, the overall sensitivity of cost is discussed for, as an example, the total yearly expenditures in 1988. Cost indicators comprise inpatient days for ARC and AIDS and outpatient cost for all three stages. Three sets of assumptions were selected as "low", "medium" and "high" cost levels. They range from very low - not to say from the lowest - plausible values to ones close to a plausible maximum, as available from the cost studies. All cost sensitivity analyses will be performed within this framework (Table 2).

Before the above economic assumptions are discussed, some results from tuning the epidemiologic parameters have to be integrated: different sets of assumptions produce almost similar useful fits up to the present state, while differing in their future spreads. Thus different basic types of spread should be used for scenarios.

The alternative basic types of spread of the HIV infection were developed by the following procedure. An exploratory universe of 31,680 sets of parameters was drawn from all possible combinations for the eight epidemiologic parameters in the two-group

Table 2. Cost assumptions for sensitivity analyses

Yearly indicator	Low	Medium[1)]	High	Increase relation[2)]
Inpatient days[3)]				
AIDS	40	60	80	$30 + 10\,i$
ARC	10	20	30	$5 + 5\,i$
Outpatient cost[4)]				
AIDS	1,500	3,000	9,000	$1{,}250 + 250 * 2^{(i-1)}$
ARCS	1,000	2,000	3,000	$500 + 500\,i$
HIV	100	300	500	$100\,i$

1) used as standard for case-mix index
2) i = 1/3/5 for low/medium/high; values 0 to 5 were checked
3) to be multiplied by a daily rate of DM 300.-
4) in DM

model, restricting them roughly to plausible ranges (e.g. restricting the number of AIDS cases in the normal-risk group below 10%). Then, the ranges were classified. For each set, the number of AIDS cases for 1981 to 1987/8 was calculated and compared with the cumulative yearly prevalences of full-blown AIDS cases officially reported by the Bundesgesundheitsamt in Berlin - omitting the problem of reporting lags. The fit was measured in terms of the mean root of square errors. In successively focussing steps, the results were screened

- According to the best fits
- According to the parameters varying with increases in fits for different high-risk group sizes
- For plausible shares of normal-risk group AIDS cases
- For redundancy
- For heterogeneity among the remaining types.

The procedure resulted in four basic types, which differ especially in the size of their high-risk group (I: 180,000, II: 100,000, III: 60,000 and IV: 20,000; for other parameters, see Appendix).

For these four basic types, cost sensitivity for yearly expenditures 1988 in the FRG was calculated. The analysis was performed for all low, all medium and all high cost parameters. The results are displayed in Fig. 1.

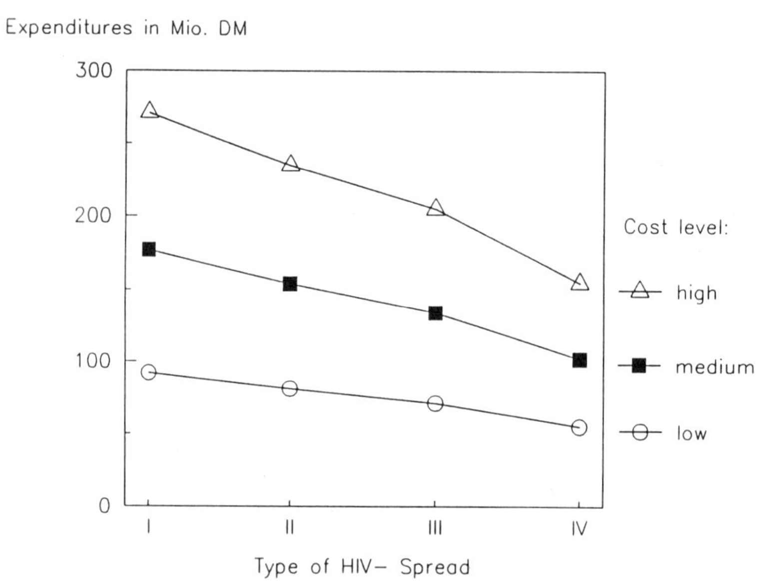

Fig. 1. Sensitivity of yearly expenditures (1988); 3 cost levels

One main source of variation in Fig. 1 stems from the number of cases in pre-AIDS stages. These cases need a considerable amount of resources for care, are empirically unknown in their extent and vary between the four basic types; i.e. the same number of AIDS cases may be observed with different numbers of cases in pre-AIDS stages. The variation between the four epidemiologic types increases with the level of cost parameters (high/medium/low) assumed. Sensitivity differences between cost level assumptions within the framework of Table 2 are more significant than between the epidemiologic types; only two scenario combinations (I/medium and IV/high) overlap across cost levels. Overall, a significant uncertainty of total 1988 AIDS expenditures is displayed.

Fig. 2 deals with the effects of two other types of variations: one is a description of the inpatient-outpatient relation in the care of ARC and AIDS patients, the other one an alternative description of resource needs in just one stage of the disease, here exemplified for the ARC cases.

Within the framework of the assumptions displayed in Table 2, descriptions of the inpatient/outpatient relation in care, which can be viewed as possible alternative treatment patterns, were operationalised in the following way:

- "High" level assumptions for the cost of outpatient care, stemming from, e.g. intensified ambulatory care
- "Low" level assumptions for inpatient days resulting from reduced hospital care

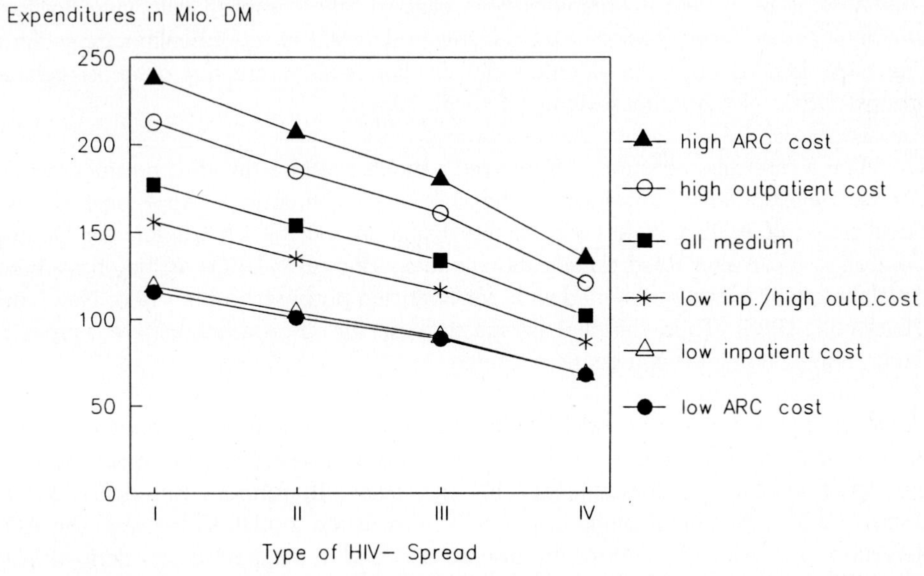

Fig. 2. Sensitivity of yearly expenditures (1988); 3 health care patterns, 2 ARC cost levels

- And a combination of both to describe a substitution of inpatient by outpatient care.

The effects of "low" inpatient costing exceed the "high" outpatient cost assumptions; combining both resulted in a decrease of overall cost as compared with the "medium" standard.

Clearly outside the range of this sensitivity picture, however, the different assumptions for just one stage of the disease, the pre-AIDS symptomatic "ARC", display an even greater variation. High cost ARC treatment within the framework of Table 2 would lead to more expenditures in all four epidemiologic types than just assuming a high level for outpatient cost. Case-specific resource needs for pre-AIDS symptomatic stages thus can be considered an especially important (sensitive) input for calculating overall cost.

4. Future case-mix developments

As shown above, total needs for care in a population for a period of time are significantly related to the specific types of disease stages. This is of course also true in a time-series perspective: during the spread of the disease, resource needs will be significantly influenced by the case-mix to be cared for. Case-mix is understood as a measure covering both medical elements (like diagnoses or functional abilities) and resource elements (like days of inpatient care needed). To describe possible developments in case-mix, an indicator for the severity of the disease within a population is proposed. It originates from case-mix tools applied with classifications that have earlier been developed for patients in different types of health care settings. The most famous case-mix oriented classification system are the diagnosis-related groups - DRGs - for hospital patients (cf. Leidl, 1987).

To define a case-mix measure, HIV infected patients must be classified by stages of the disease development. In principle, the following technique is applicable to any classification of AIDS patients, e.g. to the definitions by the US Centers for Disease Control, to the Walter-Reed classification or to specific AIDS-DRGs as they have been developed, and are experimented with, for financing purposes in the city of New York (Knickman, 1988). Thus, different perspectives on the disease and different types of medical meaningfulness can be incorporated.

However, it must be kept in mind that the classes have to be homogeneous enough in terms of resource use as to allow the identification of a representative mean value for the figure indicating resource needs in each stage. If, furthermore, definitions of disease stages differ significantly in different parts of the model, as between the ARC definition in the development of the disease part and in the parameters derived from cost studies, this may severely impede the validity of results. For the simulation examples presented here, sufficient similarity of case definitions has to be assumed.

With

- j as number of classes defined by a classification system
- p_i as the percentage of patients from a population of n HIV infected patients in class i
- r_i as the mean resource use in class i (e.g., average cost or days of hospital care per year)

the case-mix of a cohort infected at time t can be defined as

(I) $cm_t \;=\; sum\ 1..j \text{ of } (p_{it}\ r_{it}).$

cm_t denotes the average resource use needed by the population at time t. Consequently, total resources needed equal $cm_t * n$. With a reference point or a standard s (a point of time or a reference population) case-mix can be expressed by an index cmi_t, describing the difference to the standard (which equals 1)

(II) $cmi_t \;=\; cm_t / cm_s$.

Independent from the total number of cases and its development, which also has to be accounted for, this index comprises both medical severity and resource needs within the cohort of infected persons. It indicates the intensity of medical and economic problems to be coped with by society. If it increases, the average medical severity and the average resource needs of the cohort have become greater; if it decreases, problems on average have diminished.

The index refers to the total number of people infected. Thus, at the current structure of care, a reduction in the number of HIV infected people per AIDS case will increase the index, because the average need for care in the population will grow. In consequence, however, when one just thinks of AIDS cases, the only data commonly available today, the index may be misinterpreted: its "increase" may result from a reduction in the invisible number of people in pre-AIDS stages. Yet the approach proposed here is considered meaningful, since it accounts for the total number of people infected and describes - independently from data availability - the complete challenge of AIDS for the treatment system. In the future, this perspective could significantly gain weight with the emergence of standard treatment for asymptomatic HIV-infected persons (which also may make them visible).

With equation (II) and the four basic epidemiologic types that have been developed above, the long-term properties of the model can be analysed and used to describe possible future developments in case-mix. As reference point the case-mix of the year 1986 is taken, the time when cost data were collected. This means, cmi_{1986} equals 1 for all four basic epidemiologic types. As a standard for resource needs in the three classes HIV, ARC and AIDS, the "medium" option of cost assumptions in Table 2 was applied to calculate cmi_t. Experiments with other indicators of resource need, like inpatient days per year only, did not result in major deviations from patterns observed. Fig. 3 shows the development of cmi_t from 1981 to 2020. Under the assumptions made here, i.e. also for the virtually theoretical framework of an unchanged environment, e.g. with respect to behaviour or medical technology, cmi_t would be expected to stay, as compared 1986, within the range of a slight decrease and a maximum threefold increase until the year 2000. Furthermore, the analysis suggests the following hypothesis.

Case-mix is anything else but constant. Along with increasing numbers of people infected, the case-mix to be coped with by the health care system has been increasing since the beginning of the epidemic. It will continue to do so further, depending especially on the size of the high-risk groups; then it will decline for a while, and - again after a while - increase again. Possible lengths for each of these time periods can be read from Fig. 3.

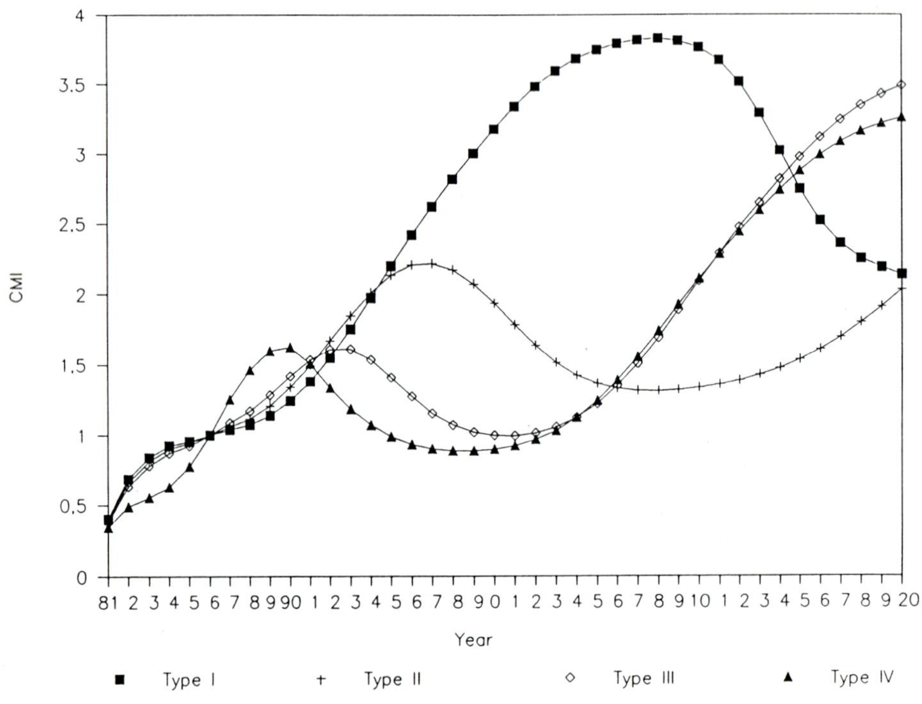

Fig. 3. Development of the case-mix index (CMI); 4 types of epidemics, 1981-2020

Furthermore, Fig. 3 clearly warns against simple extrapolations of epidemiological patterns found once: the "tip of the iceberg", as the AIDS cases are described sometimes, is not a valid picture for health care planners, since the amount below the visible part is significantly changing over time and cannot be derived from the tip as for an iceberg.

5. Conclusion

The development of a computer-based tool to describe possible futures of the economic impact of AIDS was shown, emphasising the indicator expenditures and the specific role of case-mix. At the current level theoretical and empirical knowledge of the significance of the model's elements and parameters is heavily restricted. Thus, the development of methods to assess the dynamics of the economic impact of AIDS was considered a research objective prior to exact estimation, but also for the concrete valuation of different scenario results, e.g. by attaching probabilities to scenario types.

Even in the past, considerable uncertainty about the overall treatment cost for persons with HIV infection or later stages of the disease was found by applying scenario techniques: possible ranges of total cost displayed considerable variation for different sets of assumptions concerning cost levels and, less sensitive among the scenarios compared here, types of spread. Furthermore, scenarios discussed in this paper suggest that case-mix should be thoroughly considered in cost studies and incorporated in assessments of the future economic impact of AIDS. This is first backed by the significant influence that case-specific resource needs have displayed for overall cost calculations, as has been shown for a pre-AIDS symptomatic stage, and secondly, by the significant variations of case-mix over time that can be hypothesised since the beginning of HIV spread as well as for the years to come.

6. Appendix

The infection function

It is a logistic function, derived from an exponential function E_t with growth rate w, starting at point A (the number of people infected in the beginning)

(1) $E_t = (Ae^{wt})$

and a linear weighting function g:

(2) $g = 1 - A/(A - sP) + X_t/(A - sP).$

g is 1 at A and decreases linearly to 0 at $s*P$ (the maximum rate of people susceptible to infection) in population P; the infection function X_t then is defined by

$$(3) \quad X_t = E_t g$$

(2) in (3) solved for X_t gives

$$(4) \quad X_t = \frac{E_t s P}{sP - A + E_t}$$

For each population, the infection function thus can be described by four parameters: P, A, w, s. In the two group model used here, the size of the high-risk group and its growth rate turn out to be the most sensitive parameters in time frames of about 15 years from 1980 on, accounting for the low number of people with AIDS reported from the normal-risk group so far.

In the model actually used, some minor modifications were made in the part of the low-risk group. Resulting from the tuning process (as described above), the sets of parameters selected for the four basic types of spread are displayed in Table 3 (parameters set identical for all: $P = 6 * 10^7$, $s = .2$, $s_{HR} = .9$).

The development of the disease functions

It is defined by the cases infected multiplied by the probabilities p of progression from HIV to ARC or to AIDS for 16 periods:

$$(5) \quad ARC_t = p_{arc\,1} * \mathrm{HIV}_{t-1} + \ldots + p_{arc\,16} * \mathrm{HIV}_{t-16}$$

$$(6) \quad AIDS_t = p_{aids\,1} * \mathrm{HIV}_{t-1} + \ldots + p_{aids\,16} * \mathrm{HIV}_{t-16} \; .$$

Actual parameter values are derived from epidemiological studies as far as possible. Since data are available only until year 10 for AIDS and only partly for ARC (Hessol et al., 1988), the remaining parameters are fictitious. They could, however, be fitted to

Table 3. Parameters for the four basic types of spread

Type	A	w	P_{HR} [1)]	A_{HR} [1)]	w_{HR} [1)]
I	140	10	180,000	1,300	75
II	220	40	100,000	1,300	75
III	60	70	60,000	1,500	75
IV	100	70	20,000	500	225

1) HR for parameters of the high-risk group

Table 4. Percentage distribution over disease stages for an HIV-infected cohort over 16 years

Year	1	2	3	4	5	6	7	8	9	10	11	12	13	14	15	16
HIV	91	79	66	55	46	35	24	20	17	12	9	6	4	3	2	2
ARC	9	19	29	35	39	42	43	43	43	40	36	32	28	24	21	18
AIDS	0	2	5	10	15	23	33	37	40	48	55	62	68	73	77	80

estimations of the future course of the transition function. Those parameters actually used are reported in Table 4 as a percentage distribution over disease stages for an HIV infected cohort over 16 years. Furthermore, it was assumed that of the full-blown AIDS cases 80% survive only 1 year, 15% two years and 5% three years.

Acknowledgement. Valuable and constructive comments to this paper were made by Dr. M. Postma from the Netherlands.

References

Hanpft, R., Reinecke, F., and Beske, F. (1988). Kosten für Diagnostik und Therapie HIV-Infizierter Patienten. Deutscher AIDS-Kongress, München, 8./9. January (abstract 61).

Hessol, N.A., Rutherford, G.W. et al. (1988). The natural history of HIV infection in a cohort of homosexual and bisexual men: a decade of follow-up. IV International Conference on AIDS, Stockholm.

Knickman, J. (1988). The cost of AIDS in New York City. Conference "The Economic Impact of AIDS: Research Methodology", The John Hopkins University, School of Hygiene and Public Health, Baltimore, September 27.

Koock-Walewski, A. and Stille, W. (1989). Was kostet AIDS? Eine Kosten-Leistungsanalyse stationärer Fälle. Schwer, Stuttgart.

Koock-Walewski, A., Wilke, K., Wegner, R., and Stille, W. (1988). Kostenanalysen von LAS- und AIDS-Patienten in der Universitätsklinik Frankfurt. Deutscher AIDS-Kongress, München, 8./9. January (abstracts 60).

Leidl, R. (1989). Scenarios linking epidemiology and economics: possible impacts of drug treatment of HIV infected in the F.R.G. V International Conference on AIDS, Montreal (abstract Volume # W.H.O.16).

Leidl, R. (1988). Ökonomische Aspekte. In: AIDS und HIV-Infektionen. Diagnostik, Klinik, Behandlung. Handbuch und Atlas für Klinik und Praxis (ed. H. Jäger), 1-14. Ecomed, IX-3, München-Landsberg.

Leidl, R. (1987). Die fallbezogene Spezifikation des Krankenhausprodukts. Ein methodischer und empirischer Beitrag. Springer, Berlin, Heidelberg, New York.

Reinecke, F., Hanpft, R., and Beske, F. (1988). Gesundheitsökonomische Aspekte zum erworbenen Immundefektsyndrom (AIDS), II. Diagnose und Therapie. Institut für Gesundheitssystemforschung, Kiel.

Scenarios as a Tool To Support Health Planning and Management

R.F. Schreuder

1. Introduction

Policy makers are curious people. Every future-oriented study gets their attention as long as the conclusions are in line with their expectations about future events. Those in favour of more money for AIDS campaigns will come up with studies which indicate that there will be disastrous developments as far as AIDS is concerne; those in favour of less money for AIDS will embrace studies that show a relative decline in the number of AIDS cases. It does not matter whether the study is based on mathematical-econometric models or apocalyptical visions.

Future studies are as old as the world. Over thousands of years all kinds of people have made statements on future developments. In ancient Greece the policy makers were interested in the explanations of the murmured sounds of priestesses, later on in the flights of the birds, crystal balls, how cards were laid. In the Bible the dream-explainers play an important role. The Etruscans studied the livers of slaughtered oxes. In Italy there were universities with astrology departments. Queen Elizabeth I based her strategies against the Spanish fleet on the predictions of astrologers.

Today we have more sophisticated methods for making predictions about the future. Every self-respecting company or government ministry has specialised future researchers. They are not referred to as prophets, dream explainers or astrologists, but strategic planners, policy analysts, scenario experts, etc.

In the Netherlands we had future-oriented policy units in almost every sector of government: the economy, defense, education, etc. but not in the health sector.

Nevertheless, important measures had to be taken in this sector, and information about possible future developments were lacking. Therefore the Steering Committee on Future Health Scenarios (STG) was created in 1984. I am the project coordinator of this Steering Committee.

We have now completed a number of studies, and in this paper I will focus on our experience with these projects, the structural setting and the impact of the conclusions and recommendations on the actual policy making process.

2. The Steering Committee on Future Health Scenarios

2.1 Background

The major reasons for establishing the STG were:
- Failure of traditional planning structures and methods
- Good experiences in the industry with scenario methods
- The Dutch debate on the implementation of the Health-for-all (HFA) strategies.

2.2 The terms of reference of the STG

After weighing several alternative structures for the "scenario operation" in the Dutch health care sector, it was decided to establish an independent Steering Committee for this task.

This Steering Committee is composed of people who have extensive experience in health policy-making: three former Ministers of Health, the chief Medical Officer, the chairman and the vice-chairman of the Dutch Health Council, the director of the National Institute for Health and Environment and the chairman of the Dutch Medical Society. In order to secure experience with the scenario method, a former member of the Dutch Scientific Council for Policy Development was asked to join the STG. A close link with the actual policy-makers - without interfering in the scenario-making process itself - was established by the nomination of the Director-General of Health as chairman of the Committee. Also for this reason the secretariat of the Steering Committee was incorporated in his Staff Bureau for Health Policy development. The STG got the financial support of the Ministry of Health and other organisations which regarded one or more projects as valuable.

The chief task of the Steering Committee - describing alternative futures in the field of public health - is done by commissions supported by outstanding research institutes. The members of these commissions are appointed in a personal capacity. A formal representation of interest-groups is avoided in the scenario commissions.

The first topics for scenarios were selected on the basis of social relevance and the possibility for future research. Recently, more or less spontaneously topics were suggested by the Second Chamber of Parliament, medical associations, etc. The WHO suggested the development of an international scenario project on "The Impact of AIDS on Society". The STG projects can be categorised according to diseases, determinants of health and patterns of health care facilities.

The reports of the different scenario commissions should give clear insights into future developments of disease patterns, changing concepts in the health care sector and influences of "environmental" factors on the health of the population. The conclusions of the commissions and the policy recommendations of the STG should enable policy-makers (politicians, administrative bodies, insurance companies, professional organisations) to make more rational - or less irrational - decisions about investments and priorities in the health care sector.

3. The Dutch experience

The STG completed a number of scenario studies (projects) on: aging, disease categories (cancer, cardiovascular diseases, accidents) and future medical technology. In my view all these projects provided interesting information on future developments. The most successful projects in terms of its impact on the actual policy-making process were those that focussed on disease categories.

In these projects the major questions are:

1. How will the incidence and mortality from a certain disease category develop in relation to the size of the population?
2. What development will there be in the demand for care?
3. What developments might take place in the supply of care?
4. How would it be possible to influence the developments named under 1 and 2?

For each scenario project, a number of alternative futures are drawn.

Generally, the scenario commissions draw their own conclusions at the end of each project. For instance, the cancer project produced the following results:
- It seems likely that between 1985 and 2000 there will be a sharp increase in the number of cancer patients (1.5% per annum).
- A sharp increase in the demand for diagnosis and treatment is expected.
- No real breakthroughs in cancer treatment are likely in the coming 15 years.

The results of the scenario projects are widely distributed and presented to parliament, with a governmental point of view. In the next section, a number of experiences on the impact of these projects on the actual policy-making process are presented.

4. The impact of scenarios on the actual policy-making process

Generally speaking, all scenario projects provide an interesting comprehensive data set on the topics studied. Amidst the numerous reports dealing with specific issues, the scenario reports present an overview of epidemiological and treatment trends and of expected future developments.

For this reason the reports are widely used. It is difficult to evaluate the total impact of a STG project. The number of reports sold could be calculated. The same is true for the number of articles in (health) journals, literature references, etc. Not measurable is the changing future orientation of policy-makers, the impact on new research programmes, the needs, felt for better long-term health policies, etc.

It is felt that a better link has been established between the scientific community and the policy-makers because of the activities of the Steering Committee. Without any exception the reports are used as long-term policy documents of the national health administration.

The impact of the reports in a scenario project also depends on the presentation of models, data, etc. As with other reports, the formats and presentation are of essential importance if it is to be read and acted on by busy managers. Every report contains a clear summary and in some cases an "executive summary" 1 page long.

5. Conclusions

Based on our 5-year experience with scenario projects we could draw the following conclusions.

Structure of the STG

The structure of the STG - independent but linked with the Ministry of Health - proved to be very fruitful. Much external expertise has been brought to the policy-makers. The scenario commissions have not been hampered in their work by formal representation problems of vested interests.

A relatively small disadvantage of the STG structure is the impossibility of frequent meetings of the Steering Committee itself. Much of the coordinating work has to be done by STG secretariat. Another disadvantage is the lack of direct links with the Dutch Medical Society, the Dutch Hospital Association, the insurance companies, etc. These organisations have to be involved in the various stages of a scenario project on an ad hoc basis.

Methodology for scenario projects has to be improved

All scenario projects needed to deal with the following issues:
- The demographic structure of the population now and in the future, divided according to age, sex, health status, profession, etc.
- Existing and future medical services/treatments, etc.
- Risk and exposition indicators.
- Policy measures, i.e. prevention programems, enlarging or diminishing medical facilities, etc.
- Economic forecasts.
- Social developments, attitudes towards health, etc.

These issues have been dealt with rather autonomously by all the scenario commissions. This hampered the linking of the results of different scenario exercises, for instance with respect to competing morbidity and mortality patterns. A major research effort has now been made to "streamline" the new and the already developed scenarios. A new start with scenario development for instance for AIDS will avoid this methodological problem by giving more attention to these issues in the very first stage.

It turned out that a sound "model" is absolutely essential for a successful scenario project.

Economic aspects of scenarios

Policy-making within severe financial constraints requires a thorough financial analysis of strategic alternatives. The financial translations of the conclusions of the scenario commissions and the recommendations of the STG are made extremely difficult inter alia by the lack of relevant data and the lack of resources for these cost-benefit analysis studies. Health economists, certainly in the Netherlands, are not yet familiar with this kind of scenario study. In the international scenario project "The impact of AIDS" we will try to incorporate relevant economic data.

The communication processes

A scenario project is divided into a number of phases. The report of a scenario commission is only one important step in a scenario project. This report has to be discussed in many scientific and policy-making communities. This demands articles in newspapers, scientific magazines, summary reports for a wider distribution, workshops and symposia supervised by the STG. Researchers and also the commissions are, generally speaking, very much focussed on the research aspects and not on the communication process.

From scenarios to health strategy development

The experiences with scenarios highlighted the need to increase the competence of health managers to use strategic information. In countries with pluralistic health systems like the Netherlands and the FRG, long-term policies are impossible without the support from the major actors in the health field: insurance funds, professional groups, provider organisations and the national health administrations. The scenarios are seen as an instrument to bring these groups together in order to discuss strategic issues. After this discussion the Dutch government will present a governmental point of view to parliament in order to get a kind of national consensus on major issues.

The need for strategic health policy units

A conclusion based on our experiences is that policy-oriented scenarios can thrive within an organisation only if it incorporates a department devoted to future research and or strategic policy-making. This applies not only to national health departments, but also to insurance companies, provider organisations, etc.

Monitoring systems

Conclusions and recommendations based on scenario projects have to be checked at regular intervals - for instance every two years - on their assumptions, trend analysis, high impact-low probability events, etc. Otherwise these projects have only a limited value a few years after the designing stage.

Regional scenario projects

In the Netherlands, as in many other countries, large differences exist in mortality, morbidity, demographic and many other factors between the different regions. Therefore scenario projects on a regional level may be an important feature for further action.

6. The international scenario project "The Impact of AIDS"

At the request of WHO/Euro the STG started an international scenario project on the impact of AIDS in the future. The results of the feasibility studies - based on the guidelines of the STG - will be discussed in a workshop in the Netherlands from 25th to 26th May 1989.

The main project will start September 1989. This project comprises a study on the possible epidemiological, economic and sociocultural effects of the AIDS epidemic in a number of European countries in the next decade. The first written results of this project are expected in 1991. The project will be coordinated by the WHO/Euro and the STG. This project will be closely linked with the EC-COMAC study on the Economic Aspects of AIDS and HIV infection.

Bibliography

Klein, E. (1981). The use of scenarios in corporate planning, eight case studies. Long Range Planning 5, 69.60 77.

Pannenborg, Ch.O. (1985). Scenarios as a method of probing and planning the future of health care. Paper presented in the International Meeting on Future Health Systems. Bellagio, May.

Schaars, S.P. (1987). How to develop and use scenarios. Long-Range Planning 20(1), 105 60 114.

Schreuder, R.F. (1988). Scenarios for health planning and management. The Dutch experiences. The International Journal of Health Planning and Management 3(2).

Steering Committee on Future Health Scenarios (1987). Anticipating and assessing, health care, Technology, Volume I-VIII, (eds. D. Banta and A. Geleijns), Martinus Nijhoff, Utrecht.

Steering Committee on Future Health Scenarios (1987). Growing old in the future, scenarios on health and ageing. Scenario report 1985. (eds. C.F. Hollander and H.A. Becker), Martinus Nijhoff, Utrecht.

Steering Committee on Future Health Scenarios (1987). The heart of the future, the future of the heart. Scenario-report 1986. (eds. E.J. Dunning and W.I.M. Wills), Martinus Nijhoff, Utrecht.

Steering Committee on Future Health Scenarios (1988). "Cancer in the Netherlands". In Scenarios on cancer. (ed. F.J. Cleton), Martinus Nijhoff, Utrecht.

Steering Committee on Future Health Scenarios/ WHO (1987). Scenarios and other methods to support long term health planning, (theory and practice) (eds. J.J. Brouwer and R.F. Schreuder) v. Arkel, Utrecht.

WHO/Euro (1985). Planning and management for health. Euro reports and studies 102.

WHO/Euro (1986). Health projections in Europe. WHO-publication.

Main Policy Issues of the Social and Economic Impact of AIDS from the Perspective of a Health Ministry

X. Scheil-Adlung

More than many other diseases, AIDS has a social and economic impact both on individuals and on society. These social and economic repercussions cover not only individual behaviour (sexual practices, drug abuse and the like); there is also the problem of the ability of those affected to earn a living, the question of providing them with appropriate nursing and care, as well as assistance in coping with discrimination and stigmatisation. From the point of view of a health ministry on the federal level in the Federal Republic of Germany, such AIDS-related repercussions can only be overcome in a satisfactory manner when solutions which focus on the causes of AIDS are found; in other words, when a vaccine or curative can be made available. As long as this is not the case, the number of AIDS cases will continue to rise, and the social and economic impact will persist. Since, according to the current state of medical knowledge, such a solution to the AIDS problem cannot be expected for the time being, central significance should be accorded to preventive strategies and measures to provide psychosocial and nursing care for people with HIV and AIDS.

As early as the end of 1986/beginning of 1987, the Federal Ministry for Youth, Family Affairs, Women and Health had devised and introduced the relevant strategies and accompanying measures. According to the ministry's designated responsibilities these measures are defined as those outside the social security system.

The conception of the individual measures starts from the premise that education and counselling are the key to achieving the behavioural and attitudinal changes which are necessary to maintain health. They can at least reduce the number of new cases of infection while constituting an appropriate means of handling and coping with the problem complex. The individual measures are meant to limit the repercussions of AIDS to those which are socially desirable and - economically - at least feasible under current budget constraints. One indispensable component of all measures is continuous scientific evaluation which finds its way directly into the ongoing political development of preventive strategies.

The programmes and projects of the Federal Ministry for Youth, Family Affairs, Women and Health revolve mainly around the various areas of AIDS control via the health offices, psychosocial care, out-patient care by social workers, streetwork, women's programmes, prevention among young people, children and foreigners. Other areas of focus are discrimination, drug use, sexual practices, prevention of HIV infection among the mentally retarded, as well as "AIDS and prison". Altogether, over 700 skilled personnel, scientists and practitioners are involved in these programmes. In addition, extensive education is pursued via the mass media, and personal discussions are offered and likewise evaluated. Since 1987, the Federal Ministry for Youth, Family Affairs, Women and Health has been allocating some DM 135 million per year to such programmes and projects. Additional funds are provided by the Länder (states) and the municipalities. The first politically relevant results give reason to believe that it is indeed possible to educate and advise the population and to provide care for those affected if the situation is tackled in the appropriate way. The need for the interplay of research and policy becomes clear especially in the development of preventive strategies. The following research findings serve as an illustration:

- Approximately 89% of the adult population in the Federal Republic of Germany were familiar with the way in which AIDS is transmitted, although it should be pointed out that elderly persons are less well-informed and that differences are evident depending on the level of schooling.
- Approximately half of the respondents who are actively seeking a partner, revealed that they exercised caution in their sex life. The frequency with which these persons use condoms is clearly above average.
- Emotional resistance to condoms exists among the public at large for a variety of reasons. For example, 35% of adults fear that the "mood" will be spoilt. Reservations towards the use of condoms are more widespread among men than among women; young people express the least reservations. Most reservations (44%) are expressed by those who have several partners in the course of a year. This aspect will have to be given greater consideration in safer-sex counselling in the future (Table 1).
- To date, 6% of the citizens of the Federal Republic of Germany have taken advantage of personal AIDS counselling; there was a high prevalence of persons with several partners, and persons in the 16-20 years age-group accounted for 13% (Table 2).
- In 1988, counselling was carried out to a lesser extent than in 1987 by the family doctor (30% vs. 41% in 1987) and to a greater extent by hospital physicians (16% vs. 12% in 1987). Also on the rise was the number of counselling sessions given by health offices (from 12% in 1987 to 22% in 1988) and by AIDS assistance groups (up from 3% to 9%) as can be seen from Table 3. These results point towards structural changes over time in the needs for counselling.
- On the whole, it is homosexuals who make the most use of counselling, followed by women. A trend can be observed in all pertinent models towards a strong increase in the number of women taking advantage of counselling services. In 1987, the proportion of such women in the Federal Republic of Germany was 6%, in 1988 the figure had already risen to 10%. Consequently, the content of the counselling services will have to be designed in a more sex-specific manner in the future. The same also applies to other measures aimed at providing psychosocial support for affected women. There is a need to pay greater attention, for example,

Table 1. Attitude toward condoms

	Respondents who were of the opinion that the use of condoms spoils the mood during love-making
Total no. of respondents (16 to 65 years)	35 %
Men	38 %
Women	31 %
By age-group	
16 to 20 years	27 %
21 to 29 years	35 %
30 to 44 years	37 %
45 to 59 years	35 %
60 years and over	33 %
Respondents with several sexual partners in the previous year	44 %

Source: FORSA-Institute, Dortmund

Representative survey for the FRG (n = 2,000)

Table 2. Use of AIDS counselling services

	Respondents who have received counselling on AIDS:		
	Percentage of all respondents	Percentage of respondents in need of counselling	
		1988	1987
Total no. of respondents	6	11	9
Age			
16 to 20 years	13	15	11
21 to 29 years	10	15	10
30 to 44 years	7	10	11
45 to 59 years	4	10	8
60 years and over	2	3	5
Sex			
Men	6	12	13
Women	6	10	6
School-leaving certificate			
Secondary modern school	4	7	8
Intermediate school	7	13	9
School leaving exam and university entrance qualifications, university degree	9	14	12

Source: FORSA-Institute, Dortmund

Representative survey for the FRG

Table 3. AIDS counselling centres

	No. of respondents who received counselling from:	
	1988	1987
Family doctor	30 %	41 %
Health office	22 %	12 %
Hospital physician	16 %	12 %
Lectures, school	13 %	3 %
AIDS assistance groups	9 %	
Friends and family	6 %	
Other counselling centres	5 %	
Self-help groups	2 %	

Source: FORSA-Institute, Dortmund
Representative survey for the F.R.G.

to the drug-related behaviour of women (who, in contrast to men, are more likely to become involved in prostitution than in crime in order to procure drugs) and to focus more on the desire to provide assistance to prostitutes who wish to give up their activities. Within the framework of the model programme "Women and AIDS" this is achieved, inter alia, by providing overnight accommodation under the care of social workers for drug-addicts and prostitutes, offering counselling to people with debts, creating training opportunities, giving assistance in coping with life crises, etc.

- The HIV antibody test occupies a special place in counselling. Approximately 8% of the population over 16 years of age has already taken such a test in the Federal Republic of Germany. Among persons with several sexual partners, the proportion was 22% (Table 4).
- At the health offices alone (excluding those of the Saarland and North-Rhine Westphalia) 250,000 tests had been conducted by October. An above-average number of positive test results were reported in Hessen (1.9% compared with an overall average of 0.99%). One likely explanation for this result is the fact that more people at risk avail themselves of tests in large population centers such as Frankfurt since they wish to be tested in the anonymity of a big town.

The attitude of the population to persons infected with HIV and those suffering from AIDS is of similar significance in the development of strategies against the impact: in 1988 only 7% of the adult population was in favour of isolating people suffering from the disease. This is an unmistakable decline in comparison with 1987 when 15% advocated exclusion and, above all, with 1985 when over one-third (36%) of the citizens of the Federal Republic of Germany were in support of this solution.

Table 4. Use of HIV antibody tests

	No. of respondents who have taken an HIV antibody test:	
	1988	1987
Total no. of respondents	8 %	4 %
Respondents with several sexual partners in the previous years	22 %	14 %
Age		
16 to 20 years	8 %	8 %
21 to 29 years	16 %	7 %
30 to 44 years	9 %	5 %
45 years and older	4 %	2 %

Source: FORSA-Institute, Dortmund
Representative survey for the F.R.G.

The changes in knowledge, attitude and behaviour which can be discerned already over the past two to three years facilitate an insight into the dynamics inherent in the AIDS question. Therefore, in the process of developing long-term health policy measures, we have to take into consideration changing perspectives in the social and economic impact of AIDS.

Above all, such perspectives and scenarios should provide clues about the infection potential present in various groups of the population and their economic and social characteristics. Furthermore, knowledge on the development of HIV infections and AIDS should be compiled in order to ensure sufficient medical, psychosocial and nursing care for the affected persons. Finally, a qualitative analysis of the social impact of AIDS and its dynamics in the affected groups and in society should be conducted. The aim of such an analysis would be to facilitate the quest for an appropriate solution to the problem with the aid of suitable political and administrative measures.

Policies in general - and AIDS policies in particular - need the findings generated by research to be able to devise effective strategies and implement the corresponding measures. For the AIDS policy of the Federal Ministry for Youth, Family Affairs, Women and Health, this means that research findings should constitute a tool which

- Serves to interpret the observations made
- Supports the planning and implementation of measures (including those to promote research)
- Contributes to the selection and differentiation of objectives (for example in the field of education or in interventions aimed at preventing epidemics)
- Discourses possible and predicts probable future trends.

From the point of view of the Ministry, it is of vital importance that research and the various scenarios be practice-oriented and relevant to the decision-making process. As a result, it is not sufficient for a researcher to possess only the requisite expert knowledge. He/she must also be familiar with the authority of the Ministry within the Federal Government and with the legal and political competence of the Federal Government on the one hand and the Länder on the other. The danger that findings might be misinterpreted in the press or by the public as a result of prejudice is another aspect which the researcher must bear in mind.

Particularly those researchers who deal with cost estimates and global social repercussions should be aware that although AIDS may bring with it financial burdens for the entire society, the persons most seriously affected are the victims of AIDS. Clearly, from the point of view of a health ministry, the provision of care and support for the sufferers and of prevention for the others are the top priorities. In this context economic and financial impacts are looked upon as a need to be looked after rather than a resource constraint.

Prospects

The Economic Evaluation of Care Programmes for Patients with HIV-AIDS

A. Maynard

Introduction

The purpose of this paper is to analyse economic aspects of care programmes for patients with HIV-AIDS. These programmes may extend over seven to ten years after the diagnosis of the patient's infection and will consist of alternative combinations of health care, involving varying mixes of primary and hospital care, and support in the community by a range of carers. One of the main arguments in the paper is that existing economic analysis of care programmes in HIV-AIDS has been concerned mainly with health care, and that social care networks, housing problems, labour market issues, insurance regulations and other inputs into the caring process have been relatively ignored. Yet these issues may influence the health of HIV-AIDS infected people significantly and have profound implications for the costs of health care and the cost effectiveness of total care packages. To elucidate these issues the familiar framework of topics for analysis in any economic evaluation will be used (e.g. as in Drummond et al., 1987).

1. Evaluating the care of HIV-AIDS patients

1.1 What is the question?

During the more intensive phase of the infection drug therapy is used to treat skin cancers and pneumonia. Once the infection is diagnosed, drugs such as Retrovir (AZT) can be used to maintain the efficiency of the immune system. Thus, in the health care sector the question to be answered by the evaluation may relate to the cost effectiveness of these drug therapies.

However, there are additional questions to be answered by economic evaluation. Between phases of hospitalisation and health care in primary, the HIV infected person will live in the community, and his health stock will be affected by a variety of inputs, some of which are listed in Fig. 1.

Let us review each of these. The HIV infected patient will need resources to fund dietary changes, enhanced hygiene to reduce the incidence of what for some are trivial infections, and a variety of other goods and services necessary to maintain health and

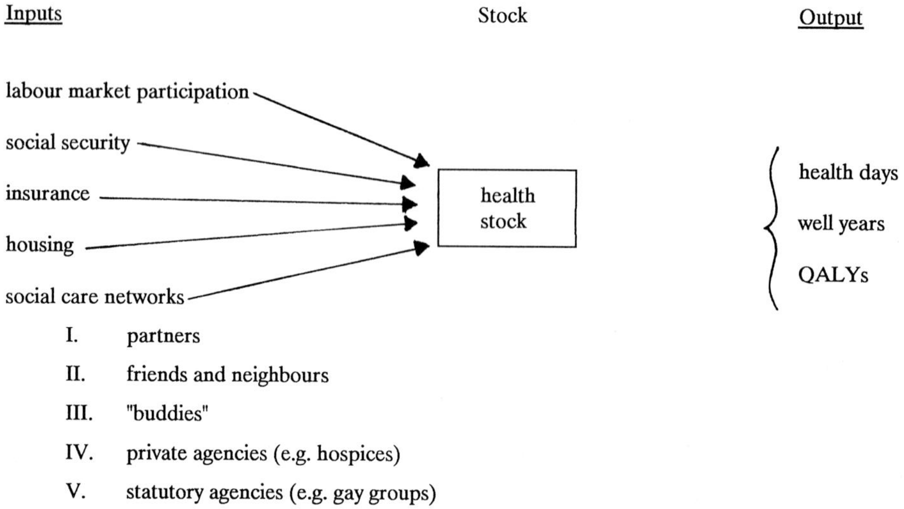

Fig. 1. The health production function of an AIDS-HIV patient

the quality of life. However, the HIV infected patient may encounter sharp discrimination in the labour force which leads to enforced job changes and reductions in disposable income. Thus, a pilot with this infection may be removed from the flight deck of planes even though the risks to passengers when HIV is non-symptomatic appears to be no different from the rest of the population.

What are the cost-effective ways of regulating labour markets so that the income of infected people is not reduced by discrimination? Such income reductions may have impacts on psychological and physical well-being which will increase the use of health care. Thus, such regulation of the labour market may reduce health care and social care costs as well as meet civil rights and ethical obligations.

Social security can replace labour market income. However, access to benefits is often related to income (labour market participation), capital and age characteristics. Thus, access to public assistance is generally means tested, and high marginal tax rates may inhibit labour market participation. Some benefits, for instance, attendance allowances in the UK, are related to significant physical or mental dependence during the day or night or, in the case of the invalid care allowance, related to minimum caring inputs (35 hours per week). Such conditions may not be met when the infection is asymptomatic or symptomatic and in its early stages.

Income from the labour market and social security may be crucial in maintaining the HIV-AIDS infected person's capacity to buy goods and services and maintain their physical, social and psychological well-being. High marginal tax rates at the boundaries of the employment and social security systems may complement the effects of labour market discrimination in reducing their capacity to maintain their health and avoid usage of the health care system.

The HIV-AIDS infected person may be a poor actuarial risk. The consequence of this may be that all policy applicants in areas of high HIV-AIDS incidence may be unable to get insurance cover. This will reduce access to life and health care insurance markets. It is the former which is important in the UK because it affects access to housing.

As in the labour market there is evidence of discrimination in the housing market: there is evidence that landlords seek to deny HIV-AIDS patients access to housing. The maintenance of the supply of stable, hygienic housing services may have significant effects on health, physical and psychological. The problems posed by loss of housing and inadequate housing may be very acute for this patient group, especially when their expected survival time is often all too short.

Perhaps the most important input into the case of HIV-AIDS infected people is the social care networks, which includes respite care. The immediate networks provided by partners, families and neighbours may dissipate after diagnosis of infection or anyway for groups such as intravenous drug users. These networks are supplemented by voluntary agencies, e.g. gay groups providing advice, support services and "buddy" arrangements.

These private sector responses to the heterogeneous social care needs of these groups are being increasingly but unevenly supplemented by statutory agencies in the UK. However, access to home help services and other local authority social service (LASS) support activities is very unequal for other clients let alone this group. The efficiency and the equity of these arrangements are largely unknown.

So what is the question to be addressed by economic evaluation? Often the question relates to that part of the care process provided by health care professionals. However, equally important questions can be asked about the efficiency of labour market policies to counter discrimination, housing market policy to improve access to good quality, secure accommodation, and social care programmes, in a wide variety of public and private forms, to support HIV-AIDS people in the community and minimise, in a cost effective fashion, their movement into high cost health care systems.

However, even if a broad range of health care, social care and other policies are evaluated, how comprehensive is the evaluation? The majority of work to date (for surveys see Drummond and Davies, 1988; Scitovsky and Over, 1988) has been merely costing studies. There has been little attempt to measure the outcomes of these expensive caring policies in terms of well years or quality adjusted life years (QALYs). The economic logic of evaluation concerned only with costs is absent: it does not supply information relevant to make choices between alternative ways of treating HIV-AIDS consumers.

Thus the questions addressed by economic evaluation of caring policies for HIV-AIDS consumers produce inadequate costings of all aspects of care and provide no evidence about outcomes. A vast amount of research activity is producing results of very limited use to decision makers.

1.2 What are the alternatives?

It is better that the health care system, especially hospital care, should be provided only for occasional, acute episodes and that the majority of care would be some combination of social care, supplemented at the margin by medical (primary care) inputs. Indeed some argue for community care only as the most appropriate means of care for HIV-AIDS people. Clearly, the alternative combinations of health and social care are numerous, and their identification must be related to the definition of the illness episode being evaluated.

1.3 How is effectiveness measured?

The objective of the economic evaluation of the effects or consequences of care is to identify its impact on physical, psychological and physical well-being. Using an index with a range of 0 (dead) to 1 (perfect health) it is possible to derive (Gudex and Kind, 1988) an estimate of the QALYs produced by alternative treatment patterns. This is illustrated in Fig. 2.

The number of QALYs (Williams, 1985) or well years (Kaplan et al., 1988) can be calculated and costed to produce estimates of the cost of producing well years with different treatments. Some cost-well year data are set out in Table 1 which reproduces data from Kaplan's work on the cost effectiveness of induced changes in the behaviour of non-insulin dependent diabetes patients (NIDDN).

Whilst single outcome measures have many attractions, there is a range of choice of such measures and of other instruments to determine the quality of life, e.g. Karnofsky and Wortman. These illustrative examples are set out in Appendix 1 together with the York quality of life measure from which Rosser QALYs can be calculated.

It is unfortunate that to date such techniques have been used rarely in conjunction with costing studies to give estimates of the cost-outcome attributes of competing policies. Until such work is done the cost effectiveness of alternative caring policies for HIV-AIDS people will be unknown, and policy choices will be based on rhetoric and guesses about the efficiency of a wide range of caring options.

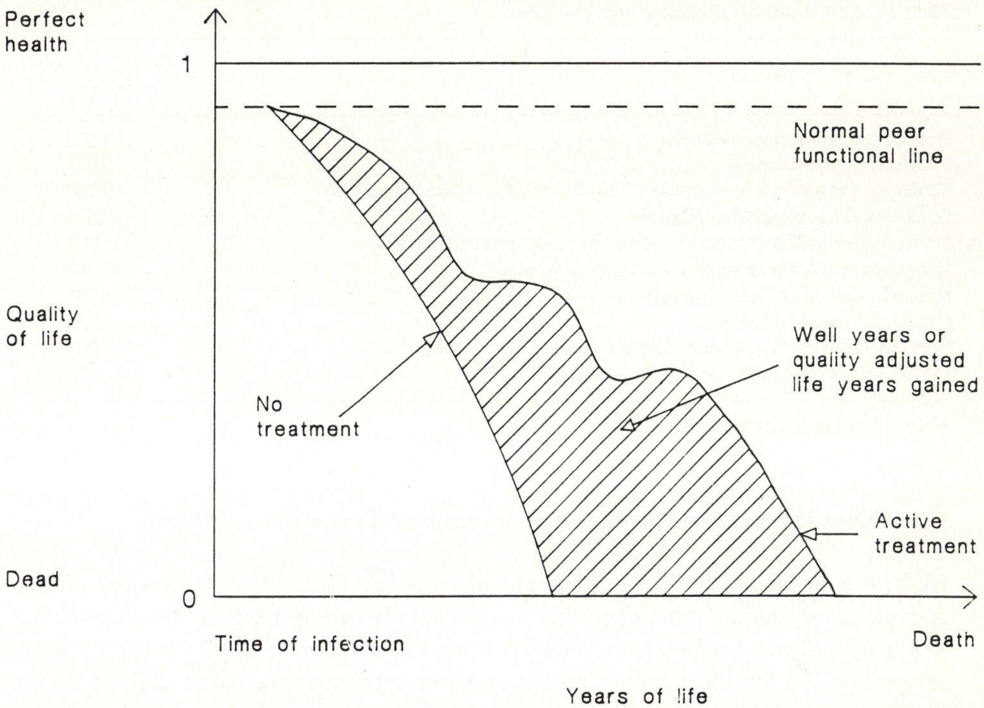

Fig. 2. Quality adjusted life years gained by treatment

1.4 How are costs to be identified, measured and valued?

Whilst it is relatively easy to identify, measure and value many of the costs in the health care system, it is less easy to identify, measure and value the costs in the informal care system. In the UK the norm is to assume that leisure time is valued at 25% of work time. However, a wide variety of circumstances and thus costs face principal carers, and the adoption from transport economics of the 25% norm is attractive from the point of view of simplicity but inappropriate in terms of its lack of accuracy. As Wright (1987) has argued, there is a need for a substantial research programme to identify the value of informal care and the opportunity cost of the work of principal carers.

Table 1. Cost utility of competing interventions

	Cost ($ US 1987) per well year
Pneumococcal vaccine, older adults	1,500
Pheylketonuria screening	7,000
Screening for severe hypertension (diastolic blood pressure above 105)	9,200
Behavioural intervention in NIDDM	10,870
Screening for mild hypertension (diastolic blood pressure 95-105)	18,600
Oestrogen replacement in post menopausal women	23,500
Rehabilitation in chronic obstructive pulmonary disease	24,600
CABG, two vessel disease	32,700
Pneumococcal vaccine, young children	114,900
CABG, single vessel disease	516,500

Source: Kaplan et al. (1988) Table 5, 337

1.5 Other issues: time preference, margins and sensitivity analysis

Whilst it is necessary to discount streams of costs and QALY to take account of time preference, to identify where possible the magnitude of the margins and to carry out sensitivity analysis, there are no special problems in attempting to do this for the social care sector. As for the health care sector these processes are made difficult by the absence of good data.

1.6 Overview

The evaluation of social care of HIV-AIDS infected people must meet the pre-requisites of a good economic study. Also it must provide the policy-maker with the results she needs. These needs may vary:

1. The policy-maker might require to know the cost per person year of treating AIDS. Drummond and Davies (1988) and Scitovsky and Over (1988) have reviewed costing studies for AIDS patients in a variety of countries. These studies tend to emphasise the health care costs, at the expense of social care costs and show that the cost of treatment is very high, e.g. £ 27,000 per patient year in the UK (Rees and Roberts, 1988). However, whilst such studies may inform bids for increased public expenditure, they tell decision makers little about the efficiency of such care.
2. The policy-maker may wish to know if such treatment is cost effective. There seem to be few studies of the cost effectiveness of AIDS treatment. The cost-QALY data shown in Table 2 indicate that the most inefficient therapy generated a QALY for £ 14,000. Treatment of AIDS patients appears to be less efficient than this.

2. Efficiency and ethics

A Benthamite approach to the use of the data in Table 2, and ignoring for the moment the issue of the identification of marginal values, would lead to advice to the policy-maker to create the greatest benefit from the finite health care budget by putting resources into those activities which have the lowest cost per QALY (or well year). This would result in the treatment of end stage renal failure and AIDS being deprived of funds: such investments are inefficient use of resources.

The Benthamite would argue that inefficient resource allocation deprives potential patients of care from which they could benefit. Thus, the £ 27,000 spent to treat an AIDS patient for one year could produce over 160 QALYs if spent on GP advice to stop smoking.

But can patients with HIV-AIDS be deprived of care? The final decision is for the politician to take. Humanitarian responses, even if inefficient, will always influence resource allocation in health care. The results of economic evaluation inform but do not decide resource allocation in health care. Such results show clearly that the opportunity cost of humane treatment of these patients is high. Of course such behaviour begs the question of why act inefficiently towards this group? and the answer may be that some relevant costs and benefits which are difficult to measure, for instance the social and political consequences of behaving differently, are excluded from economic evaluations.

Table 2. UK data on costs and QALYs (Williams)

GP advice to stop smoking	167
Pacemaker implantation for atrioventricular heart block	700
Hip replacement	750
Valve replacement for aortic stenosis	900
CABG for severe angina with LMD	1,040
CABG for severe angina with 3VD	1,270
CBAG for moderate angina with LMD	1,330
GP control of hypertension	1,700
GP control of total serum cholesterol	1,700
CABG for severe angina with 2VD	2,280
CABG for moderate angina with 3VD	2,400
CABG for mild angina with LMD	2,520
Kidney transplant	3,200
Breast cancer screening	3,309
Heart transplant	5,000
Hospital haemodialysis	14,000

Source: Williams (1985, 1986); Department of Health and Social Security (1987)

3. Conclusions

1. Much of the economic work concerning HIV-AIDS has consisted of costing studies which emphasise the resource consequences of treatment provided by the statutory and private (e.g. hospices) community agencies. There is a relative neglect of the informal care element of social care because these services are difficult to identify, measure and value.
2. Many policies other than those in the health and social care sectors affect the well-being of HIV-AIDS infected people. Furthermore, factors such as discrimination in labour and housing markets and difficulties in accessing the social security system may influence the use of statutory health and social care programmes, well-being and survival to a considerable extent.
3. Although many HIV-AIDS treatment packages have been evaluated incompletely, it is clear that AIDS treatment is costly. As yet the systematic evaluation of the costs and outcomes (e.g. cost per QALY) of competing treatments for HIV-AIDS people is absent, and so the efficiency of care is unclear but in all probability relatively cost ineffective. Is it ethical to be efficient? Efficient resource allocation might leave AIDS patients untreated. Is inefficiency unethical? Treating AIDS patients deprives other patients of care from which they could benefit. These questions have economic answers, but economics does not always, and perhaps should not always, determine resource allocation.

References

Department of Health and Social Security (1987). Breast cancer screening. The report of the Forrest Committee, HMSO, London.

Drummond, M. and Davies, L. (1988). Treating AIDS: the economic issues. Health Policy 10, 1-19.

Drummond, M., Stoddart, G., and Torrance, G. (1987). Methods of economic evaluation of health care programmes. Oxford University Press, Oxford.

Gudex, C. and Kind, P. (1988). The QALY toolkit. Discussion paper 38. Centre for Health Economics, University of York.

Kaplan, R.M., Atkins, C.J., and Wilson, D.K. (1988). The cost-utility of diet and exercise interventions in non-insulin-dependent diabetes mellitus. Health Promotion 2(4), 331-340.

Rees, M. and Roberts, B. (1988). Quality adjusted life years (QUALYs) and the costs of AIDS patients. IV International Conference on AIDS, Stockholm (abstract 9586).

Scitovsky, A. and Over, M. (1988). AIDS: the economic issues. Health Policy 10, 1-19.

Williams, A. (1985) Economics of coronary artery bypass grafting. British Medical Journal 291, 326-329.

Williams, A. (1986). Screening for risk of CHD: Is it a wise use of resources? In: Screening for risk of coronary heart disease (eds. M. Oliver, M. Ashley-Miller, and D. Wood). John Wiley & Sons.

Wright, K. (1987). The economics of informal care of the elderly. Discussion paper 23, Centre for Health Economics, University of York.

Appendix Quality of life measures in social care

(1) Karnofsky performance status index

Definition	%	Criteria
Able to carry on normal activity and to work	100	Normal; no complaints; no evidence of disease
	90	Able to carry on normal activity; minor signs or symptoms of disease
	80	Normal activity with effort; some signs or symptoms of disease
Unable to work. Able to live at home, care for most personal needs	70	Cares for self. Unable to carry on normal activity or to do active work. A varying amount of assistance is needed
	60	Requires occasional assistance but is able to care for most of needs
	50	Requires considerable assistance and frequent medical care
Unable to care for self Requires equivalent of institutional or hospital care Disease may be progressing rapidly	40	Disabled; requires special care and assistance
	30	Severly disabled; hospitalisation is indicated although death not imminent
	20	Very sick; hospitalisation necessary; active supportive treatment necessary
	10	Moribund; fatal processes progressing rapidly
	0	Dead

(2) The York quality of life questionnaire

General mobility

Which one of these statements best describes your situation?

I can move round indoors and outdoors on my own with no aids or help	☐
I can get about indoors and outdoors on my own but I have to use a walking aid e.g. stick, frame, crutch, wheelchair, etc.	☐
I can move around the house without anyone's help but I need someone's help to get outdoors	☐
I spend nearly all my time confined to a chair (other than a wheelchair)	☐
I have to spend nearly all my time in bed	☐

Self care

Do you have difficulty with any of the activities listed below?

If you do, do you also need help from someone else to do them?

	no difficulty at all	some difficulty but cope on my own	such difficulty that I need someone's help
Washing yourself	☐	☐	☐
Dressing yourself	☐	☐	☐
Eating or drinking	☐	☐	☐
Using the toilet	☐	☐	☐

Usual activities

1. Tick the activity below that best describes your present situation.

In paid employment (at work or from home)	☐	Retired	☐
Housework or looking after family	☐	Unemployed	☐
Studying	☐	Other (please specify)	☐

2. Does your current state of health make you cut down on, or use special aids for this activity?

yes ☐ no ☐

3. Have you had to change from a different activity that you were doing before, because of your state of health?

yes ☐ go to Q.4 no ☐ go to Q.5

4. What was this activity that you were doing before?

In paid employment (at work or from home)	☐	Retired	☐
Housework or looking after family	☐	Unemployed	☐
Studying	☐	Other (please specify)	☐

5. If your present state of health has made you cut down or change your usual activity, how seriously does this affect your life?
Mark a cross on the line.

not at all ____________________ extremely seriously
0 10

This question does not apply to me because my usual activity is not affected by my health ☐

Feelings

Over the last two weeks has your state of health led you to experience any of these feelings?

If so, how much distress have they caused you? Mark a cross on the line.

	no	yes	no distress at all ... extreme distress
Feeling sad or depressed	☐	☐	______________________
Feeling anxious or worried	☐	☐	______________________
Pain	☐	☐	______________________
Feeling sick	☐	☐	______________________
Breathlessness	☐	☐	______________________
Difficulty sleeping	☐	☐	______________________
Lack of energy	☐	☐	______________________
Dissatisfaction with your appearance	☐	☐	______________________
Incontinence (i.e. lack of control over bladder or bowel movements)	☐	☐	______________________
Embarrassment	☐	☐	______________________
Uncertainty about the future	☐	☐	______________________
Anger or resentment	☐	☐	______________________
Guilt	☐	☐	______________________
Loneliness	☐	☐	______________________
Loss of self-confidence	☐	☐	______________________
Feeling dependent on a machine for my health	☐	☐	______________________
Inability to concentrate	☐	☐	______________________
Poor memory	☐	☐	______________________
Difficulty in speaking	☐	☐	______________________
Difficulty in hearing	☐	☐	______________________
Difficulty in writing	☐	☐	______________________
Difficulty in seeing	☐	☐	______________________
Any other problems that cause you distress?	☐	☐	______________________

Please specify

____

How much does your state of health distress you overall?

Mark a cross on the line.

no distress at all ______________________________ extreme distress

Summary

How would you rate your overall quality of life?

Mark a cross on the line.

extremely good ______________________________ extremely bad

What aspect of your state of health most upsets you?

....

....

Social and personal relationships

Does your state of health seriously affect any of the following?

Your social life	yes ☐	no ☐
Seeing friends or relatives	yes ☐	no ☐
Your hobbies or leisure activities	yes ☐	no ☐
Your sex life	yes ☐	no ☐

Has your financial situation been affected by your state of health?

yes ☐ no ☐

If **yes**, please indicate how severely.

not at all ______________________________ extremely severely

(3) The social support scale

Social support scale developed by Dr. Camille Wortman for coping and change: a study of Chicago men.

The next questions are about how things are currently going between you and the people in your personal life - lovers, friends, relatives, etc. Please answer in terms of how things have been going for you in the past month.

Note: Questions 1-12 are rated as never (1), rarely (2), sometimes (3), frequently (4), or all the time (5).

In the past month:

1. Did you feel that the people in your life let you down by not showing you as much love and concern as you would have liked?
2. Have the people in your personal life really got on your nerves?
3. Did the people in your personal life make you feel respected?
4. Have you felt loved and wanted?
5. Have you felt isolated from others?
6. Have you felt that no one really knows you well?
7. Have you felt as though you were part of a group of friends?
8. Have you felt tense from arguing or disagreeing with people in your personal life?
9. Have you felt irritated or resentful towards people in your personal life?
10. Have you wished for more friends?
11. Have you kept pretty much to yourself?
12. Did you feel misunderstood by the people in your personal life?

Next, we would like to ask whether people would be available to help you deal with different problems or situations that might arise.

Note: Questions 13-23 are rated as definitely not (1), probably not (2), possibly (3), probably (4), or definitely (5).

13. Is there someone who would help take care of you if you were confined to bed for several weeks?
14. Is there someone you could turn to if you needed to borrow 5, a lift to the doctor, or some other small, immediate help?
15. Is there someone you could turn to if you needed to borrow several hundred pounds for a medical emergency?

16. Would the people in your personal life give you information, suggestions or guidance if you needed it?

17. Would someone be available to talk to you if you were upset, nervous or depressed?

18. Is there someone you could turn to if you needed advice to help make a decision?

19. Is there someone you could contact if you wanted to talk about an important personal problem you were having?

20. Is someone around to confide in or talk to about yourself and your problems if you want to?

21. Do the people in your personal life approve of the way you do things?

22. Do the people in your personal life tend to size up things and people the same way you do?

23. Is there someone you feel you can tell just about anything to, someone you can count on for understanding and support? If so, how many such people are there?

    No one 1
    1 person 2
    2 or 3 people 3
    4 or 5 people 4
    6 or more people 5

Now we'd like to ask you a number of questions about your interactions with friends and relatives and about your social activities.

24. About how often do you get together with friends or relatives (for example, visiting each other's homes, going out together, or participating together in recreational activities)?

    Every day 1
    Several days a week 2
    About once a week 3
    2 or 3 times a month 4
    About once a month 5
    5 to 10 times a year 6
    Less than 5 times a year 7

25. During the past month, about how often were you involved in a social interaction or exchange that was unpleasant or distressing? Please include interactions with your lover, your friends and family, your co-workers, people in shops, etc.

    Every day 1
    Several days a week 2
    About once a week 3
    2 or 3 times a week 4
    About once during the month 5
    Not at all 6

26. About how many groups or organizations do you belong to just because you want to -- like clubs, church groups, lodges etc?

(write in number. If none, enter "0" and go to question 28 below).

Number: ____________________

If you belong to any groups or organizations:

[For gay men only]

a. How many of these are gay organizations or groups?

(write in number. If none, enter "0").

Number: ____________________

b. How active are you in the groups or clubs you belong to?
(If you belong to a great many, just count those you feel closest to.)

Very active; I attend most meetings 1
Fairly active; I attend fairly often 2
Not active: I belong but hardly ever go 3

27. In the past year, of the times you got together with friends and relatives, how often were you the one who planned or initiated the activity and invited others to participate?

<u>Not applicable:</u> Hasn't gotten together with
friends and relatives in the past year 8

Never 1
Not too often 2
Sometimes 3
Pretty often 4
Almost every time.. 5

International Research Needs for AIDS

S. Wayling, H. Zöllner

Health-for-all targets in Europe

Health for all - global, regional and in countries - is the most ambitious health policy ever set. The member states of WHO have chosen a far-reaching goal: health for all people by the year 2000. At the heart of the health-for-all movement is a new look at health with a broader perspective.

The European member states have taken the first steps towards their revolutionary goal. Through their representatives in the Regional Committee for Europe, the parliament of the Regional Office, they adopted 38 regional targets as concrete goals to work towards, and 65 regional indicators by which to measure their progress. Briefly put, the targets describe how present conditions must be changed to reach health for all. Most countries reflect health for all in their national health policies.

The structure of the targets suggests six broad tasks:

- Describing every aspect of the health of the population so that progress towards the targets can be monitored (target 32)
- Finding out what biological factors determine health (targets 1-12)
- Assessing the part that lifestyles play in maintaining or endangering health (targets 13-17)
- Studying the ways in which the physical, biological and social environments (including the basic prerequisites for health) determine the health of individuals and populations (targets 13-25)
- Developing effective and efficient methods of providing people with appropriate care (targets 26-31)
- Improving policy-making, planning and management in programmes for health for all (targets 32-38).

Target 4 specifically includes AIDS although it is realised that AIDS is implicitly addressed in all groups of targets, and especially lifestyles and health (targets 13-17).

WHO European regional programme on AIDS

In Europe the infection continues to spread, and the number of cases has doubled each year, with a total of 16,960 cases reported by 30 European Region member states by the end of December 1988 (Albania and San Marino have no detected AIDS cases so far), and an estimated 500,000-1,000,000 asymptomatic people are infected with the human immunodeficiency virus (HIV).

In September 1987 the Thirty-seventh Session of the Regional Committee for Europe, by Resolution EUR/RC37/R5, called on the Regional Office for Europe to expand its involvement in AIDS activities along the lines set forth in the Global Programme and the suggested an European Regional Programme on AIDS.

The Regional Programme on AIDS is directed by a medical officer and a social scientist, reflecting the duality of the disease. They are supported by other professional staff with expertise in the subject areas. These include public policy, education for health, counselling, care, media and national programme support.

The Regional Office Programme forms an integral part of the overall WHO Global Programme on AIDS (GPA). The team works in close cooperation with headquarters and makes use of the expertise available from various related Regional Office units. Since its inception in January 1988, the Regional Programme on AIDS has become the largest technical unit in the Regional Office.

In 1988 the European Regional Programme on AIDS focused mainly on further improving the existing regional AIDS surveillance system, on various AIDS prevention activities, and on assisting member states in the development of comprehensive national programmes on AIDS prevention and control through information, education and counselling. For 1989, the objective is to build upon the momentum generated in 1988 with increased emphasis on supporting the development of comprehensive and integrated AIDS/HIV policies and programmes in the European region.

The Regional Programme on AIDS continues to work within four broad subject areas.

1. Epidemiological surveillance

The WHO collaborating centre in Paris has established a European regional epidemiological surveillance system for AIDS. Thirty European member states send regular quarterly information on AIDS to the centre, which processes it and redistributes it to the countries in the form of a detailed epidemiological analysis on various aspects of HIV infection characterising the trends of the AIDS epidemic in Europe - a prerequisite to evaluating the efficacy of European programmes and policies.

The AIDS reporting forms were revised and endorsed for use as "WHO European regional surveillance forms for AIDS cases" at a WHO consultation on information support for the AIDS surveillance system held in Czechoslovakia, in February 1988. At this meeting, it was agreed that the existing surveillance system in Europe was functioning well and that significant problems of underreporting had not been encountered. Countries of the Region have established testing facilities for HIV seropositivity at a national level; most also have them at a regional level, and although some do not have them at district level, this may reflect the geographical size of the country and the distribution of its population.

To facilitate reporting in a timely manner, a uniform computerised system in Europe is under review. Meanwhile, a faster system of electronic mail is being established between European countries for reporting data on surveillance of AIDS and HIV seroprevalence. An agreement has been reached between member states that reports of total numbers of AIDS cases should be made available at monthly intervals to the WHO Regional Office so as to minimise the unavoidable delays in reporting the information collected by the WHO collaborating centre. Information on the total numbers of AIDS cases in Europe is now available at monthly intervals, and the figures are published regularly by the GPA secretariat in Geneva.

Surveillance of HIV seropositivity is rapidly becoming both an important and a difficult issue. There is an urgent need for sentinel HIV seroprevalence studies, covering both general population groups and at-risk groups. Draft guidelines for a standardized methodology of HIV serosurveys specifically aimed at the installation of sentinel HIV serosurveillance have been distributed to all member states.

2. National programme support

Since AIDS cannot be stopped in any one country unless it is stopped in all countries, every Member State needs a comprehensive national AIDS programme, to be implemented under the direction of a national committee on AIDS. The Regional Office was the first WHO entity to react to the AIDS epidemic when, together with the Danish Cancer Society, it convened in 1983 a first European meeting on AIDS with the participation of 17 European member states. Since then, at the Regional Office's suggestion, national committees on AIDS prevention and control have been formed in almost all European member states, and activities on surveillance, reporting, health education and public information have been developed. Close collaboration between national AIDS committees and the Regional Office through initial assessment visits or exchange of information has been established with more than 25 member states.

In 1988, WHO provided general assistance to Albania and Turkey, including the assignment of teams of experts for initial assessment and development of a short-term plan. In close collaboration with the governments, the Regional Office is now developing a cooperative medium-term programme for a period of 2-3 years on various aspects of health, taking into account WHO's objectives regarding health for all by the year 2000 as set forth in the European Strategy and the resources available, including in those programmes provision for AIDS activities. Preparation of such programme components for Bulgaria, Greece, Poland, Romania and Spain has been completed.

In 1989, the Regional Office continues to evaluate the European activities in support of the member states. WHO guidelines for the development of national AIDS prevention and control programmes have previously been distributed to all national AIDS committees. And as the next step, the Regional Office will promote the evaluation of such programmes according to further guidelines now being developed by the programme.

A National AIDS Policy study of all member states is underway to support member states in meeting the pre-existing objectives. The study integrates the activities within the regional programme so that a comprehensive overview and data base is available. Specific areas of interest are:

- The different and evolving aspects of National AIDS Committees, their membership and roles
- The need and availability of integrated, comprehensive medical and psychosocial care services
- The special role of counselling and counsellors, both professional and lay persons, in prevention, management and care services.

3. Prevention of the spread of HIV infection

In the absence of vaccine and effective chemotherapeutic drugs for AIDS prevention and treatment, intensive and frank health education remains the way of attacking the problem.

Two international consultations on public education and AIDS prevention and AIDS education in the workplace, respectively, were organized in Cologne, Federal Republic of Germany, by the Federal Centre for Health Education in 1987 and 1988. They were attended by participants from 20 European countries and the USA who, among many other points, stressed the importance of developing an international health education network oriented to AIDS prevention. A third meeting is planned in autumn 1989.

A pilot study of AIDS prevention among male homosexuals, including an examination of the attitudes and behaviour of the general population towards homosexuality has now been completed. This study incorporates experience gained in those European countries in which the disease is spread mostly among homosexual and bisexuals, including Denmark, Federal Republic of Germany, Norway and Sweden.

In cooperation with the WHO Collaborating Centre for Health Information, a study on the impact of the media on the prevention of HIV transmission is being initiated by the

Regional Office for Europe. The study will also consider the social attention given to HIV seropositives and AIDS patients.

A review of the present situation in Europe concerning the management of neuropsychiatric aspects of AIDS is being undertaken and will be followed by the development of a proposal for European countries.

To cope with the growing dilemma of health legislation and ethics in the prevention of HIV transmission and treatment of AIDS patients, a joint WHO/Norwegian Government meeting on this issue was held in Oslo in April 1988. Participants reviewed the legislative situation of AIDS and HIV infection in Europe and noted that control of biological products is now being practised in all European member states. They strongly recommended not to use compulsory HIV screening of the general population or particular groups, or testing without consent.

There was a consensus that AIDS should not be considered as a separate category of infectious disease and that it does not require a separate legislative approach. Thus, the existing national laws for control and prevention of infectious diseases will be reexamined as to whether they are appropriate for the new epidemic and are adequate to protect individual and community rights.

To promote appropriate counselling and social and medical care services for HIV-positive individuals, AIDS patients and their contacts, the Regional Office has organised an analysis of counselling and care services for these people, which is being undertaken in 12 European member states. A protocol for country contributions has been developed and distributed to the national AIDS committees. The data received through this analysis were reviewed at the meeting of a working group on counselling and care services for HIV-infected people at the end of November. These activities are aimed at developing a model for counselling for use in European member states and at determining rational health care settings for AIDS patients at various stages of disease progression.

To estimate future developments with regard to the health, social, cultural and economic impact of AIDS on individual member states and on the region as a whole, a first meeting on the development of scenarios for this purpose was organized by the Regional Office in Kiel, Federal Republic of Germany, at the end of 1987. A second meeting, on the development of scenarios, took place in August 1988 in Geneva. A European regional meeting on the financial implications of the growing problem of AIDS is now being prepared by the Regional Office in close collaboration with the global programme.

4. Cooperation with intergovernmental organisations

Close cooperation is being maintained with the European Community, the Council of Europe and the Nordic Council through exchange of information and joint participation in meetings. Efforts have been made to coordinate the AIDS control activities undertaken by WHO, the European Community's research working party on AIDS and the Council of Europe in the fields of AIDS among intravenous drug abusers, HIV surveillance and counselling.

Regional staff have participated in various meetings organized by the global programme as well as in various meetings organised by countries or the European Community, including meetings on clinical manifestations of AIDS, on HIV variability, and on progress in the development of HIV vaccines.

A joint meeting of the Regional Office's Standing Committee on AIDS and global staff was convened so as to review progress in developing the European regional component of the global programme and to outline the activities that can be delegated to the Regional Office in 1989.

A report on the current situation of the HIV epidemic in the region and on activities of the Regional Programme since the last session in September 1987 were presented at the thirty-eighth session of the Regional Committee and widely discussed by the delegations, who affirmed the importance of AIDS prevention and acknowledged the progress made by the member states and the WHO Regional Office for Europe in AIDS prevention and control.

On the occasion of the World AIDS Day an international day of awareness and education about AIDS was held in the Regional Office, drawing attention to a comprehensive care model, including medical as well as psychosocial support to those affected by HIV/AIDS. There was an exhibition, panel discussion and moving deliberations of HIV-infected people. All these events made the day outstanding in our struggle with stigmatisation and discrimination of HIV/AIDS sufferers.

Health-for-all research policy in Europe

Target 32 of the European health-for-all strategy specifically demands that all member states should have formulated, before 1990, research strategies to stimulate investigations which improve the application and expansion of knowledge needed to support their health-for-all developments.

A common research strategy was approved by the Regional Committee at its thirty-seventh session in 1987. The following sections are excerpted from the resulting publication "Priority research for health for all", Copenhagen, WHO Regional Office for Europe, 1988 (European health for all series, No. 3).

Priority areas for research are those that are

- Highly likely to contribute to the attainment of the regional targets
- Closely linked to the Regional Committee's suggested solutions for attainment
- Likely to yield results that can be translated into health policy and action
- Unfortunately, likely to be neglected otherwise, despite their importance.

The regional targets share common themes, vital elements of their success: equity, disease prevention, health promotion, primary health care, community participation, and intersectoral and international cooperation. Similar themes run through research for health for all. They include three areas of research:

- Health policy and organizational behaviour
- Inequities
- Community participation and intersectoral collaboration

and two essential tools:

- Better information systems and indicators for the targets
- International comparative studies.

Many concrete research questions can touch several themes. The importance of the themes will vary from country to country.

To provide the necessary knowledge, health research must venture for the first time into fields that lie outside its traditional domain. To succeed, health researchers must seek cooperation with people in all the disciplines that can contribute the expert knowledge necessary. This will especially involve the biomedical, behavioural and social sciences.

As regards targets 1-12, they aim at reducing health inequities, morbidity and mortality from specific causes, and at improving the quality of life.

Increased research is needed:

- To improve the data base
- To redirect research towards public health needs
- In the forms of longitudinal studies and small area data.

Setting up a reliable data base on inequities, morbidity, mortality and the quality of life is of primary importance. It is needed to provide information for the monitoring of progress towards the targets.

Priority should be given to research projects aimed at prevention of treatment or rehabilitation for common diseases. Research that offers chances of improving the quality of life is equally important. Research objectives should not therefore be limited to issues affecting only selected target populations, such as hospital patients, but should extend to problems of morbidity in primary care and the community. While better, broader assessments of high-powered modern technology are urgently needed, more attention should also be paid to diagnostic and therapeutic strategies and evaluative research in primary health care.

To give a wider focus to health policy, health surveys should include people's perceptions of their health and that of their families. Both retrospective and, in most cases, prospective longitudinal studies will also be necessary. Small area data on the need for health services and their provision and results are required to plan and evaluate intervention programmes. These data should be collated with relevant community or regional data.

With regards to AIDS under target 4, epidemiological studies on people with AIDS and those who have human immunodeficiency virus (HIV) are required, especially innovative research into the psychosocial and economic aspects of the problem. Member states should develop educational programmes for health personnel and the general public to prevent or limit the spread of HIV. These programmes should be monitored for effectiveness.

European research activities on AIDS in 1989-1990

The number of AIDS cases in Europe continues to increase at approximately the same rate as in the last few years, and this calls for an intensified effort to combat the disease throughout the region. Considerable progress has been made in the implementation of the regional programme on AIDS; however, it is a priority to continue the efforts of the past years. A carefully monitored surveillance system for AIDS together with the system planned for HIV infection in Europe is making it possible to keep the European community aware of the growing magnitude of the epidemic and hence to take collective action.

Important issues such as HIV serosurveillance and uniform computerized systems are under scrutiny, legislative and ethical issues inherent in AIDS/HIV are a major concern and are being carefully reviewed as are strategies to evaluate various approaches and components policies and programmes. This is being accomplished through intensive efforts in the Regional Office for Europe and with close cooperation between WHO, member states and the major European intergovernmental organisations.

There are seven social science research foci for 1989-1990:

1. Programme direction

This includes the continuing collection of country-specific AIDS information in order to establish a comprehensive data base. Of particular interest is the question of seroprevalence data and the legal, medical and ethical questions implicit in this subject. Seroprevalence, in itself, is considered a good indicator of the efficacy of programmes and as such deserves investigation.

New initiatives also include establishing closer links with non-governmental organisations, evaluating the role and impact of the media and reviewing AIDS discrimination particularly as applied to insurance.

2. Initiatives on intravenous drug abusers (IVDA)

The forecast is that by mid-1990, over 50% of new AIDS cases will be intravenous drug users with the added consideration that an associated increase in paediatric AIDS through neonatal transmission can also be expected. Social and psychosocial IVDA issues in terms of risk reduction programmes and further development of possible interventions are priorities.

3. Health and social services

Developing strategies for a comprehensive and integrated care continuum form a priority for 1989. As a starting point, an evaluation and assessment of care practices in the European region will be undertaken. The needs of people with AIDS/HIV, their families and the providers of care will be addressed. Following this activity, two projects are planned - one oriented to nursing care practices and the other meeting the concerns of health care professionals.

4. Epidemiological support and research

To use better the improving epidemiological data base, workshops will be convened on the evaluation of prevention programmes with emphasis on resource allocation methods. Additionally, national participants will be trained and evaluations initiated.

5. Health promotion

Building on the work of the Regional Office and the inroads made in the development of health promotion as a policy focus, the AIDS unit will initiate projects to develop models in a series of venues. The results will help train national participants in appropriate health promotion methods and how best to implement programmes in different locations including schools and the workplace, and for target groups including adolescents, women and illiterates.

6. Social and behavioural research

Counselling became a priority in 1989, starting with an evaluation of counselling services in selected countries. These outcomes are to be added to existing knowledge and implemented through a series of three sub-regional workshops which also include an evaluative component. Health workers' roles and response to this responsibility are also to be evaluated.

7. Economic impact assessment

As regards the economic aspects, a study has been initiated in cooperation with the Health Services Management Centre, The University of Birmingham, England. The objectives of the study are twofold. First, to collect essential economic data from a number of countries as an input to the scenario project described in the next section. Second, to specify the contribution that economic analysis can make to the development of policies for this important public health problem. The study comprises the collection of existing data on the costs of programmes for preventing and treating AIDS and the development of appropriate methodologies for the economic analysis of AIDS policies.

A meeting was held in Tewkesbury, United Kingdom, 5-7 July 1989, addressing the key economic issues. The topics considered at the meeting included:
- The economic burden of AIDS
- Cost-effectiveness of treatment strategies for AIDS
- Economics of prevention programmes
- Costs of safety measures and subjective assessment of risks from AIDS
- Social security effects of AIDS
- Priority setting for AIDS and other health care programmes.

The meeting demonstrated that economists were actively studying aspects of the AIDS epidemic. Most of the work has been on estimating the direct costs to the health care sector, and economists are beginning to overcome the methodological problems involved in generating such estimates. Nevertheless, this work is in danger of becoming too narrowly focussed and lacking integration with other relevant disciplines. Priorities for further economic analysis of AIDS and HIV would include:
- Cost-effectiveness studies of treatment options, based on controlled or natural experiments
- The analysis of prevention strategies, using assumptions generated by consensus approaches when firm data do not exist
- The identification of the main needs for better epidemiological data, as judged by the sensitivity of estimates of economic impact to these data
- The development of more dynamic approaches to economic evaluation, to facilitate the study of rapidly changing treatment patterns

- The exploration of the incentives and disincentives facing key people, particularly at risk of AIDS, as a first step towards designing better interventions to change behaviour
- The identification of the wider economic effects of AIDS, particularly when the policy objectives of different ministries/sectors may conflict
- The exploration of the distributional consequences of the AIDS epidemic and the equity aspects of the various intervention strategies.

8. Multi-national study on scenarios on social and economic impact of AIDS

This activity has special relevance in view of the EC-COMAC-HSR Conference. The Office has initiated an international scenario on the psychosocial and economic impacts of AIDS. This is a coordinated research project which integrates activities related to AIDS with a special emphasis on the psychosocial and economic implications. The project is being coordinated by the Steering Committee on Future Health Scenarios, Ministry of Welfare, Health and Cultural Affairs, the Netherlands.

There are at present five countries with an official institutional commitment in this project: Federal Republic of Germany, Italy, the Netherlands, Spain and Switzerland. The United Kingdom is considering joining the project as are several other countries. This component of the project is designed to serve as an information exchange forum regrouping the interested member states to review AIDS developments in shared scenarios for the future.

It may sometimes be difficult to identify common denominators among projects because of their country specificity, but it is considered essential to compare methodological approaches and results as the country projects develop.

The choice of topics is being made according to

- Common interests as a policy priority topic of the countries participating in the project
- The possibility of developing both the economic and psychosocial facets of the topic
- Minimum information available.

A meeting of national coordinators was held in May 1989 to refine the two-year plan of work and review presentations from participating countries. In addition, a preparatory meeting on the social indicators advisory group was held. Its role and relationship with the economic advisory group were reviewed. A meeting to review developments of these country-based activities is planned for autumn 1989.

A preliminary list of key issues is included as the appendix.

The scenario study will receive technical input from two advisory groups, one on the economic implications and the other on the psychosocial implications.

Close collaboration will be maintained with other international organisations working in this field, such as the European Communities and the Organization for Economic Co-operation and Development.

The main task ahead will be the coordination of the various aspects of research: medical and social science research, basic and applied research, positivistic research and action research, research on facts and research on values and perception.

WHO strategy for AIDS - the global challenge

The Fortieth World Health Assembly (May 1987) defined a Global AIDS Strategy which was supported by the United Nations General Assembly. The World Summit of Ministers of Health, which took place in London on 28 January 1988, stressed the need for urgent action by all governments and people the world over to implement this strategy.

The World Health Organization global AIDS plan, which has the generous financial support of governments and industry, rests on five key concepts.

1. HIV infection and AIDS can be stopped; concerted action, coordinated at global level, can prevent its spread.
2. In the absence of a vaccine and a cure, the developments of which are in hand but cannot be expected to be available for at least five years in the case of vaccines, education is the key. Changes in behaviour, directed away from risk activities, will prevent the spread of the virus. This requires messages that will convince people that they themselves hold the answer and thereby persuade them to change their behaviour.
3. Behavioural change will not happen overnight and therefore the commitment must be a long-term one.
4. Programmes to prevent and control the epidemic must be developed and implemented at national level.
5. Because the epidemic is truly worldwide, worldwide coordination is necessary. Guidance and leadership at global level can ensure that we learn as quickly as possible, and the resources coordinated and channelled appropriately. In order to be most effective, moreover, all AIDS control and prevention programmes should be integrated into national health systems and national health plans.

Within this conceptual framework, the Global Programme on AIDS has established the following objectives:

- Prevention of infection
- Care of people with HIV/AIDS and
- Unification of efforts against AIDS at international and national levels.

To meet these objectives, programme strategies include the following.

Prevention of sexual transmission

As already described, this depends on education and behavioural changes, combined with provision of appropriate health and social services, in the context of a supportive social environment.

Prevention of transmission through blood

Increasingly, blood is being tested and blood products treated to avoid transmission. Similarly, donations of semen and organs can be screened. Where risks lie in the use by more than one person of unsterilised skin-piercing equipment, those risks can be minimised by education, and by the availability of suitable sterile equipment.

Action on perinatal transmission

This difficult area should emphasise prevention and the provision of advice to prospective, but HIV-infected or high-risk mothers and to women of child-bearing age whose partners are infected on the likelihood of bearing an infected child. Success will depend on a number of factors including: the sensitivity with which the advice is handled; the pressure on families to go on having children, especially in areas of high infant mortality; social beliefs, attitudes and legislation on contraception or abortion.

Impact reduction

This involves the individual, his or her family, friends and community, as well as the tangible and intangible costs borne by society at large. Direct financial costs can be overwhelming at the family level; they will also significantly affect health care systems. Indirect costs include the political and social as well as economic ramifications in lives and productivity loss. Psychological crises arising from HIV infection and disease need particularly sensitive responses. The discrimination that is increasing in parallel with the epidemic is counterproductive, alienating the very people that need to be reached and involved in programmes, as well as undermining the fundamental values on which society is founded. Reduction of these impacts will require a massive, conscious and coordinated response around the world and across boundaries of nationality, race, sex, religion, sexuality and political belief.

Therapeutic agents

As therapeutic agents become more available, their use will become an increasingly important part of programmes for the prevention of AIDS-related morbidity and mortality. At present and in the foreseeable future, such agents are expensive, far from being universally available and limited in their efficacy.

Vaccines

The development of a vaccine is still at least five years away and probably more. Even when developed, distribution and use will require formidable logistic arrangements, and such a vaccine will not be of use to persons already infected. Strategies involving the widespread use of vaccines and therapeutic drugs are currently in a different category of priorities in the WHO global programme. Research in these areas is a high priority and is coordinated at global level.

APPENDIX

Key socio-economic issues in AIDS

1. Effect on attitudes

- attitude change to other vulnerable groups
- services to other vulnerable groups
- risk perception (individual and society)
- human rights
- ethics/legislation
- discrimination and tolerance
- attitude towards dying
- social networks

2. Effects on the economy

- productivity
- employment - job qualification
- distribution
- local economy (geographical pockets)
- participation (lost earnings, individual, societal)
- international exchange (goods and services)
- social security schemes
- dependents/family - support system

3. Effects on technology

- diagnostic and treatment equipment
- management insurance schemes
- safety standards
- information technology

4. Effects on health care

- health
- manpower - staffing
- quality of services (positive effect on safety regulations, blood circuit, confidentiality mechanisms)
- hospital management and planning
- efficiency
- pharmaceutical (industry)
- infectious diseases

- health insurance schemes
- alternative resource allocation
- take-home technologies
- research
- epidemiologic pattern (e.g. mortality notification bias)
- attitude towards health professionals
- comparative effect on other public health authorities
- public/private mix
- alternative care

5. Effects on demography

- age sub-division of society (age-divided society)
- immigration
- rural/urban

6. Effects on education/prevention

- education and values (openness and explicitness of previously concealed matters)
- health education approaches
- prevention/promotion strategies

Future Research Policies

H. Stein

This paper intends to point to some aspects that might be important for future research on AIDS. Doing that I shall, however, not restrain myself to research policies. Indeed, it would be more appropriate to put this word of my paper's title - research - into brackets. I shall try to outline frame, content and purpose of EC cooperation in fighting AIDS and to show what effective contribution this meeting, the COMAC-HSR and a "concerted action" will possibly be able to make. In addition, this is an attempt to give at least part of an answer to the question what objectives research on the economic aspects of AIDS should try to attain.

Research is of course an integrated part of EC cooperation; in fact, as happens so often, research was there from the very beginning, and was the first field of EC cooperation; all the others - policy, public health administration, etc. - followed years later. Nevertheless, even in fighting AIDS, research - especially "health services research" - cannot be a goal in itself; it does not exist for its own purpose but must aim at improving public health and public health policy - and nobody can deny the need for that.

In this context I would like to thank Dr. Zöllner and Prof. Maynard for having pointed out and stressed the importance of the social aspects of AIDS and of the measures taken, something that up to their contribution played too small a role in this conference and was sometimes even neglected.

We always have to keep in mind that economic aspects, important as they may be in some respects, cannot and must not be the main concern of AIDS policy. Its main aim (at least here in the Federal Republic of Germany) is not to minimise costs, but to prevent people from getting infected and to care for those who have been infected or are already ill and are going to die. And this has to be done at whatever costs - "reasonable" or not.

In order to make an acceptable and accepted contribution to improving public health policy in this respect, research has to know - and to try and influence! - what is going on, has to make its results and findings known to policy-makers and administrators in an understandable way, has to build bridges between research and politics.
It is the purpose of this paper to assist in building this bridge or - should it already exist - to fortify it. I feel legitimised to do so because I helped not only to create the COMAC HSR in 1980 but also the council's ad-hoc group on AIDS in 1986.

The general prospect for the future can be summed very briefly:
Economic aspects of AIDS - and these go far beyond the costs of treatment - and, even more, social aspects of AIDS are so important and have such manifold political implications that research on them cannot and should not be a "one day event" but must be continuous.

The questions however are:

- Who shall define the tasks of research?
- Who shall perform them?
- Who is going to finance all that?

In order to address these questions, I would like to make a few remarks about the general EC background in health policy and health research policy.

EC health policy

As the EC's legal basis - the treaty of Rome of 1957 or the "European Single Act" of 1986 - does not provide the EC Commission with any competence for health matters as such, it is a very open question how far EC activities can go in this field. The situation is quite similar to the one in the FRG where the constitution, the Grundgesetz, gives very little competence in health matters to the federal government. However, as far as AIDS is concerned, the Länder, i.e. the regional governments (which otherwise watch the central government very closely to see that it does not exceed its constitutional competence) were in this case quite glad to accept federal money for several AIDS programmes.

AIDS, therefore, has had an impact on the constitutional division of power between central and regional governments in West Germany. I believe the same is happening in Brussels. Officially, however, there has been up to now no common EC health policy. Yet a great number of health and health related activities are going on as, for instance, the programme "Europe against cancer" or the "EC strategy against AIDS".

EC strategy against AIDS

As early as 1984, the European Parliament demanded EC activities against AIDS. First steps were taken in the field of medical research when, within the Third Medical and Public Health Research Programme, a special group on AIDS was created. Cooperation started in medical and epidemiological research.

The political and economic implications of AIDS were grossly underestimated at that time. This is clearly shown by the fact that the budget proposed for AIDS by the Commission, was cut by 50% by the Council. The advisory body of the Commission being asked how high it rated the political importance of AIDS, agreed to these cuts - it did not give AIDS a very high research priority.

I can easily call this a very poor judgement and a gross underestimation of a tremendous problem since, at that time, I was the chairman of that body. But, as always, there is an explanation if not an excuse: we had, then, very few facts and figures at hand, especially concerning the potentially fearsome economic and social implications of that disease; we just had to guess, and our guess was a bad one.

It has been argued that resource allocation and proper criteria for it are one of the main reasons for doing research on the economic aspects of AIDS. At the moment, lack of money is not a problem as far as AIDS is concerned - at least not in the FRG. Yet, there is a need for this kind of research work because there is not only the danger of giving too little money, but also the danger of allocating too much, which I have the feeling is sometimes the case with AIDS research. AIDS at a national as well as international level - this includes the EC - seems to be the magic word to open treasurers' chests. However, the time will come - and it may not be far away - when researchers and others have to give account of for what purpose and with what success all that money was spent.

To return to the EC situation:

Only a few years later, in 1987, a common EC AIDS strategy was agreed upon by the member states in the Health Council. AIDS was declared to be an international health problem of the utmost importance. A number of general policy principles were set up:

- The prime importance of information and education
- The refusal of systematic and compulsory screening
- the creation of a rapid communication system for epidemiological data
- No discrimination of affected people
- Need for guaranteeing complete freedom of movement.

It is my assumption - but I may be wrong - that this sudden interest in AIDS at the EC level was not caused by a deep concern for health matters. If that had been the case, action against cardiovascular diseases would have been much more appropriate. Rather, the motive seems to have been the fear of uncontrollable consequences of an economic, social and political nature of AIDS, of the effects of measures taken to fight this spreading disease, and of its impact on the production of goods and services, on gross national product, trade and tourism.

This argument is strengthened by the fact that at practically the same time, in June 1987, the World (Trade) Summit in Venice agreed upon a very strong statement on AIDS, describing it as being the biggest potential health problem in the world - needless to say that the truth of that may very well be questioned.

Here again we can note the strange phenomenon that, although it was the economic and social implications which led to the interest of the heads of state in Venice or the health ministers in Brussels, this background and motivation were not mentioned in the statements; instead, the latter as well as the measures and actions proposed were of a purely medical nature.

This, of course, is not surprising for two simple reasons:

1. Since AIDS is considered a health problem, the solution to overcome it must in the end be a medical one: a therapy, a vaccine or - as at the moment - health education.
2. Very little is up to now known about the possible and feared economic and social effects of AIDS, including the side effects of measures taken to prevent or slow down the further spreading of the disease.

Despite this deplorable lack of knowledge, not enough has so far been done to improve the situation. First and notable steps in this direction are the WHO activities for multi-national studies on the social and economic impact of AIDS and this EC-HSR meeting.

New and more knowledge is very definitely needed to prevent politicians and administrators from taking steps into wrong directions. This, however, does not mean that I am demanding a complete reorientation of the AIDS strategy towards a much more economic direction. This again would be wrong and inappropriate. Economic and financial impacts of AIDS are not of prime relevance, but they cannot be neglected either. And in order to avoid ill-conceived policies, the decision makers must be supplied with more and substantial information on the socio-economic effects of AIDS. It is research that has to provide it.

Having remained very general so far, I will now draw some rather concrete conclusions for the future work on AIDS at the EC level:

1. The EC should continue its endeavours according to the political decisions of the Health Council prepared by the Council ad-hoc group on AIDS and by the Commission. The new topics to be taken up - AIDS and the work-situation, AIDS and health personnel, AIDS and social discrimination, etc. - should generally be more oriented towards economic and social issues.
2. The ad-hoc group and the Commission need help and assistance; they cannot produce all the results by themselves. They need research results.
3. At the moment the only field of cooperation between the Council's ad-hoc group on AIDS and the research groups on AIDS is the epidemiology data base at the Paris centre.
4. Concerted research activity could very well serve as a "think-tank" for the Council's group and provide data, facts, findings and proposals even for political action.

5. For the resulting future activities, direct working relationships between the administration and the research groups should be considered.

References

Adler, M.W. (1987). Care for patients with HIV infection and AIDS. British Medical Journal 295, 27-30.

Alameda Lozada, J.I. and González Martinez, A. (1989). Economic analysis of AIDS of Puerto Rico. Paper presented at the V International Conference on AIDS, Montreal.

Alderman, M.H., Drucker, E., Rosenfield, A., and Healton, C. (1988). Predicting the future of the AIDS epidemic and its consequences for the health care system of New York. Bulletin of the New York Academy of Medicine 64(2), 175-183.

Anderson, R.M. (1988). The possible demographic impact of AIDS in developing countries. First International Conference on The Global Impact of AIDS, Barbican Centre, London, 8-10 March (abstract S2.2).

Andrulis, D.P. and Beers, V.S. (1988). Coordinating hospital and community-based care for AIDS patients. Journal of Ambulatory Care Management 11(2), 5-13.

Andrulis, D.P., Beers Weslowski, V., and Gage, L.S. (1989). The 1987 US hospital AIDS survey. Journal of the American Medical Association 262(6), 784-794.

Andrulis, D.P., Beers, V.S. et al. (1987). The 1985 NAPH/COTH AIDS survey: final report. National Association of Public Hospitals, November 1.

Andrulis, D.P., Beers, V.S., Bentley, J.D., and Gage, J.D. (1987). The provision and financing of medical care for AIDS patients in US public and private teaching hospitals. Journal of the American Medical Association 258, 1343-1346.

Arno, P.S. (1986). The nonprofit sector's response to the AIDS epidemic: community-based services in San Francisco. American Journal of Public Health 76, 1325-1330.

Arno, P.S. (1987). The economic impact of AIDS. Journal of the American Medical Association 258, 1376-1377.

Arno, P.S. and Lee, P.R. (1986). Economic costs of AIDS. In: AIDS. Facts and Issues (eds. V. Gong and N. Rudnick). Rutgers University Press, New Brunswick, London, 167-178.

Arno, P.S., Shenson, D., Siegel, N., Franks, P., and Lee, P.R. (1989). The economic impact of early intervention in HIV disease. Paper presented at the V International Conference on AIDS, Montreal.

Ball, J.K., Kelly, J.V. et al. (1988). Distribution of the financial burden for AIDS hospitalizations among third-party payors in New York. IV International Conference on AIDS, Stockholm (abstract 9520).

Barrett, T. (1986). AIDS myths. California Nurse 82(4).

Bateson, M.C. and Goldsby, R. (1988). Thinking AIDS. Addison-Wesley Publishing Company, Inc. Reading, MA.

Bayer, R., Levine, C. et al. (1986). HIV antibody screening. Journal of the American Medical Association 256(13), 1768-1774.

Bennett, C.L., Garfinkle, J.B., Greenfield, S., Draper, D., Rogers, W., Mathews, C., and Kanouse, D.E. (1989). The relation between hospital experience and in-hospital mortality for patients with AIDS-related PCP. Journal of the American Medical Association 261(20), 2975-2979.

Berger, R. (1985). Cost analysis of AIDS cases in Maryland. Maryland Medical Journal 34(12), 1173-1175.

Berliner, H. (1987). AIDS - casting a long shadow. The Health Service Journal, June, 644-645.

Beske, F. and Hanpft, R. (1987). Gesundheitsökonomische Auswirkungen des erworbenen Immundefektsyndroms (AIDS) im Bereich des Blutspendewesens. Das Öffentliche Gesundheitswesen 49, 99-101.

Bilheimer, L. (1989). AIDS cost modeling in the US: a pragmatic approach. Health Policy 11(2), 147-168.

Blanchet, K.D. (ed.) (1988). AIDS - a health care management response. Aspen Publishers, Inc. Rockville, Maryland.

Blattner, W., Gallo, R.C. et al. (1988). HIV causes AIDS. Science 24, 515-516.

Bloom, D.E. and Carliner, G. (1988). The economic impact of AIDS in the United States. Science 239, 604-610.

Bloom, D.E. and Glied, S. (1989). The evolution of AIDS economic research. Health Policy 11(2), 187-196.

Booth, W. (1987). A frustrating glimpse of the true AIDS-epidemie. Science 238, 747.

Buchanan, R.J. (1988). State medicaid coverage of AZT and AIDS-related policies. American Journal of Public Health 78(4), 432-436.

Bulkin, W., McNnally, L. et al. (1987). Hospice care of intravenous drug abuser AIDS patients in a skilled nursing facility. III International Conference on AIDS, Washington DC (abstract 162).

Burkhard, J. (1986). AIDS - Arbeitsmedizinische Aspekte eines aktuellen Krankheitsbildes. Arbeitsmedizin Sozialmedizin Präventivmedizin (1), 7-11.

Carballo, M. and Carael, M. (n.y.). Impact of AIDS on social organization. Manuscript, Global Programme on AIDS, World Health Organization, Geneva.

Carbine, M.E. and Welsing, M. (eds.) (1988). AIDS reference guide a sourcebook for planners and decision makers. Atlantic Information Services, Inc. Washington DC.

Chidiac, C., Houriez, S. et al. (1988). First episode of PCP in AIDS patients: evaluation of the cost of the medical care in an AIDS reference center. IV International Conference on AIDS, Stockholm (abstract 9598).

Choukroun, G., Lons Danic, D. et al. (1988). Cost of medical care for inpatients with full blown AIDS in a french suburban hospital. First International Conference on The Global Impact of AIDS, Barbican Centre, London, 8-10 March (abstract W.16).

Clark, J. and McCallum, D.B. (1987). The adequacy of hospital reimbursement for AIDS Patient Care. Paper presented at the conference Socioeconomic Impact of AIDS on Health Care Systems, Washington DC, March.

Clarke, L.K. and Potts, M. (eds.) (1988). The AIDS reader. Documentary history of a modern epidemic. Branden Publishing Company, Boston, MA.

Cleary, P.D., Barry, M.J. et al. (1987). Compulsory premarital screening for the human immunodeficiency virus. Technical and public health considerations. Journal of the American Medical Association 258(13), 1757-1762.

Clifford, K.A. and Iuculano, R.P. (1987). AIDS and insurance: the rationale for AIDS-related testing. Harvard Law Review 100, 1806-1825.

Corless, I.B. and Pittman-Lindeman, M. (eds.) (1988). AIDS: principles, practices, & politics. Hemisphere Publishing Corporation, Washington.

Covell, R.G. (1987). HIV infection and adoption in Scotland. Scottish Medical Journal 32, 117-118.

Crimp, D. (ed.) (1987). AIDS cultural analysis cultural activism. The MIT Press Cambridge, Massachusetts, London.

Cunningham, D. and Griffith, S.F. (1987). AIDS: counting the costs. British Medical Journal 295, 921-922.

D'Intignano, B. (1988). La facture du SIDA en 1990. Informations Professionelles No 4202.

Dalton, H.L. and Burris, S. (eds.) (1987). AIDS and the law - a guide for the public. Yale University Press New Haven and London, 185-200.

Davachi, F., Ndoko, K. et al. (1988). Economic impact on families of children with AIDS in Kinshasa, Zaire. First International Conference on The Global Impact of AIDS, Barbican Centre, London, 8-10 March (abstract S3.10).

Des Jarlais, D.C. (ed.) (1988). AIDS & Public Policy Journal.

Deutscher AIDS-Kongreß (1988). Programm und Abstracts. München - 8. und 9. Januar. Futuramed Verlagsgesellschaft, München.

Deutscher AIDS-Kongreß (1989). Programm und Abstracts. Berlin - 23. und 24. Januar. Futuramed Verlagsgesellschaft, München.

Dickens, B.M. (1988). Legal rights and duties in the AIDS epidemic. Science 239(4840), 580-585.

Dondero, T.J. (1989). Current estimates of HIV prevalence and incidence: source and data. Health Policy 11(2), 115-124.

Dondero, T.J., Pappaioanou, M. et al. (1988). Monitoring the levels and trends of HIV infection: the public health service's HIV surveillance program. Public Health Report 103(4), 213-219.

Dornette, W.H.L. (ed.) (1987). AIDS and the law. Wiley Law Publications, John Wiley & Sons, New York.

Downs, A.M., Ancelle, R.A., Jager, J.C, and Brunet, J.-B. (1987). AIDS in Europe: current trends and short-term predictions estimated from surveillance data, January 1981-June 1986. AIDS 1(1), 53-57.

Drager, N. and Kingma, S. (1988). Money and AIDS: financing national AIDS programmes. IV International Conference on AIDS, Stockholm (abstract 9585).

Drucker, E. and McMaster, P. (1987). Hospital utilization patterns and charges for the care of inner city AIDS patients: by risk group, sex & race/ethnicity. Paper presented at the III International Conference on AIDS, Washington DC.

Drucker, E., Rothschild, J. et al. (1988). IV drug users with AIDS in New York City: a study of dependent children, housing and drug addiction treatment. New York Academy of Sciences, July.

Drucker, E., Webber, M.P. et al. (n.y.). Increasing rate of pneumonia hospitalizations in the Bronx: a sentinel indicator for human immunodeficiency virus. Background Paper. Montefiore Medical Center Bronx, New York.

Drummond, M. and Davies, L. (1988). Treating AIDS: the economic issues. Health Policy 10, 1-19.

Duesberg, P. (1988). HIV is not the cause of AIDS. Science 24, 514-515.

Duncan, C. (1989). A national strategy designed to reduce barriers hindering the implementation of effective HIV education for youth: first year's achievements. Paper presented at the V International Conference on AIDS, Montreal.

Eastwood, A. and Maynard, A. (1987). Treating AIDS patients: Is it ethical to be efficient? Paper presented at the IRISS Conference 'Quality of Life: Perspectives and Policies', University of York, 11-12 November.

Eberbach, W. (1986). Rechtsprobleme der HTLV-III-Infektion (AIDS). Straf- und zivilrechtliche Aspekte gefährlicher ansteckender Krankheiten. Springer Verlag, Berlin, Heidelberg, New York, Tokyo.

Eisenstaedt, R.S. and Getzen, T.E. (1988). Screening blood donors for human immunodeficiency virus antibody: cost-benefit analysis. American Journal of Public Health 78(4), 450-454.

Exner-Freisfeld, H. and Helm, E.B. (1989). Ambulante und stationäre Kosten für Diagnostik und Therapie eines AIDS-Patienten der Frankfurter Universitätsklinik, unter Berücksichtigung der zunehmenden Sozialproblematik, einschließlich der Sozialhilfeleistungen von der Diagnosestellung bis zum Tod. Das Öffentliche Gesundheitswesen 51(1), 12-16.

Faden, R.R. and Kass, N.E. (1988). Health insurance and AIDS: the status of state regulatory activity. American Journal of Public Health 78(4), 437-438.

Fanning, M.M. and Harmon, T. (1987). Influence of disease and casemix severity on the hospital cost of caring for AIDS Patients. III International Conference on AIDS, Washington DC (abstract 45).

Fauci, A.S. (1987). Scientific issues in developing a strategy for dealing with the acquired immunodeficiency syndrome. Paper presented at a Colloquium for the 100 Years Anniversary of the NIH, Munich, 31 July.

Figueroa, J.P. and Brathwaite, A. (1988). AIDS in Jamaica: epidemiology and economic impact. First International Conference on The Global Impact of AIDS, Barbican Centre, London, 8-10 March (abstract W.11).

Fineberg, H.V. (1988). Education to prevent AIDS: prospects and obstacles. Science 239, 592-596.

Fischl, M.A., Richman, D.D. et al. (1987). The efficacy of Azidothymidine (AZT) in the treatment of patients with AIDS and AIDS-related complex. New England Journal of Medicine 317(4), 185-191.

Flandre, P. and Valleron, A.J. (1988). Impact démographique de la mortalité par SIDA en France en 1990: le SIDA devant le suicide et proche des accidents de la circulation. La Revue D'Epidemiologie et de Santé Publique, 1-12.

Flatten, G. and Allhoff, P.G. (1988). AIDS - Informationen für niedergelassene Ärzte. Deutscher Ärzte-Verlag, Köln.

Foster, J. (1986). AIDS and politics. California Nurse, May.

Fox, D.M. and Thomas, E.H. (1987/88). AIDS cost analysis and social policy. Law, Medicine & Health Care 15(4), 186-211.

Francis, D. and Chin, J. (1987). The prevention of acquired immunodeficiency syndrome in the United States. Journal of the American Medical Association 257, 1357-66.

Frierson, R.J., Lippmann, S.B. et al. (1987). AIDS: psychological stresses on the family. Psychosomatics 28(2), 65-28.

Frösner, G.G. (o.J.) Unterschiedliche Inzidenz der AIDS-Erkrankungen und Schätzung der Prävalenz der HIV-Infektion in verschiedenen Teilen der Bundesrepublik Deutschland im Vergleich zu den USA. Max-von-Pettenkofer-Institut der Universität München.

Gallup Report (ed.) (1988). AIDS: America's most important health problem. The Gallup Report. Report No. 268-269, January-February.

Garry, R.F., Witte, M.H. et al. (1988). Documentation of an AIDS virus infection in the United States in 1968. Journal of the American Medical Association 260(14), 2085-2087.

Gillon, R. (1987). Refusal to treat AIDS and HIV positive patients. British Medical Journal 294, 1332-1333.

Gloy, S. (1986). Insurance costs related to AIDS. Kansas Medicine, March, 76-77.

Gong, V. (ed.) (1985). Understanding AIDS: a comprehensive guide. Cambridge University Press, Cambridge.

Graves, E.J. and Moien, M. (1988). Hospitalizations for AIDS, United States 1984-1986. IV International Conference on AIDS, Stockholm, (abstract 9523).

Green, J. and Arno, P. (1989). The "medicaidization" of AIDS. Poster presented at the V International Conference on AIDS, Montreal.

Green, J., Singer, M. et al. (1987). Projecting the impact of AIDS on hospitals. Health Affairs 6(3), 119-131.

Griffiths, A. (1988). Evaluating the economic impact of AIDS. IV International Conference on AIDS, Stockholm (abstract 9579).

Griggs, J. (ed.) (1987). AIDS public policy dimensions. United Hospital Fund of New York.

Groopman, J.E. and Detsky, A. (1983). Epidemic of the acquired immunodeficiency syndrome: a need for economic and social planning. Annals of Internal Medicine 99(2), 259-261.

Grönfors, M. and Stalström, O. (1987). Power, prestige, profit: AIDS and the oppression of homosexual people. Acta Sociologica 30(1), 53-66.

Gutzwiller, F., Martin, J., Mombelli, G., Somaini, B., and Steffen, R. (eds.) (1989). AIDS in der Schweiz. Die Epidemie, die Folgen, die Maßnahmen. Ein Bericht der Eidgenössischen Kommission für AIDS-Fragen und des Bundesamtes für Gesundheitswesen.

Hammond, J.D. and Shapiro, A.F. (1986). AIDS and the limits of insurability. The Milbank Quarterly 64, Suppl. 1, 143-167.

Hanpft, R., Reinecke, F., and Beske, F. (1988). Ausgaben für und Kosten der Diagnostik und Therapie HIV-infizierter Patienten. Paper presented at: Deutscher AIDS-Kongreß, München, 8 January.

Harding, T.W. (1987). AIDS in prison. Manuscript. University Institute of Legal Medicine, Geneva, October.

Hardy, A., Rauch, K. et al. (1986). The economic impact of the first 10,000 cases of acquired immunodeficiency syndrome in the United States. Journal of the American Medical Association 255, 209-211.

Hardy, A.M. (1986). Planning for the health care needs of patients with AIDS. Journal of the American Medical Association 256(22), 3140.

Hatziandreou, E., Graham, J.D., and Stoto, M.A. (1987). AIDS and biomedical research funding: a comparative analysis. Reviews of Infectious Diseases 10(1), 159-167.

Hausser, D. and Lehmann, P. (1987). Evaluation des campagnes de prévention contre le SIDA en Suisse. Institut Universitaire de Médecine Sociale et Préventive, Lausanne, IUMSP No 23, Decembre.

Hay, J.W. (1989). Econometric issues in modeling the costs of AIDS. Health Policy 11(2), 125-146.

Hay, J.W. and Osmond, D.U. (1988). Projecting the future medical costs of AIDS in the United States. IV International Conference on AIDS, Stockholm (abstract 9578).

Hegarty, J.D. and Abrams, E.J. (1988). The medical care costs of human immunodeficiency virus-infected children in Harlem. Journal of the American Medical Association 260(13), 1901-1905.

Hellinger, F.J. (1988). Forecasting the personal medical care costs of AIDS from 1988 through 1991. Public Health Reports 103(3), 309-319.

Helm, E.B., Brodt, R. et al. (1987). Spontan-Verlauf der HIV-Infektion. Eine Bilanz 5 Jahre nach den ersten AIDS-Erkrankungen in Frankfurt/Main. AIDS-Forschung 2, 567-572.

Herlitz, C. and Brorsson, B. (1988). The AIDS epidemic in Sweden: estimates of costs, 1986, 1987, and 1990. IV International Conference on AIDS, Stockholm (abstract 9594).

Heseltine, P.N.R., Leedom, J.M. et al. (1987). Comprehensive outpatient-based health care reduces inpatient stay for persons with AIDS or ARC: the Los Angeles County Model. III International Conference on AIDS, Washington DC (abstract 161).

Hessol, N.A., Rutherford, G.W. et al. (1988). The natural history of HIV infection in a cohort of homosexual and bisexual men: a decade of follow-up. Paper presented at the IV International Conference on AIDS, Stockholm.

Hopkins, K.R. and Johnston, W.B. (1988). The incidence of HIV infection in the United States. Hudson Institute Indianapolis, Indiana, August.

Hopkins, S., Lafferty, W.E. et al. (1988). Charges for AIDS compared to non-AIDS hospitalizations within the same diagnosis-related group. IV International Conference on AIDS, Stockholm (abstract 9600).

House of Commons (1987). Problems associated with AIDS. Third Report from the Social Services Committee, London, Volume II.

Hummel, R.F., Leavy, W.F. et al. (eds.) (1986). AIDS. Impact on public policy. Plenum Press, New York, London.

Iglehart, J.K. (1987). Financing the struggle against AIDS. New England Journal of Medicine 317(3), 180-184.

Iglehart, J.K., Leighton, R.J. et al. (1987). The socioeconomic impact of AIDS on health care systems. Health Affairs 6(3), 137-147.

Info-Börse (1988). US-Versicherer beteiligt sich an AIDS-Forschung. Pharm. Ind. 50(8), 893-894.

Institute of Actuaries (ed.) (1987). AIDS working party. Bulletin No. 1 and 2, London.

Institute of Medicine (ed.) (1986). Confronting AIDS. Directions for public health care and research. National Academy Press, Washington DC.

Jackson, M.M., Healy, S.A. et al. (1986). The AIDS epidemic: dilemmas facing nurse managers. Nursing Economic 4(3), 109-116.

Jager, H.C. and Ruitenberg, E.J. (1988). Statistical analysis and mathematical modelling of AIDS. Oxford University Press, Oxford.

Jager, J.C, Borleffs, J.C.C., Geels, R.M.A., Heisterkamp, S.H., Jong, J.T.L., and Ruitenberg, E.J. (1988). A method for monitoring hospital costs related to AIDS and HIV-infection. Poster presentation at the IV International Conference on AIDS, Stockholm.

Jenke, A., Reinkemeier, A.-M., and Beske, F. (1989). Gesundheitsökonomische Aspekte zum erworbenen Immundefektsyndrom (AIDS). III. Prävention, psychosoziale Betreuung und Beratung, Forschung. Schriftenreihe des Instituts für Gesundheitssystemforschung, Kiel.

Jillson-Boostrom, I., Figueroa, P. et al. (1988). Assessing the social and economic impact of AIDS in developing countries: a simplified methodology. IV International Conference on AIDS, Stockholm (abstract 9584).

Johnson, A.M., Adler, M.W., and Crown, J.M. (1986). The acquired immune deficiency syndrome and epidemic of infection with human immunodeficiency virus: costs of care and prevention in an inner London district. British Medical Journal 293, 489-492.

Johnson, J.A. (1987). Federal funding for AIDS research. Issue Brief. Congressional Research Service. The Library of Congress, Washington DC, February.

Jones, N.L. (1987). Acquired immune deficiency syndrome (AIDS): a brief overview of the major legal issues. Congressional Research Service. The Library of Congress, Washington DC, February.

Jones, P. (1986). AIDS Conference - 1986: Newcastle Upon Tyne -. Intercept Limited Ponteland, Newcastle Upon Tyne, 153-174.

Kelly, J.V., Ball, J.K. et al. (1988). Severity of illness in use of hospital resources by AIDS patients. IV International Conference on AIDS, Stockholm (abstract 9596).

Kirby, M.D. (1986). AIDS legislation - turning up the heat? Journal of Medical Ethics 12, 187-194.

Kizer, K.W. (1986). A quantitative analysis of AIDS in California. Department of Health Services. State of California, March.

Kizer, K.W. (1987). A updated quantitative analysis of AIDS in California. Department of Health Services. State of California, April.

Knickman, J.R., Gibson, G. et al. (1988). The cost of AIDS in New York City. New York City Strategic Plan for AIDS, Abstract, May.

Koizumi, L.S. and Sorian, R. (1986). The AIDS epidemic: crisis or challenge? 'Perspectives' Medicine & Health, Supplement, November.

Koock-Walewski, A. and Stille, W. (1989). Was kostet AIDS? Eine Kosten-Leistungs-Analyse stationärer Fälle. Schwer Verlag, Stuttgart.

Kosterlitz, J. (1987). AIDS strains the system. National Journal Health Report 6(27), 1650-1654.

Kourouma, A. (1989). Les assureurs-vie africains face au SIDA. Paper presented at the V International Conference on AIDS, Montreal.

Kuthy, L. (1988). Die klare AIDS-Diagnose erfolgt häufig immer noch zu spät. Frankfurter Rundschau 16.1.

Lafferty, W.E., Hopkins, S.G., Honey, J., Harwell, J.D., Shoemaker, P.C., and Kobayashi, J.M. (1988). Hospital charges for people with AIDS in Washington State: utilization of a statewide hospital discharge data base. American Journal of Public Health 78(8), 949-952.

Lafferty, W.E., To, T.K. et al. (1988). Inpatient hospital utilization by people with AIDS: a 30 month study in Washington State. IV International Conference on AIDS, Stockholm (abstract 9599).

Lakhani, A. et al. (1988). The cost of care - planning comprehensive health care for HIV/AIDS in district health authority. Paper presented at the First International Conference on The Global Impact of AIDS, Barbican Centre, London, 8-10 March (abstract W.18).

Landesman, S.H., Ginzburg, H.M. et al. (1985). The AIDS epidemic. New England Journal of Medicine 312(8), 521-525.

Lee, P.R. (1986). AIDS: allocating resources for research and patient care. Issues in Science and Technology 2(2), 66-73.

Lee, P.R. and Moss, A.R. (1987). AIDS prevention: is cost-benefit appropriate? Health Policy 8, 193-196.

Lehmann, P., Hausser, D., Somaini, B., and Gutzwiller, F. (1987). Campaign against AIDS in Switzerland: evaluation of a nationwide educational programme. British Medical Journal 295, 1118-1120.

Leidl, R. (1988). Ökonomische Aspekte. In: AIDS und HIV-Infektionen. Diagnostik, Klinik, Behandlung. Handbuch und Atlas für Klinik und Praxis (ed. H. Jäger). Ecomed, Landsberg, IX-3, 1-14.

Leidl, R. (1989). Scenarios linking epidemiology and economics: possible impacts of drug treatment of HIV-infected in the FRG. Paper presented at the V International Conference on AIDS, Montreal (abstract W.H.O.16).

Leopold, D. (1987). AIDS - aus der Sicht der gesetzlichen Krankenkassen. Das Öffentliche Gesundheitswesen 49, 181-184.

Lock, F. (1989). Les assureurs europeéns et le SIDA. Compagnie Suisse de Réassurances, Zurich, juin.

Loewy, E.H. (1988). AIDS and the human community. Social Science and Medicine 27(4), 297-303.

Long, D.L. (1987). AIDS - fighting the economic epidemic. Nursing Management 18(9), 66-71.

Löw, R. (1988). Die ethische Problematik von AIDS aus philosophischer Sicht. AIDS-Forschung 8, 470-478.

Marasca, G., Abeni, D. et al. (1988). Hospital care of AIDS patients in Italy. IV International Conference on AIDS, Stockholm (abstract 9518).

Matheny, S., Hostetter, C. et al. (1988). An emergency assistance program for low income AIDS patients under treatment with Zidovudine. IV International Conference on AIDS, Stockholm (abstract 9588).

McCallum, D.B. and Higgins Radany, M. (1986). Financing the AIDS epidemic: problems and policy issues. Paper presented at the Conference on Responding to the AIDS Epidemic: Constitutional, Legal and Social Policy Issues, Arizona State University Tempe, Arizona, 7 April.

McHugh, L.B. (1987). AIDS: international problems and issues. Issue Brief. Congressional Research Service. The Library of Congress, Washington DC, October.

Miller, D., Weber, J. et al. (eds.) (1986). The management of AIDS patients. The Macmillan Press ltd. Houndmills Basingstoke, Hampshire and London.

Miller, R. and Bor, R. (1988). AIDS - a guide to clinical counselling. Science Press, London.

Milleson, S. (1987). Social issues in workplace - involving AIDS patients. Paper presented at the conference The Socio-Economic Impact of AIDS on Health Care Systems, Project Hope, Washington DC, March.

Ministère de la Solidarité, de la Santé et de la Protection Sociale (1988). La Frequentation Hospitalière Liée au VIH. Informations Rapides No 128, 5 Octobre.

Moatti, J.P., Manesse, L., Le Galès, C., Pagès, J.P., and Fagnani, F. (1988). Social perception of AIDS in the general public: a French study. Health Policy 9, 1-8.

Moffatt, B.C., Spiegel, J. et al. (eds.) (1987). AIDS: a self-care manual. AIDS Project Los Angeles. IBS Press, Santa Monica.

Moien, M. and Kozak, L.J. (1989). Hospital utilization and hospital expenditures for patients with HIV diagnoses, United States, 1984-87. Poster presented at the V International Conference on AIDS, Montreal.

Moja Jauregui, F. (1987). Consideraciones sobre los costes sociales causados por el SIDA. Economía y Salud, Año 1(1), 10-11.

Morbidity and Mortality Weekly Report (MMWR) (1987). Human immunodeficiency virus (HIV) infection classification. MMWR 36(S-7), 1-20.

Morbidity and Mortality Weekly Report (MMWR) (1987). Public health service guidelines for counseling and antibody testing to prevent HIV infection and AIDS. AIDS-Forschung 9, 534-536.

Morbidity and Mortality Weekly Report (MMWR) (1988). AIDS and Human immunodeficiency virus infection in the United States. 1988 update. MMWR 38(S4).

Morbidity and Mortality Weekly Report (MMWR) (1988). HIV seroprevalence in migrant and seasonal farmworkers - North Carolina, 1987. Journal of the American Medical Association 260(13), 1852.

Morbidity and Mortality Weekly Report (MMWR) (1988). Number of sex partners and potential risk of sexual exposure to human immunodeficiency virus. Journal of the American Medical Association 260(14), 2020-2021.

Morbidity and Mortality Weekly Report (MMWR) (1988). HIV-related beliefs, knowledge, and behaviors among high school students. MMWR 37(47), 717-721.

Möri, Th. and Hofmann, C. (1988). AIDS: Übersicht über die Massnahmen von Bund, Kantonen und nichtstaatlichen Institutionen. (SIDA: Vue d'Ensemble sur les Mesures Prises par la Confédération, le Cantons et les Institutions Privées.). Schweizerisches Institut für Gesundheits- und Krankenhauswesen SKI, Aarau.

Myatt, A. (1987). Health care economics and AIDS. The Humanist July/August, 18-45.

Myers, P.S. (1987). Pooling the AIDS risk. Best's Review, Life/Health Insurance Edition 87(9), 36-40.

National Center for Health Services Research and Health Care Technology Assessment (1988). AIDS health services research, Rockville MD, May.

National Center for Health Services Research and Health Care Technology Assessment (1988). Research activities - will AIDS treatment costs be less than expected? Rockville MD, No 6, June.

National Center for Health Services Research and Health Care Technology Assessment (1988). Selected bibliography on AIDS for health services research. Rockville, September.

National Center for Health Services Research and Health Care Technology Assessment (NCHSR) (1989). Health services research on HIV-related illnesses. Program note, Rockville MD, May.

National Center for Health Services Research and Health Care Technology Assessment (NCHSR) (1989). Extramural research on HIV-related illnesses. 4/21/89.

National Swedish Board of Health and Welfare (1988). HIV and AIDS in care. An analytical survey for the health care and medical services. Socialstyrelsen 5-7, 32-36.

Ndilu, M., Sequeira, D. et al. (1988). Medical, social and economic impact of HIV infection in a large african factory. IV International Conference on AIDS, Stockholm (abstract 9583).

Nees, A. (1987). AIDS aus der Sicht der Sozialhilfeträger. Das Öffentliche Gesundheitswesen 49, 273-277.

Niehoff, J.U. and Sönnichsen, N. (1987). AIDS - Eigenschaften einer echten Epidemie. Zeitschrift für Klinische Medizin 42(24), 2141-2145.

Novello, A., Wright, A., and Sondheimer, D. (1989). Potential impact of HIV/AIDS on the future labor force. Choc potentiel du HIV/SIDA sur la main d'œuvre future. Paper presented at the V International Conference on AIDS, Montreal.

Office of Technology Assessment (1987). The cost of AIDS and other HIV infections: review of the estimates. Staff Paper, May.

Office of Technology Assessment (1988). AIDS-related issues. AIDS and health insurance. An OTA Survey. Staff Paper, February.

Office of Technology Assessment (ed.) (1985). Review of the public health service's response to AIDS (acquired immunodeficiency syndrome). A technical memorandum. Congress of the United States, Office of Technology Assessment, Washington DC, February.

Office of the New York State Comptroller (ed.) (1987). Projected costs of the treatment of acquired immune deficiency syndrome in New York City. Report 11-88, July 8.

Ohi, G., Kai, I. et al. (1987). AIDS prevention in Japan and its cost-benefit aspects. Health Policy 8, 17-27.

Olesen, B., Gøtzsche, P.C., Bygbjerg, I.C., Møller, L.H., and Faber, V. (1988). Hospitalsomkostninger ved diagnostik og behandling af AIDS-patienter. Ugeskr Læger 150/38, 2250-2252.

Oppenheimer, G.M. and Padgug, R.A. (1986). AIDS: the risks to insurers, the threat to equity. Hastings Center Report 16(5), 18-22.

Osborn, J.E. (1986). AIDS and the world of the 1990s: here to stay. Aviation, Space, and Environmental Medicine, December 1208-1214.

Osborn, J.E. (1988). Sounding board AIDS: politics and science. The New England Journal of Medicine 318(7), 444-447.

Over, M. (1988). The indirect cost of HIV infection in the developing world: a case study. First International Conference on The Global Impact of AIDS, Barbican Centre, London, 8-10 March (abstract S3.1).

Over, M., Bertozzi, S., and Chin, J. (1989). Guidelines for rapid estimation at the direct and indirect costs of HIV infection in a developing country. Health Policy 11(2), 169-186.

Panem, S. (1988). The AIDS bureaucracy. Harvard University Press, Cambridge, Massachusetts, London, England.

Parrish, J,A., Lumley, C.E. et al. (1988). Survey of research and development expenditure for AIDS by the UK pharmaceutical industry. First International Conference on The Global Impact of AIDS, Barbican Centre, London, 8-10 March (abstracts TU.28).

Pascal, A. (1987). The costs of treating AIDS under medicaid: 1986-1991. RAND Corporation, Santa Monica, May.

Pascal, A. (1989). Conceptual issues in assessing the economic effects of the HIV epidemic. Health Policy 11(2), 105-114.

Pedergnana, M., Schmid, H., and Wartburg von, N.P. (eds.) (1988). AIDS: Zur Entwicklung in der Schweiz bis 1995. Hans Huber, Bern, Stuttgart, Toronto.

Pindaro, C.M. (1985). Alternatives to hospitalization: AIDS home care. Journal of the Lousiana State Medical Society 137(9), 57-59.

Pine, P.L. (ed.) (n.y.) Current or planned AIDS research activities in the health care financing administration. Department of Health and Human Services, USA, Baltimore, MD.

Piot, P., Plummer, F.A., Mhalu, F.S., Lamboray, J.-L., Chin, J., and Mann, J.M. (1988). AIDS. An international perspective. Science 239(4840), 573-579.

Pockell, O.G. (1987). The impact of the AIDS crisis on a large private health care organization. Paper presented at the conference The Socio-Economic Impact of AIDS on Health Care Systems, Project Hope, Washington DC, March.

Presidential Comission (1988). Human immunodeficiency virus epidemic. Report of the Presidential Commission, 24 June.

Rees, M. and Roberts, B. (1988). Quality adjusted life years (QUALYs) and the cost of AIDS patients. IV International Conference on AIDS, Stockholm (abstract 9586).

Rees, M., Hawkins, D.A., Gazzard, B.G., Roberts, B. (1988). The impact of AIDS/HIV on the activities and costs of St. Stephen's Hospital, London. IV International Conference on AIDS, Stockholm (abstract 9601).

Reinecke, F. (1988). Gesundheitsökonomische Aspekte zum Erworbenen Immundefektsyndrom (AIDS). II. Diagnose und Therapie. Institut für Gesundheits-System-Forschung (GSF), Kiel.

Ritter, D.B. and Turner, R. (1987). AIDS: employer concerns and options. Labor Law Journal 38(2), 67-83.

Rosemeier, H.P. (ed.) (1987). Psycho-social aspects of AIDS and HIV-infection. (Paper has been adopted at the 20th meeting of the COMAC-HSR on 13th November 1987.) Institute of Medical Psychology Free University Berlin, Germany.

Rowe, M.J. and Ryan, C.C. (1988). Comparing state-only expenditures for AIDS. American Journal of Public Health 78(4), 424-429.

Ruiz González, C. and Ponce de León, S. (1987). Perfil socioeconómico y costo del tratamiento de pacientes con síndrome de inmunodeficiencia adquirida atendidos en el Instituto Nacional de la Nutrición "Salvador Zubirán". La Revista de Investigación Clínica 39, Suplemento, 139-141.

Ruiz, C. and Ponce de Leon, R.S. (1988). Socioeconomic profile and treatment cost in patients with AIDS - a mexican experience. First International Conference on The Global Impact of AIDS, Barbican Centre, London, 8-10 March (abstract W.14).

Schatz, B. (1987). The AIDS insurance crisis: underwriting or overreaching? Harvard Law Review 100(7), 1782-1805.

Schäublin, C. (1987). AIDS-Kompendium Hoechst 1987. Ausgabe Bundesrepublik, Basel.

Schietinger, H. (1986). A home care plan for AIDS. American Journal of Nursing. September, 1021-1028.

Schwefel, D. (1988). Gesundheitsökonomische Aspekte von AIDS. AIDS-Forschung 3, 341-350.

Scitovsky, A.A. (1988). The economic impact of AIDS in the United States. Health Affairs, Fall, 33-45.

Scitovsky, A.A. (1989). The costs of AIDS: an agenda for research. Health Policy 11(2), 197-207.

Scitovsky, A.A. and Rice, D.P. (1987). AIDS: the cost in dollars. The Internist 28(4), 9-15.

Scitovsky, A.A. and Rice, D.P. (1987). Estimates of the direct and indirect costs of acquired immunodeficiency syndrome in United States 1985, 1986 and 1991. Public Health Reports 102, 5-17.

Scitovsky, A.A., Cline, M. et al. (1986). Medical care costs of patients with AIDS in San Francisco. Journal of the American Medical Association 256, 3103-3106.

Seage, G.R. and Landers, S. (1988). Medical costs of ambulatory patients with the AIDS-related complex (ARC) and/or generalized lymphadenopathy syndrom (GLS) related to HIV infection, 1984-85. American Journal of Public Health 78(8), 969-970.

Seage, G.R., Landers, S. et al. (1986). Medical care costs of AIDS in Massachuesetts. Journal of the American Medical Association 256(22), 3107-3109.

Shepard, D.S. and Eichner, J. (1988). Cost-effectiveness of screening to reduce transfusion-related AIDS in developing areas. Paper presented at the IV International Conference on AIDS, Stockholm.

Shepard, D.S. and Kouri, Y. (1988). A model for assessing the costs of AIDS in Puerto Rico. Harvard Institute for International Development, Cambridge, MA, September.

Sherrard, M. and Gatt, I. (1987). Human immunodeficiency virus (HIV) antibody testing. Guidance from an opinion provided for the British Medical Association. British Medical Journal 295, 911-912.

Shilts, R. (1987,1988). And the band played on. Politics, people, and the AIDS epidemic. Penguin Group Viking Penguin Inc. New York.

Shultz, J.M., Danila, R.N. et al. (1987). The predicted disease impact of acquired immunodeficiency syndrome in Minnesota: five-year projection models for a low-incidence state. Minnesota Medicine 70, 203-209.

Siegel, J.E., Graham, J.D. et al. (1988). Allocating resources among AIDS research strategies. Draft, June.

Sisk, J.E. (1987). The costs of AIDS: a review of the estimates. Health Affairs, Summer, 5-21.

Slutkin, G., Leowski, J. et al. (1988). Effects of AIDS on the tuberculosis problem and national and global tuberculosis programmes. First International Conference on The Global Impact of AIDS, Barbican Centre, London, 8-10 March (abstract S3.9).

Smith, R.W. (1988). Mathematical and heuristic models of the impact and costs of HIV infections. IV International Conference on AIDS, Stockholm (abstract 9602).

Somers, A.R. (1986). The changing demand for health services: a historical perspective and some thoughts for the future. Inquiry 23, 395-402.

State AIDS Policy Center (ed.) (1988). State AIDS reports. Intergovernmental health policy project. George Washington University, Washington DC, March-April.

Symposium International (ed.) (1987). Symposium International de Réflexion sur le SIDA. Paris 22/23 Octobre.

Thomsen jr., D.L. (1989). SIMS four-year study: statistical methodology for study of the AIDS epidemic. Announcement of technical reports series. Societal Institute of the Mathematical Sciences (SIMS), June.

Tresalti, E., Ortona, L. et al. (1988). Economic aspects of an integrated system of AIDS related hospital care. IV International Conference on AIDS. Stockholm (abstract 9519).

Turner, B.J., Kelly, J.V., and Ball, J.K. (1989). A severity classification system for AIDS hospitalizations. Medical Care 27(4), 423-437.

United Hospital Fund (ed.) (1987). AIDS: its impact on New York City. Blueprint, United Hospital Fund of New York, Fall.

Walters, L. (1988). Ethical issues in the prevention and treatment of HIV infection and AIDS. Science 239(4840), 597-603.

Wayling, S. (1989). AIDS policies and programmes in the European region. Regional programme on AIDS. World Health Organization Regional Office for Europe.

Weinstein, M.C. and Graham, J.D. (n.y.). Cost-effectiveness analysis of AIDS prevention programs: concepts, complications, and illustrations. Harvard School of Public Health, Boston, Massachusetts.

Weinstein, M.C., Siegel, J. et al. (1988). Cost-effectiveness evaluation of interventions to prevent or treat AIDS. IV International Conference on AIDS, Stockholm (abstract 9589).

Weitz, R. (1987). The interview as legacy: a social scientist confronts AIDS. Hastings Center Report, June, 21-23.

Wells, N. (1986). The AIDS virus forecasting its impact. Office of Health Economics, London.

Wilkie, P.A. (1987). Life assurance, HIV seropositivity and haemophilia. Scottish Medical Journal 32, 119.

Winkenwerder, W. and Roper, W.L. (1988). Federal government spending on AIDS in the United States. IV International Conference on AIDS, Stockholm (abstract 9580).

World Health (1988). AIDS: a shadow in our world. The Magazine of the World Health Organization, March.

World Health Organization (1988). AIDS prevention and control. Pergamon Press Oxford, New York, Beijing, Frankfurt, Sao Paulo, Sydney, Tokyo, Toronto.

World Health Organization (1988). Guidelines for the development of a national AIDS prevention and control programme. Geneva WHO AIDS Series 1.

World Health Organization (1988). The global epidemiology and projected impact of AIDS. Special Programme on AIDS. A technical document for the OECD consultation of January 1988 in preparation for the meeting of OECD social policy ministers, Juli 1988, Paris.

Wormser, G.P., Stahl, R.E. et al. (eds.) (1987). AIDS- acquired immune deficiency syndrome - and other manifestations of HIV infection. Noyes Publications Park Ridge, New Jersey.

Wu, A.W., Mathews, W.C. et al. (1988). Quality of life measures in AIDS clinical trials. IV International Conference on AIDS, Stockholm (abstract 9557).

Wykoff, R.F., Conway, G. et al. (1988). Cost-effectiveness of HIV-screening proposals. IV International Conference on AIDS, Stockholm (abstract 9566).

Wyszewianski, L. (1986). Financially catastrophic and high-cost cases: definitions, distinctions, and their implications for policy formulation. Inquiry 23, 382-394.

Zeugin, P. (1988). Repräsentative Befragung bei Personen zwischen 17 und 30 Jahren zur Kondom-Benuetzung (Evaluation des Campagnes de Prevention contre le SIDA en Suisse). Institut Universitaire de Médecine Sociale et Préventive Lausanne, IUMSP No 23.1, Januar.